CLINICAL DECISION MAKING SERIES™

PEDIATRIC DECISION MAKING

STEPHEN BERMAN, M.D.

Associate Professor of Pediatrics
University of Colorado School of Medicine
Head, Section of General Pediatrics
University of Colorado Health Sciences Center
Denver, Colorado

1985

B. C. DECKER INC. • Philadelphia • Toronto
The C. V. MOSBY COMPANY • Saint Louis • Toronto • London

Publisher: **B.C. Decker Inc.**
3228 South Service Road
Burlington, Ontario L7N 3H8

B.C. Decker Inc.
P.O. Box 30246
Philadelphia, Pennsylvania 19103

North American and worldwide sales and distribution:

The C.V. Mosby Company
11830 Westline Industrial Drive
Saint Louis, Missouri 63141

In Canada: **The C.V. Mosby Company, Ltd.**
120 Melford Drive
Toronto, Ontario M1B 2X5

Pediatric Decision Making

ISBN 0-941158-17-9

Library of Congress catalog card number: 83-72417

Last digit is print number: 10 9 8 7 6 5 4 3 2 1

To my family, Elaine, Seth, and Ben, for all the weekends that they let me work on this book.

To my parents, Shirley and Syd, for their endurance in raising three boys.

To my brothers, Jim and Ed, for being there when we lost 103 to 36.

CONTRIBUTORS

STEPHEN BERMAN, M.D.

Associate Professor of Pediatrics, University of Colorado School of Medicine; Head, Section of General Pediatrics and Medical Director, University Hospital Pediatric Ambulatory Care Center, Denver, Colorado

EDWARD R. BERMAN, M.D.

Fellow in Neonatology, Department of Pediatrics, University of Colorado School of Medicine, Children's Hospital, Denver, Colorado

MICHAEL S. KAPPY, M.D., Ph.D.

Associate Professor of Pediatrics, University of Florida at Gainesville College of Medicine; Division of Endocrinology, J. Hillis Miller Health Center, Gainesville, Florida

PETER A. LANE, M.D.

Fellow in Hematology-Oncology, Department of Pediatrics, University of Colorado School of Medicine, Denver, Colorado

BARTON D. SCHMITT, M.D.

Associate Professor of Pediatrics, University of Colorado School of Medicine, University Hospital, Denver, Colorado

PREFACE

Pediatric Decision Making presents an algorithmic approach to the diagnosis and management of common clinical problems. A well done history and physical examination form the essential foundation upon which all subsequent clinical decisions are based. The findings of the history and physical must be integrated with diagnostic studies, therapeutic trial, and careful follow-up. In the management algorithms, four clinical decision points are reviewed: (1) Does the patient require immediate therapeutic intervention? (2) Should the patient be hospitalized? (3) Does the patient require diagnostic studies of specific therapy? (4) What is the appropriate follow-up for the patient? The answers to the above questions are based on an assessment of the degree of illness. Severely ill patients require immediate supportive care and hospitalization. Moderately ill patients need a further work-up or clinical trial to decide whether hospitalization or specific therapy is indicated. Mildly ill patients can be managed as outpatients with minimal diagnostic studies. Follow-up and reassessment are necessary in order to document the development of new symptoms or persistent symptoms that require additional intervention.

Clinical decision making will always remain difficult because a single disorder can present with a wide spectrum of signs and symptoms, and many different disorders can present with similar signs and symptoms. This means that clinical decision making should be structured in a manner that is both risk- and cost-beneficial. This book rather than being a comprehensive pediatric textbook seeks to provide medical students, pediatric housestaff, and practitioners with a reasonable guide to clinical problem-solving which takes into account quality of care and cost containment considerations.

Writing this book would not have been possible without the encouragement and support of medical students, pediatric housestaff, and my colleagues in the University of Colorado Department of Pediatrics, especially Frederick C. Battaglia, Department Chairman. Several individuals deserve special acknowledgement for reviewing sections of this book. They include Arnold Silverman for reviewing gastroenterology, Gary Lum and Brad Warday for renal, Paul Francis and James Wiggins for cardiology, Frank Accurso and Ernest Cotton for pulmonary, Bill Weston for dermatology, Bill Hathaway and Jack Githens for hematology, Dennis Deitrich and David Stumpf for neurology, David Kaplan for adolescent gynecology, and Ron Gotlin and Georganna Klingensmith for endocrine and metabolic sections. I would also like to thank two pediatric residents, Steve Marsocci and David Elkayam, for reviewing the manuscript and Mary K. Maudsley for her assistance in editing and Brian Decker for his support. Helen Coffin, Sharon Lawson, and Carol Webb provided invaluable secretarial assistance. I appreciate greatly the excellent effort, encouragement, and enthusiasm of my contributors, Ed Berman, Mike Kappy, Peter Lane, and Bart Schmitt.

Stephen Berman, M.D.

CONTENTS

NEONATAL DISORDERS

How To Use This Book

Depending on its complexity, each clinical topic is discussed in one or more algorithms. Essential baseline data are described before the point at which the first decision must be made. The algorithm branches at crucial decision points. Notes on the page facing the algorithm elucidate points that require further discussion or debate. The approach presented reflects each author's clinical experience and his understanding of the literature; the references provide further background reading.

Each algorithm is meant to address the decision making *process* more than the *content*. As such, it is a skeleton upon which the flesh of more detailed clinical and theoretical knowledge can grow. The greatest benefit will therefore be obtained when the reader focuses on his or her own broad approach to a clinical problem, comparing and contrasting it with that of the chapter's author. Since each decision tree focuses more on the structure of a clinical decision than on its contents, additional reading is necessary to develop a well rounded understanding of each clinical problem.

FEVER IN EARLY INFANCY

A. Assess the degree of illness. Moderately to severely ill infants have altered mental status (apnea, seizures, coma, irritability, or lethargy), gastrointestinal symptoms (poor feeding, abdominal distension, or vomiting), or signs of vascular instability (hypotension or pale mottled extremities with poor capillary refill). Consider infants with a temperature of ≥ 40°C moderately to severely ill; 18 percent of these have meningitis.

B. The bacterial infections identified on physical examination are acute otitis media (10%), pneumonia (7%), impetigo (4%), adenitis (2%), cellulitis (1%), omphalitis (1%), bacterial enteritis (bloody diarrhea) (1%), and septic arthritis/osteomyelitis (1%). The risk of an associated bacteremia is greater than 50 percent in infants with cellulitis, adenitis, and omphalitis. An associated bacteremia occurs in 10–30% of cases with bacterial enteritis and pneumonia. Less than 5% of cases with acute otitis media are bacteremic.

C. Fever during the first 2 weeks of life is an uncommon occurrence, accounting for only 5 percent of infants under 2 months who present with fever. Hospitalize all infants under 2 weeks of age who present with fever because asymptomatic group B streptococcus bacteremia occurs in infants at this age. A WBC count > 15,000 and a sedimentation rate > 30 are only useful as indicators for possible bacteremia in infants older than 1 month.

D. Perform a lumbar puncture as part of a septic workup in infants who appear moderately to severely ill or who have a temperature of ≥ 40°C, regardless of appearance. Approximately two–thirds of the cases of meningitis are viral, and one–third are bacterial. Organisms causing bacterial meningitis are *group B streptococcus, Listeria monocytogenes, S. pneumoniae, H. influenzae, Salmonella, N. meningitidis*, and *E. coli*.

E. Blood cultures will be positive in 18% of infants with fever who appear ill and in 1–5% of infants who appear well (including infants under 2 weeks of age). The organisms causing bacteremia are *group B streptococcus, S. aureus, Salmonella, E. coli, N. meningitidis, N. Gonorrhea*, and *H. influenzae*. For cases of suspected sepsis without meningitis, initiate IV antibiotic therapy with ampicillin 200 mg/kg/day given in 4 divided doses and gentamicin 7.5 mg/kg/day given in 3 divided doses, pending culture results.

REFERENCES

Baker CJ. Group B streptococcal cellulitis-adenitis in infants. Am J Dis Child 1982; 136:631.

Bruhn FW, McIntosh K. Fever under three months. Pediatr Res 1976; Abstract 269.

Caspe WB, Chamudes O, Louie B. The evaluation and treatment of the febrile infant. Pediatr Inf Dis 1983; 2:131.

Crain EF, Shelov SP. Febrile infants: Predictors of bacteremia. J Pediatr 1982; 101:686.

McCarthy PL, Dolan TF. The serious implications of high fever in infants during their first three months. Clin Peds 1976; 15:794.

Roberts KB, Borzy MS. Fever in the first eight weeks of life. Johns Hopkins Med J 1977; 141:9.

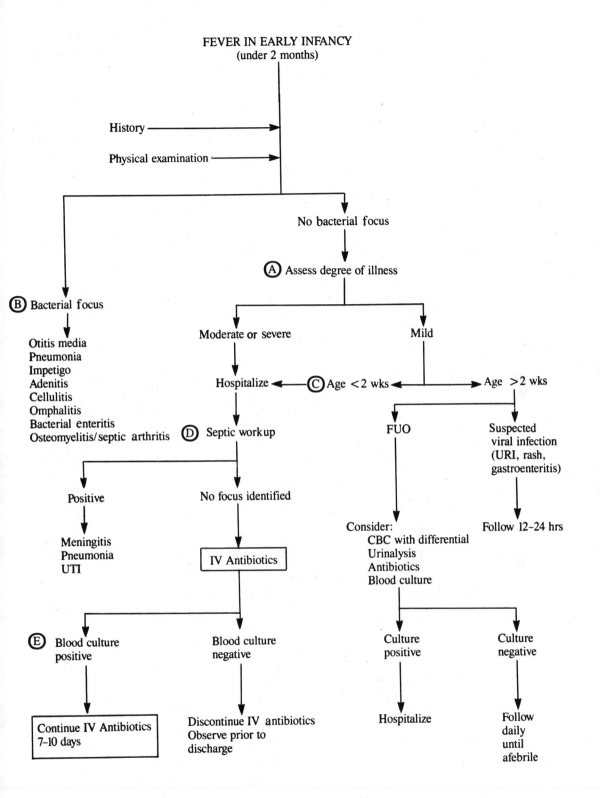

FEVER IN EARLY INFANCY
(under 2 months)

History

Physical examination

No bacterial focus

(A) Assess degree of illness

(B) Bacterial focus

Otitis media
Pneumonia
Impetigo
Adenitis
Cellulitis
Omphalitis
Bacterial enteritis
Osteomyelitis/septic arthritis

Moderate or severe

Mild

Hospitalize ← (C) Age <2 wks ← → Age >2 wks

(D) Septic workup

FUO

Suspected
viral infection
(URI, rash,
gastroenteritis)

Positive

No focus identified

Meningitis
Pneumonia
UTI

IV Antibiotics

Consider:
CBC with differential
Urinalysis
Antibiotics
Blood culture

Follow 12–24 hrs

(E) Blood culture
positive

Blood culture
negative

Culture
positive

Culture
negative

Continue IV Antibiotics
7–10 days

Discontinue IV antibiotics
Observe prior to
discharge

Hospitalize

Follow
daily
until
afebrile

3

FEVER AND OCCULT BACTEREMIA

A. The level of fever is useful in predicting occult bacteremia or meningitis. Fewer than 1% of children with temperature below 39°C are bacteremic. However, 4% of children with temperatures between 39° and 40.4°C, 13% of children with temperatures between 40.5° and 41°C, and 23% of children with temperatures higher than 41°C are bacteremic. The risk of bacterial meningitis is 3% in children under 24 months of age who present with fever of 38.5°C or higher and 10% in children with temperatures higher than 41°C.

B. Consider using a complete blood count with differential and erythrocyte sedimentation rate as a screen for occult bacteremia or significant bacterial disease. An abnormal screen consists of a total white blood cell count >15,000, an absolute neutrophil count >10,000, an absolute band count >500, or a sedimentation rate >30. A normal screen makes the possibility of occult bacteremia unlikely. Twenty-eight percent of young children with fever of unknown origin who appear moderate to severely ill and have an abnormal CBC with differential or a sedimentation rate >30 will have bacteremia. When obtained routinely in all febrile cases, urine cultures are positive in 5% of cases, and stool and chest x-rays are positive in 18%.

C. Assess the child's degree of illness. Mildly ill children have temperatures less than 40°C, appear alert, active, and playful, and can be consoled by their parents. Moderately ill children have temperatures of 40°C or higher, or have an altered mental status and an altered activity level. They appear irritable or lethargic, eat poorly, refuse to play, and are difficult to console. Consider immunocompromised children (as a result of sickle cell disease, splenectomy, immunosuppressive therapy, malnutrition, or immune deficiency diseases) moderately to severely ill, regardless of their temperature or clinical state. Severely ill children have a temperature higher than 41°C or appear toxic, hypotensive, have meningeal signs or a markedly altered mental status.

D. Adequate follow-up of children at risk for bacteremia and delayed–onset meningitis is essential. Contact the parents of children with mild to moderate illness within 12 hours; when fever persists, schedule a revisit. At the 48–hour revisit, one-half of the children will be afebrile, one-fourth will have a focus of infection identified, and one-fourth will have persistent fever. Initiate a diagnostic workup for occult infection in children whose fever persists longer than 4 or 5 days.

E. The two most common organisms causing bacteremia are *S. pneumoniae* (40–60%) and *H. influenzae* (11–40%). Other less frequent causes of bacteremia are *Salmonella, N. meningitidis, N. gonorrhoeae* and *S. aureus*. Occult bacteremia can persist and cause meningitis, periorbital cellulitis, pneumonia, epiglottitis, septic arthritis, and pericarditis. Oral antibiotic therapy reduces the sequelae in bacteremia caused by *H. influenzae* and *S. pneumoniae*. Treat cases of suspected bacteremia with amoxicillin 75–100 mg/kg/day as a *tid* dose. Follow patients closely; oral antibiotic therapy does not prevent delayed–onset meningitis. The risk of delayed–onset meningitis is 15% in children with H. influenzae bacteremia, regardless of oral antibiotic therapy. Oral antibiotic therapy may reduce the 2% risk of delayed–onset meningitis which complicates S. pneumoniae bacteremia. Untreated bacteremic children under the age of 1 year, in whom a lumbar puncture is performed, may be at high risk for delayed–onset meningitis. Therefore, treat children under 1 year of age with fever of unknown origin who have undergone lumbar puncture. Evaluate children with occult bacteremia with *N. meningitidis* or *N. gonorrhoeae* for complement deficiencies.

REFERENCES

Baron MA, Fink HD. Bacteremia in private pediatric practice. Pediatrics 1980; 66:171.

McCarthy PL, Jekel JF, Dolan TF. Temperature greater than or equal to 40°C in children less than 24 months of age: a prospective study. Pediatrics 1977; 59:663.

Murray DL, Zonana J, Seidel JS, et al. Relative importance of bacteremia and viremia in the course of acute fevers of unknown origin in outpatient children. Pediatrics 1981; 68:157.

Teele DW, Dashefsky B, Rakusan T, et al. Risk of LP in bacteremic children. New Engl J Med 1981; 305:1079.

Teele DW, Marshall R, Klein JO. Unsuspected bacteremia in young children. Pediatr Clin N Am 1979; 26:773.

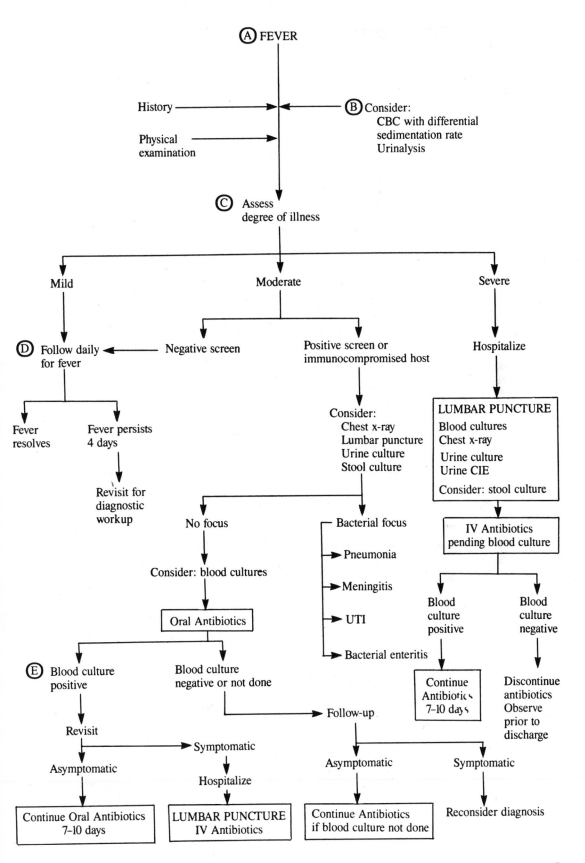

PROLONGED FEVER OF UNKNOWN ORIGIN

A. In pediatrics, prolonged fever of unknown origin is an unexplained fever that persists beyond 7 to 10 days. The fever may resolve, and the etiology often remains unclear. Many cases (50%) are infectious. The remainder are related to collagen vascular disease (15%), neoplasms (7%), inflammatory bowel disease (4%), and other causes (12%). Infections include: viral syndromes (2–18%), URI (2–10%), LRI (4–8%), UTI (3–4%), gastroenteritis (<2%), osteomyelitis (<2%), CNS infections (3–4%), TB (<3%), bacteremia (<2%), SBE (<2%), mononucleosis (<2%), abscess (<1%), brucellosis (<1%), (<2%), and malaria (<1%). Associated collagen vascular diseases are: rheumatoid arthritis (10%), SLE (3%), HSP (1%), and vasculitis (1%). Associated malignancies are: leukemia, lymphoma, and neuroblastoma.

B. The characteristics of the fever (onset, duration, and pattern) and nonspecific symptoms such as anorexia, fatigue, chills, headache, and mild abdominal pain are rarely helpful in diagnosis. Ask about animal exposures: ticks (lyme disease, relapsing fever), rats (plague, rat-bite fever, leptospirosis), hamsters (LCM virus), rabbits, (tularemia), cattle, goats, dogs, (brucellosis), birds, (psittacosis), and cats (cat scratch fever). Also note any history of pica, travel or foreign contacts, and drug exposure (salicylism). Nonspecific symptoms such as anorexia, fatigue, chills, headache, and mild abdominal pain are rarely helpful in diagnosis. Specific symptoms referable to organ system dysfunction are more helpful. Note predisposing conditions such as sickle cell disease, malignancies, immune deficiency states, diabetes mellitus, and dysautonomia.

C. The presence of arthralgia, arthritis, myalgia, or localized limb pain suggests collagen vascular disease, neoplasms, or infections (osteomyelitis/septic arthritis). Significant heart murmurs suggest bacterial endocarditis. Note signs of GI involvement; abdominal pain, bloody stools/diarrhea, or weight loss suggest inflammatory bowel disease. Abdominal pain or mass may be present with a ruptured appendix. Jaundice is consistent with hepatitis; a rash may indicate collagen vascular disease, neoplasms, or infection. Pharyngitis, tonsillitis, or peritonsillar abscess can be caused by the usual bacteria or infectious mononucleosis, CMV, tularemia, or leptosporosis. Respiratory distress may relate to an underlying neoplasm, collagen vascular disease, or infection. Work up children with meningeal or focal neurologic signs for encephalitis, meningitis, or neoplasm. While lymphadenopathy and hepatosplenomegaly are nonspecific findings which may be related to multiple infectious or noninfectious causes, obtain a consultation to rule out malignancy.

D. The CBC with differential may occasionally help guide in the workup. Pancytopenia, unexplained neutropenia with thrombocytopenia, or the presence of lymphoblasts on the peripheral smear requires a hematology/oncology consult and bone marrow test. Reactive lymphocytes on differential suggest mononucleosis or other viral infections. Severe neutropenia in a mild-to-moderately ill patient is consistent with many infections. Leukocytosis and elevated sedimentation rate suggest infection and collagen vascular disease. Hemolytic anemia suggests collagen vascular disease or endocarditis. Nonhemolytic anemia suggests chronic illness or malignancy. Pyuria and bacteriuria suggest urinary tract infection; hematuria suggests endocarditis.

E. Inappropriate antibiotics may alter typical signs of occult infections (especially abdominal abscess or osteomyelitis) and delay diagnosis and appropriate therapy. Resolution of fever with antibiotics may also result in an inappropriate search for an occult bacterial focus when none exists. The best approach to prolonged fever is a conservative, rational workup based on the severity of illness in the child utilizing careful follow-up and periodic reassessments rather than the indiscriminate use of expensive radiographic studies and scans. With the exception of aspirin in cases of suspected juvenile rheumatoid arthritis (JRA), avoid therapeutic trials of antibiotics and other drugs. Exploratory laparotomy without signs of intra-abdominal pathology is not indicated in children.

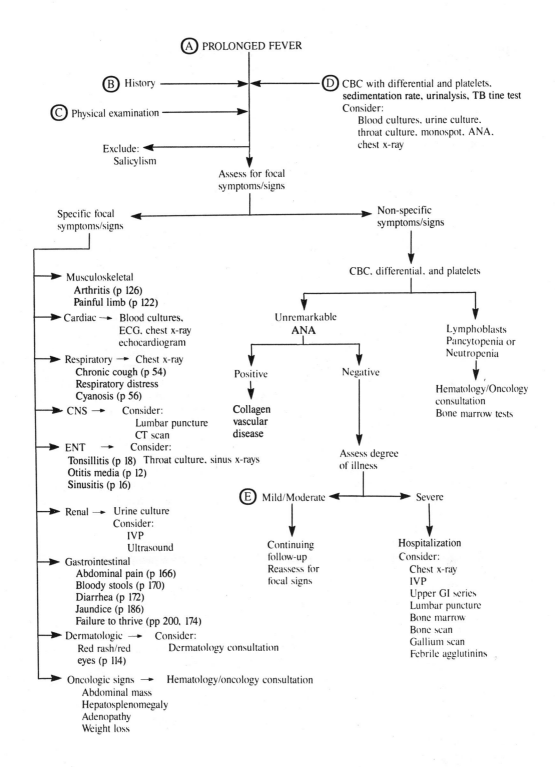

(A) PROLONGED FEVER

(B) History

(C) Physical examination

(D) CBC with differential and platelets, sedimentation rate, urinalysis, TB tine test
Consider:
Blood cultures, urine culture, throat culture, monospot, ANA, chest x-ray

Exclude:
Salicylism

Assess for focal symptoms/signs

Specific focal symptoms/signs

Non-specific symptoms/signs

CBC, differential, and platelets

Musculoskeletal
Arthritis (p 126)
Painful limb (p 122)

Cardiac → Blood cultures, ECG, chest x-ray echocardiogram

Respiratory → Chest x-ray
Chronic cough (p 54)
Respiratory distress
Cyanosis (p 56)

CNS → Consider:
Lumbar puncture
CT scan

ENT → Consider:
Tonsillitis (p 18) Throat culture, sinus x-rays
Otitis media (p 12)
Sinusitis (p 16)

Renal → Urine culture
Consider:
IVP
Ultrasound

Gastrointestinal
Abdominal pain (p 166)
Bloody stools (p 170)
Diarrhea (p 172)
Jaundice (p 186)
Failure to thrive (pp 200, 174)

Dermatologic → Consider:
Red rash/red   Dermatology consultation
eyes (p 114)

Oncologic signs → Hematology/oncology consultation
Abdominal mass
Hepatosplenomegaly
Adenopathy
Weight loss

Unremarkable
ANA

Positive

Negative

Collagen vascular disease

Assess degree of illness

(E) Mild/Moderate

Severe

Continuing follow-up
Reassess for focal signs

Hospitalization
Consider:
Chest x-ray
IVP
Upper GI series
Lumbar puncture
Bone marrow
Bone scan
Gallium scan
Febrile agglutinins

Lymphoblasts
Pancytopenia or
Neutropenia

Hematology/Oncology consultation
Bone marrow tests

REFERENCES

Fulginiti VA. Pediatric Clinical Problem Solving. Baltimore: Williams & Wilkins, 1981.

Lohr JA, Hendley JO. Prolonged fever of unknown origin: a record of experiences with 54 childhood patients. Clin Pediatr 1977; 16:768.

McClung HJ. Prolonged fever of unknown origin in children. JAMA 1972; 124:544.

Pizzo PA, Lovejoy FH, Smith DH. Prolonged fever in children: review of 100 cases. Pediatrics 1975; 55:468.

FREQUENT INFECTIONS

A. Note the type, frequency, pattern, and outcome of frequent infections. Review results of prior radiologic studies and cultures of the throat, eye, middle ear fluid, stool, urine, blood, and spinal fluid. Rule out allergies, immunosuppressive therapy, splenectomy, sickle cell disease, cystic fibrosis, neonatal tetany (DiGeorge's syndrome), malignancy, and other known immune disorders. Note family size and composition and the type of day care. Ask about the family history for early, unexplained infant deaths and known immune disorders.

B. Perform a complete physical examination. Note the presence of lymphoid tissue (lymph nodes and tonsils); assess growth and development.

C. Children under 6 years of age may experience 6 to 12 viral infections per year. These episodes of URIs and diarrhea are usually mild and self-limited. Children who attend nursery school or day care centers are more likely to experience frequent viral infections. Causes of recurrent bacterial infections include recurrent exposures, anatomic defects, allergy, and constitutional host factors. Recurrent tonsillitis may relate to recurrent *S. pyogenes* exposures in the family or day-care setting. Anatomic conditions that cause obstruction can produce recurrent otitis media (eustachian tube), recurrent sinusitis (nasal obstruction), recurrent lower respiratory infections, and recurrent urinary tract infections. Atopic children with reactive airway disease, allergic rhinitis, and eczema are predisposed to develop recurrent respiratory infections (bronchitis, pneumonia, otitis media, and sinusitis), and secondary bacterial infection of eczema.

D. Patients at risk for an immune problem include children with recurrent pyogenic infections including acute otitis media, sinusitis, and bacterial pneumonia, bacteremia, meningitis, and osteomyelitis, (disorders of B cells or complement), chronic and recurrent infections of lymph nodes, skin, liver, lungs, and GI system (disorders of neutrophils), and infections caused by herpes viruses, fungi (*Candida*) and unusual opportunistic bacteria (disorders of T cells).

E. Consider the following studies in the initial immune workup: a CBC with differential to identify lymphopenia or neutropenia; serum immunoglobulins to measure IgG, IgA, IgM and IgE and serum complement (C3 and total hemolytic complement); a chest x-ray and lateral neck x-ray to document thymus size and nasopharyngeal lymphoid tissue skin tests for *Candida*, streptokinase, tokinase, streptodornase, and mumps to evaluate cell-mediated immune function. Consider an NBT test to assess phagocytosis and killing ability, other neutrophil functions tests, isohemagglutinin titers or antibodies after immunization with diphtheria or tetanus toxoid, and a determination of the percentage of T and B cells of peripheral lymphocytes.

F. Disorders of B cells (antibody synthesis) include hereditary agammaglobulinemia (Bruton's disease), a sex-linked disorder in which IgG and all other immunoglobulins are deficient. Rarely, agammaglobulinemia can also occur as a non-sex-linked disease. Isolated immunoglobulin deficiencies have been described for IgG, IgA, IgM, IgE, and IgD. Abnormalities of neutrophils include deficient number (congenital or cyclic neutropenia) and functions such as adherence to vascular endothelium, chemotaxis (lazy leukocyte syndrome), ingestion, and microbial killing (chronic gramulomatous disease). Disorders of complement may result in recurrent bacteremia and meningitis especially with gonorrhea or meningococcus.

G. Specific immune deficient syndromes include severe combined immunodeficiency (Swiss type A gammaglobulinemia), DiGeorge's syndrome, Wiskott-Aldrich syndrome, ataxia telangectasia, chronic mucocutaneous candidiasis, Leiner's disease, staphylococcal abscesses (Job's syndrome), chronic granulomatous disease, and Chediak-Higashi syndrome.

REFERENCES

Fulginiti VA. Pediatric Clinical Problem Solving. Baltimore: Williams & Wilkins, 1981.

Johnston RB. Defects in neutrophil function. New Engl J Med 1982; 307:434.

Moffet HL. Pediatric Infectious Disease: A Problem Oriented Approach. Philadelphia: JB Lippincott, 1981.

Ward DW. Laboratory diagnosis of immunodeficiency disease. Pediatr Clin North Am 1977; 24:329.

FREQUENT INFECTIONS

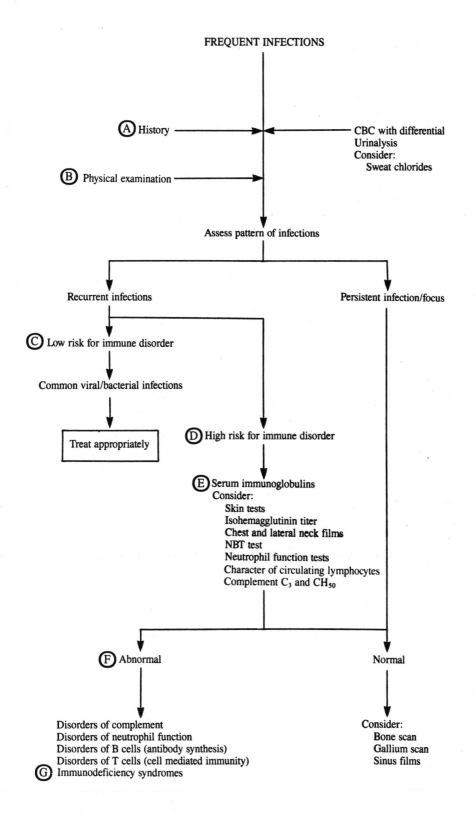

NECK MASS

Peter A. Lane, M.D.

A. Note the duration of the mass and determine whether or not it has been changing in size or character. If painful, determine whether salivation worsens the pain (salivary gland enlargement). Record any treatment already undertaken (i.e., antibiotics) and its effect on the size and character of the mass. If the mass is thought to be a lymph node, inquire specifically about previous local infections in the area drained by the node. Note travel and exposure to animals. If there has been exposure to cats, inquire about scratches, papules, or pustules in the area drained by the node (cat scratch disease). Note the presence or absence of systemic symptoms such as fever, unexplained weight loss, night sweats, irritability, skeletal pain, cough, or wheezing.

B. Perform a complete physical examination. The finding of lymph node enlargement in more than 2 noncontiguous lymph node regions or of hepatosplenomegaly suggests generalized lymphadenopathy (p 162). Characterize the mass: note location, mobility, consistency, fluctuation, warmth, erythema, tenderness, or fixation to the skin. Record accurate measurements in 2 dimensions. Parotid gland enlargement characteristically obscures the angle of the mandible, with at least one-half of the mass palpable above the angle. Examine the scalp, ears, nose, and oral pharynx for evidence of local infection or neoplasm. Look for sinus tract openings in the skin if the mass is midline (thyroglossal duct cyst) or anterior to the sternocleidomastoid muscle (branchial cleft cyst). Consider transillumination of any mass suspected to be cystic, particularly if it is lobulated and located in the supraclavicular fossa of a young child (cystic hygroma). Signs of acute inflammation suggest acute bacterial lymphadenitiis or an infected congenital cyst.

C. Children with supraclavicular or scalene lymphadenopathy or with unexplained systemic symptoms, especially weight loss or prolonged fever, are considered at significant risk. Additional worrisome characteristics of an undiagnosed mass may include a diameter >3 cm, onset during the neonatal period, history of rapid or progressive growth (especially in the absence of any inflammation) or lack of mobility. Most children with a neck mass fall into the low-risk group.

D. Frequently, clues provided in the history and physical will allow a presumptive diagnosis. In the absence of severe caries or dental infections (anaerobes), acute unilateral cervical adenitis can be treated with an antibiotic effective against both *S. aureus* and streptococci. Fluctuant adenitis may require surgical drainage. Closed aspiration with an 18-gauge needle may hasten the resolution of cat scratch disease.

E. When no presumptive etiology is apparent for a neck mass in a child determined to be at low risk for serious disease, a 7–10 day course of an oral antibiotic (to cover both *streptococcus* and *staphylococcus*) is warranted. Consider aspirating an enlarged lymph node since positive bacterial cultures may be obtained in the absence of inflammation or fluctuance. Place a PPD on young children with unilateral tonsillar or submandibular adenopathy.

F. Perform a PPD, CBC with differential, monospot, and chest x-ray. These studies are frequently normal in the face of a lymphoma, so an excisional biopsy is warranted if no etiology is apparent (particularly if the mass has continued to enlarge on antibiotics).

G. Obtain an oncology consult. An excisional biopsy is necessary in most cases. Ultrasound examination of the mass may detect cystic components. Gallium avidity suggests infection or neoplasm. Young children, especially those with irritability, fever, skeletal pain, or anemia should have a urine collection for VMA and catecholamines. The serum LDH is typically elevated by nonHodgkins lymphoma but often normal in Hodgkins disease.

REFERENCES

Knight PJ, Mulne AF, Vassay LE. When is lymph node biopsy indicated in children with enlarged peripheral nodes? Pediatrics 1982; 69:391.

Knight PJ, Reiner CB. Superficial lumps in children: what, when, and why? Pediatrics 1983; 72:147.

Marcy SM. Infections of lymph nodes of the head and neck. Pediatr Infect Dis 1983; 2:397.

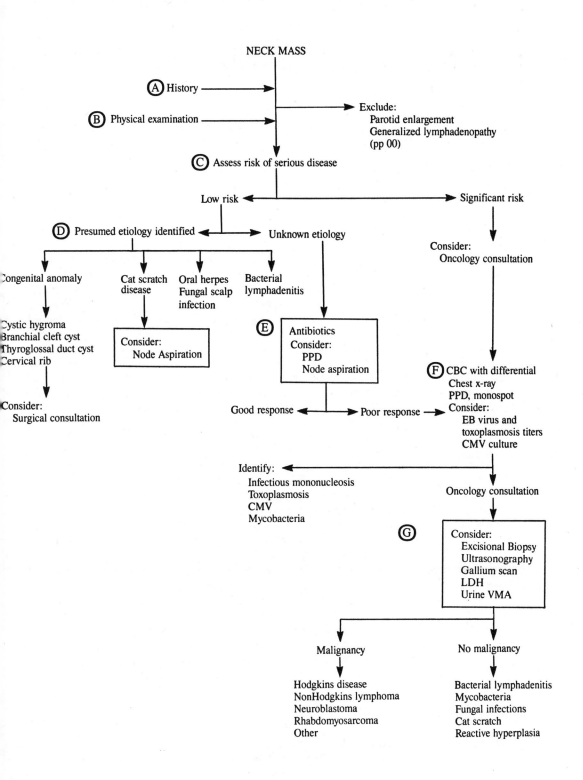

NECK MASS

(A) History ⟶

(B) Physical examination ⟶

Exclude:
Parotid enlargement
Generalized lymphadenopathy
(pp 00)

(C) Assess risk of serious disease

Low risk ⟵⟶ Significant risk

(D) Presumed etiology identified ⟵⟶ Unknown etiology

Consider:
Oncology consultation

Congenital anomaly | Cat scratch disease | Oral herpes Fungal scalp infection | Bacterial lymphadenitis

Cystic hygroma
Branchial cleft cyst
Thyroglossal duct cyst
Cervical rib

Consider:
Node Aspiration

(E) Antibiotics
Consider:
PPD
Node aspiration

(F) CBC with differential
Chest x-ray
PPD, monospot
Consider:
EB virus and
toxoplasmosis titers
CMV culture

Consider:
Surgical consultation

Good response ⟵⟶ Poor response ⟶

Identify: ⟵
Infectious mononucleosis
Toxoplasmosis
CMV
Mycobacteria

Oncology consultation

(G) Consider:
Excisional Biopsy
Ultrasonography
Gallium scan
LDH
Urine VMA

Malignancy | No malignancy

Hodgkins disease
NonHodgkins lymphoma
Neuroblastoma
Rhabdomyosarcoma
Other

Bacterial lymphadenitis
Mycobacteria
Fungal infections
Cat scratch
Reactive hyperplasia

Pounds LA. Neck masses of congenital origin. Pediatr Clin North Am 1981; 28:841.
Zitelli BJ. Neck masses in children: adenopathy and malignant disease. Pediatr Clin North Am 1981; 28:813.

ACUTE OTITIS MEDIA

A. Note symptoms suggestive of acute otitis media such as earache, draining ear, irritability, decreased feeding, vomiting, fever, and ataxia. Ask about respiratory symptoms, alteration in mental status, or conjunctivitis. Inquire as to frequency of past episodes of acute otitis media and their outcome. Identify predisposing conditions such as allergic rhinitis, cystic fibrosis, immune deficiency disorders, or Kartagener's syndrome.

B. Note signs of acute otitis media including abnormal color of the tympanic membrane (red or yellow), a bulging contour, diminished or absent tympanic membrane mobility. Also note signs of chronic or recurrent episodes such as tympanosclerosis, severe retraction, atelectatic pockets, or cholesteatoma (yellow, greasy mass). Evaluate the patient's mental status and note the presence of neurological signs such as focal neurologic findings, seizures, or ataxia.

C. Treat acute otitis media with amoxicillin (50 mg/kg/day in 3 divided doses). Acute otitis media is caused by *S. pneumoniae* in 31% of cases, *H. influenzae* 27%, *group A streptococci* 2%, *S. aureus* 2%, and others (including gram–negative enterics, *B. catarrhalis*, and anaerobes) in 4%. Middle ear aspirates are either sterile or grow presumed nonpathogens (*S. epidermidis* and diptheroids) in 33% of cases. Treat children who are allergic to penicillin derivatives with trimethoprim sulfamethoxazole (TMP/SMZ), or erythromycin/sulfisoxazole combination. A return visit at 36–48 hours is necessary, when fever, earache, irritability, vomiting, or lethargy fail to improve, in order to identify resistant infections or serious occult disease such as bacteremia or meningitis. At 2 weeks approximately 50% of treated cases will have resolution of the middle ear effusion, 40% will have a residual serous effusion, and 10% will have persistent acute infection. Middle-ear aspirates from children who fail to respond to therapy with amoxicillin, TMP/SMZ, or erythromycin/sulfisoxazole most often have sterile effusions (57%). Organisms resistant to the initial therapy are identified in 19% of repeat middle-ear aspirates. Resistant isolates from children treated initially with amoxicillin respond to TMP/SMZ or erythromycin/sulfisoxazole and vice versa.

D. Perform a tympanocentesis or myringotomy as part of a septic workup in a child with suspected sepsis or meningitis, when suppurative labyrinthitis or mastoiditis is identified, in an immunocompromised host, and in an infant < 6 weeks of age with a past neonatal intensive care hospitalization. Consider tympanocentesis for persistent acute otitis media which has failed to respond to 2 courses of antibiotic therapy.

E. Treatment of residual serous effusion is unnecessary; spontaneous resolution occurs in 85% of cases within 6 weeks. The use of decongestants, antihistamines, or myringotomy will not prevent residual effusions or result in more rapid resolution of the effusion. Consider gantrisin prophylaxis (75 mg/kg/day *bid*) in children with a history of recurrent otitis; residual effusions predispose to recurrent acute episodes.

F. Refer for ventilating tubes children < 3 years of age with unilateral or bilateral persistent effusions associated with a documented hearing loss for ≥ 3 months, persistent acute otitis media unresponsive to antibiotics, and children who have recurrent acute otitis (≥3 episodes per 6-month period) despite antibiotic prophylaxis.

REFERENCES

Gebhart DE. Tympanostomy tubes in the otitis media prone child. Laryngoscope 1981; 91:849.

Healy GB, Smith HG. Current concepts in the management of otitis media with effusion. Am J Otolaryngol 1981; 2:138.

Howie VM, Schwartz RH. Acute otitis media, one year in general pediatric practice. Am J Dis Child 1982; 137:155.

Perrin JM, Charney E, MacWhinney JB Jr et al. Sulfisoxazole as chemoprophylaxis for recurrent otitis media: A double-blind crossover study in pediatric practice. New Engl J Med 1974; 29:664.

Schwartz RH. Bacteriology of otitis media: A review. Otolaryngol Head Neck Surg 1981; 89:444.

Teele DW, Pelton SI, Klein JO. Bacteriology of acute otitis media unresponsive to initial antimicrobial therapy. J Pediatr 1981; 98:537.

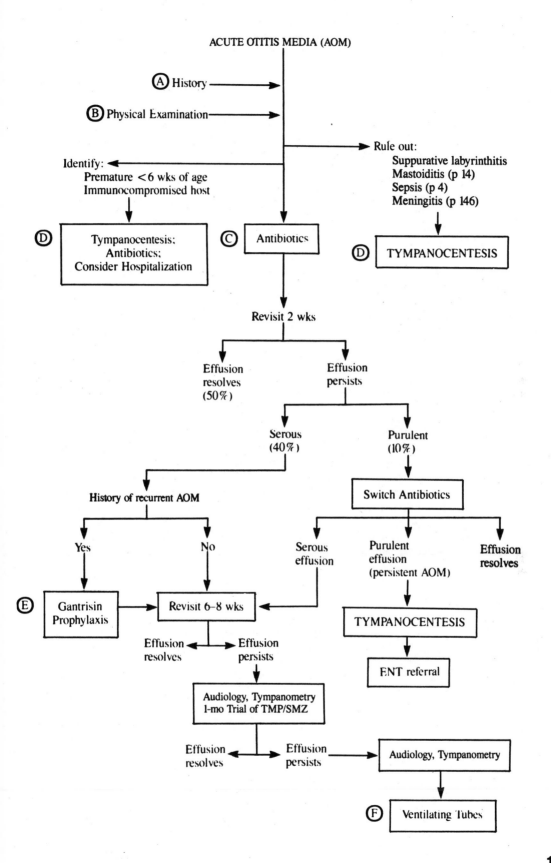

ACUTE OTITIS MEDIA (AOM)

(A) History

(B) Physical Examination

Rule out:
    Suppurative labyrinthitis
    Mastoiditis (p 14)
    Sepsis (p 4)
    Meningitis (p 146)

Identify:
Premature <6 wks of age
Immunocompromised host

(D) Tympanocentesis;
Antibiotics;
Consider Hospitalization

(C) Antibiotics

(D) TYMPANOCENTESIS

Revisit 2 wks

Effusion resolves (50%)

Effusion persists

Serous (40%)

Purulent (10%)

History of recurrent AOM

Yes

No

Serous effusion

Switch Antibiotics

Purulent effusion (persistent AOM)

Effusion resolves

(E) Gantrisin Prophylaxis

Revisit 6–8 wks

TYMPANOCENTESIS

Effusion resolves

Effusion persists

ENT referral

Audiology, Tympanometry
1-mo Trial of TMP/SMZ

Effusion resolves

Effusion persists

Audiology, Tympanometry

(F) Ventilating Tubes

ACUTE MASTOIDITIS

A. Ask about earache, ear discharge, and fever. Identify predisposing conditions such as chronic or recurrent otitis media, cystic fibrosis, Kartagener's syndrome, and immune deficiency syndromes. Note signs of CNS complications such as headache, vertigo, vomiting, ataxia, stiff neck, weakness, changes in sensorium, or seizures.

B. Note any swelling over the mastoid area with overlying erythema. Infants under 1 year of age with mastoiditis present with swelling superior to the ear with the pinna pushed down rather than out. Examination of the tympanic membrane reveals swelling of the external ear canal and signs of acute otitis media. Evaluate the child's mental status and level of activity, and identify neurologic signs such as meningeal signs, facial palsy, cranial nerve deficits, focal seizures, and ataxia.

C. Meningitis complicates approximately 9% of cases with acute mastoiditis. This infection should be suspected when the child has a high fever, stiff neck, severe headache, or other meningeal signs. A lumbar puncture should be performed to accurately diagnose this infection. Brain abscess (occurring in 2% of cases) may be associated with persistent headache, recurring fever, or changes in sensorium. A CT scan should be performed to identify these cases.

D. Mastoid x-rays will determine the presence of subperiosteal abscess with bony destruction, which occurs in approximately 18% of cases. Some otolaryngologists consider the destruction of septal bone (osteitis) in the mastoid air cells (coalescent mastoiditis) an indication for immediate surgery.

E. Assess the degree of illness. Severely ill children who require immediate surgery appear toxic or present with acute suppurative labyrinthitis, facial palsy, coalescent mastoiditis, or a CNS complication. In a simple mastoidectomy, the mastoid air cells are removed while both the inner table of bone over the dura and the middle ear space are left intact.

F. The initial management of uncomplicated, acute mastoiditis includes IV antibiotic therapy and possible surgery. The results of the Gram stain of an initial tympanocentesis may help in selecting antibiotics. Use amoxicillin and nafcillin; the most common etiologic agents are *S. pneumoniae*, *S. aureus* and Group A β–hemolytic streptococci. *H. influenzae* causes mastoiditis much less frequently than expected. Other agents which can cause this disease include pseudomonas, tuberculosis, and enteropathic gram–negative rods. Anaerobic organisms appear to play a role in chronic mastoiditis; there are no data regarding their role in acute mastoiditis. Surgery is indicated by failure to respond to 24–48 hours of antibiotic therapy or the development of complications on therapy.

REFERENCES

Brook I. Aerobic and anaerobic bacteriology of chronic mastoiditis in children. Am J Dis Child 1981; 135 (5):478.

Ginsburg CM, Rudoy R, Nelson JD. Acute mastoiditis in infants and children. Clin Pediatr 1980; 19 (8):549.

Macadam AM, Rubio T. Tuberculous otomastoiditis in children. Am J Dis Child 1977; 131 (2):152.

Venezio FR, Naidich TP, Shulman S. Complications of mastoiditis with special emphasis on venous sinus thrombosis. J Pediatr 1982; 101:509.

ACUTE MASTOIDITIS

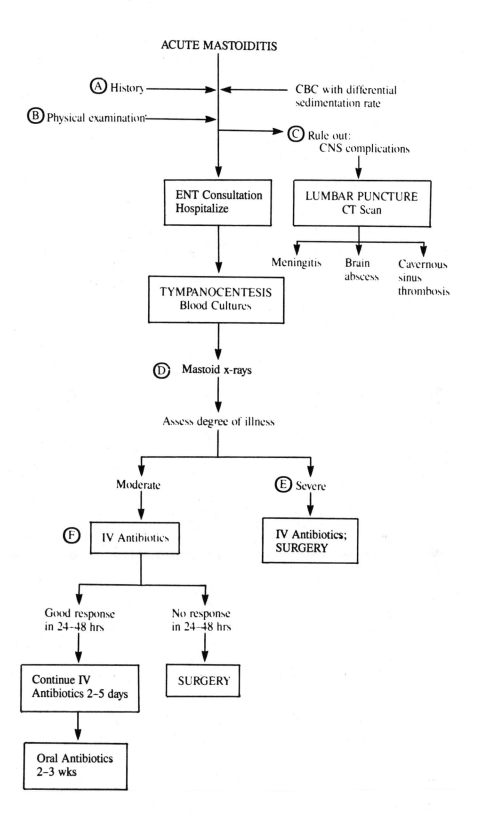

Ⓐ History ⟶⟶ ⟵⟵ CBC with differential
sedimentation rate

Ⓑ Physical examination ⟶⟶

⟶ Ⓒ Rule out:
CNS complications

| ENT Consultation Hospitalize | LUMBAR PUNCTURE CT Scan |

Meningitis   Brain abscess   Cavernous sinus thrombosis

TYMPANOCENTESIS
Blood Cultures

Ⓓ Mastoid x-rays

Assess degree of illness

Moderate   Ⓔ Severe

Ⓕ IV Antibiotics   IV Antibiotics; SURGERY

Good response   No response
in 24–48 hrs   in 24–48 hrs

Continue IV   SURGERY
Antibiotics 2–5 days

Oral Antibiotics
2–3 wks

PARANASAL SINUSITIS

A. Paranasal sinusitis results from infections of the ethmoid, maxillary, or frontal sinuses. The ethmoids are present at birth, the maxillary sinuses become clinically important by 18–24 months of age, and the frontal sinuses become pneumatized at 7–10 years of age.

B. Note congestion, cough, purulent rhinorrhea, malodorous breath, and fever. Headache, facial pain, and an altered sense of smell are indicative of paranasal sinusitis but are found infrequently in children. Identify predisposing conditions such as a history of allergies, recurrent respiratory tract infections, dental infections, anatomic conditions (nasal malformation, nasal trauma, tumors, polyps, foreign bodies, cleft palate), cyanotic congenital heart disease, and barotrauma secondary to swimming and diving.

C. Note tenderness or swelling overlying the sinuses, especially the frontal sinus (Potts puffy tumor), dental problems including tooth abscess, caries, or apical abscess, and the presence of a nasal foreign body. Evaluate the child's mental status and identify neurologic signs such as cranial nerve deficits, seizures, and meningeal signs. Identify signs of periorbital or orbital cellulitis including periorbital swelling, redness, proptosis, or paralysis of extraocular movements.

D. Assess the degree of illness. Severely ill patients appear toxic, have severe persistent headache, signs of periorbital or orbital cellulitis, facial swelling, or signs of CNS complication. Moderately ill children present with fever greater than 39°C, headache, facial pain, or marked irritability. Mildly ill patients have a low grade fever or no fever and a chronic cough, but no headache or mental status changes.

E. The initial management of acute paranasal sinusitis in children with mild or moderate illness is amoxicillin 50 mg/kg/day in 3 divided doses combined with a topical and/or systemic decongestant. In children allergic to penicillin, use trimethoprim/sulfisoxazole or erythromycin/sulfisoxazole. Reviews of the bacteriology of sinus aspirates in pediatric cases of acute maxillary sinusitis show that *S. pneumoniae* causes 25–45% of cases, *H. influenzae* 13–30%, *B. catarrhalis* 10–15%, Group A β–hemolytic streptococcus 2–6%, *S. aureus* 0–10%, and others (including gram-negative enteric organisms and anaerobes) 0–10%. In 20–30% of cases, aspirates are sterile or contain nonpathogens.

F. Switch antibiotics when symptoms such as fever, facial pain, or headache fail to improve after 36–48 hours of therapy or when milder symptoms persist after a 7–14 day course of therapy. Consider covering β-lactamase producing organisms such as *H. influenzae* or *B. catarrhalis* as well as *S. aureus* by switching antibiotics to TMP/SMZ, erythromycin/sulfisoxazole, or cefaclor. Obtain sinus films. Evidence for sinusitis includes the presence of air fluid levels, complete opacity, or mucosal thickening >5 mm. Sinus films in children under one year of age are often difficult to interpret.

G. Treat severely ill children with a combination of ampicillin and either moxolactam or chloramphenicol. Suspect a CNS complication when the patient presents with an altered mental status or neurologic signs; do a CT scan and lumbar puncture. The valveless opthalmic venous system allows for free communication among the cavernous sinus, orbit, and paranasal sinuses, and predisposes the patient to a CNS infection.

REFERENCES

Brook I, Friedman EM, Rodriguez WJ. Complications of sinusitis in children. Pediatrics 1980; 66:568.

Sable NS, Hengerer A, Powell KR. Acute frontal sinusitis with intracranial complications. Pediatric Infect Dis 1984; 3:58.

Wald ER. Acute sinusitis in children. Pediatr Infect Dis 1983; 2:61.

Wald ER, Milmoe GJ, Bowen AD et al. Acute maxillary sinusitis in children. N E J M 1981; 304:749.

Wald ER, Reilly JS, Casselbrant M, et al. Treatment of acute maxillary sinusitis in childhood: A comparative study of amoxicillin and cefaclor. J Pediatr. 1984; 104:297.

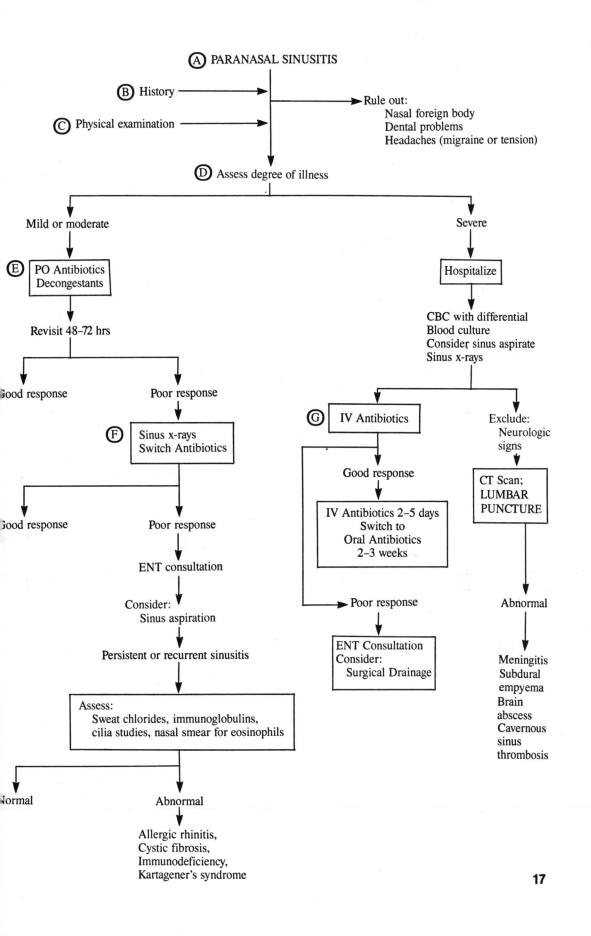

(A) PARANASAL SINUSITIS

(B) History

(C) Physical examination

Rule out:
Nasal foreign body
Dental problems
Headaches (migraine or tension)

(D) Assess degree of illness

Mild or moderate

Severe

(E) PO Antibiotics
Decongestants

Hospitalize

Revisit 48–72 hrs

CBC with differential
Blood culture
Consider sinus aspirate
Sinus x-rays

Good response

Poor response

(F) Sinus x-rays
Switch Antibiotics

(G) IV Antibiotics

Exclude:
Neurologic
signs

Good response

Good response

Poor response

IV Antibiotics 2–5 days
Switch to
Oral Antibiotics
2–3 weeks

CT Scan;
LUMBAR
PUNCTURE

ENT consultation

Consider:
Sinus aspiration

Poor response

Abnormal

Persistent or recurrent sinusitis

ENT Consultation
Consider:
 Surgical Drainage

Meningitis
Subdural
empyema
Brain
abscess
Cavernous
sinus
thrombosis

Assess:
 Sweat chlorides, immunoglobulins,
 cilia studies, nasal smear for eosinophils

Normal

Abnormal

Allergic rhinitis,
Cystic fibrosis,
Immunodeficiency,
Kartagener's syndrome

17

SORE THROAT

A. Determine the onset, duration, severity (ability to swallow or talk) of the sore throat. Note symptoms of upper respiratory obstruction such as stridor, drooling, inability to swallow, inability to lie down, air hunger, or restlessness. Identify associated symptoms including fever, rhinorrhea, nasal congestion, cough, earache, fatigue, malaise, vomiting, diarrhea, headache, abdominal pain, and rash.

B. Note the size of the tonsils, the presence of exudate or petechiae, cervical adenitis, deviation of the uvula, or a sandpaper rash suggesting scarlet fever. Identify signs of acute otitis media, a mucopurulent rhinorrhea (sinusitis), or abnormalities of the pharynx. Note signs of mononucleosis such as lymphadenopathy, hepatosplenomegaly, edema of the eyelids, or a rash (frequently associated with ampicillin).

C. Acute pharyngitis can be caused by multiple agents. Signs such as tonsillar exudate with petechiae on the palate, cervical adenitis, and a sandpaper rash increase the probability of infection with *S. pyogenes* from 33% to 75%. Viral agents which can cause acute pharyngitis include Epstein-Barr virus (mononucleosis), enterovirus (herpangina), adenovirus, and influenza virus. Consider *N. gonorrhoeae* in a sexually active adolescent.

D. The goals of antibiotic therapy for *S. pyogenes* pharyngitis include the prevention of rheumatic fever and, possibly, glomerulonephritis and the prevention of suppurative sequelae such as peritonsillar abscess, parapharyngeal abscess, or cervical adentitis. It is unclear whether antibiotics modify acute symptoms. Therapy given within 9 days of the infection will prevent rheumatic fever. Early treatment may not prevent glomerulonephritis. Penicillin (50 mg/kg/day *qid*) for 10 days or 1 shot of benzathine penicillin IM (<30 lbs—300,000 units, 31-60 lbs—600,000 units, 61-90 lbs—900,000 units, >90 lbs—1,200,000 units) will prevent rheumatic fever related to *S. pyogenes* pharyngitis. Erythromycin (20-40 mg/kg/day *qid*) can be used for penicillin–allergic patients but resistance is emerging. Trimethoprim/sulfamethoxazole is not an acceptable antibiotic for *S. pyogenes*.

E. Peritonsillar swelling with deviation of the uvula indicates spread of infection to the peritonsillar space between the tonsillar capsule and the superior constrictor pharyngeal muscle. Needle aspiration confirms the presence of an abscess. In the nontoxic child, cellulitis can initially be managed with penicillin (IM or oral) or amoxicillin. Incision and drainage of the abscess or acute tonsillectomy are recommended for peritonsillar abscess. Recurrence of the abscess is uncommon (7%) in children treated with only incision and drainage. Anaerobes are associated with 65% of cases and *S. pyogenes* with 30%. *H. influenzae*, *S. aureus*, or *S. pneumoniae*, rarely cause a peritonsillar abscess.

REFERENCES

Haddy RI, Gordon RC, Shamiyeh L. Erythromycin resistance in Gp A beta–hemolytic streptococci. Pediatr Infect Dis 1982; 1:236.

Holt GR, Tinsley PP. Peritonsillar abscesses in children. Laryngoscope 1981; 91:1226.

Pantell RH. Pharyngitis: Diagnosis and management. Pediatr Rev 1981; 3:35.

Sugita R, Kawamura S, Icikawa G et al. Microorganisms isolated from peritonsillar abscess and indicated chemotherapy. Arch Otolaryngol 1982; 108:65.

Todd JK. Throat cultures in the office laboratory. Pediatr Infect Dis 1982; 1:265.

SORE THROAT

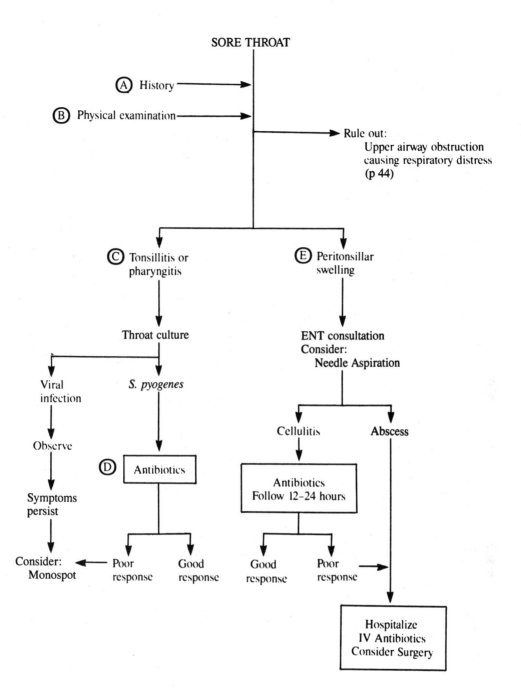

(A) History

(B) Physical examination

Rule out:
Upper airway obstruction
causing respiratory distress
(p 44)

(C) Tonsillitis or
pharyngitis

(E) Peritonsillar
swelling

Throat culture

ENT consultation
Consider:
Needle Aspiration

Viral
infection

S. pyogenes

Cellulitis

Abscess

Observe

(D) Antibiotics

Antibiotics
Follow 12–24 hours

Symptoms
persist

Consider:
Monospot

Poor
response

Good
response

Good
response

Poor
response

Hospitalize
IV Antibiotics
Consider Surgery

RED, PAINFUL EYES

A. Evaluate the severity of the inflammation by asking about the amount of exudate, the degree of swelling, the presence of pain, and the effect on vision. Inquire as to the onset and duration of the inflammation, pattern of symptoms, and prior episodes. Note associated symptoms including fever, rash, cough, rhinorrhea, nasal congestion, malodorous breath, headache, vomiting, or malaise. The presence of severe headache, protracted vomiting, seizures, focal neurologic signs, or an altered mental status suggest CNS involvement. Identify precipitating factors or predisposing conditions such as trauma, insect bites, exposure to allergens, or sinusitis.

B. Note the degree of conjunctival injection, periorbital swelling, presence of purulent discharge, evidence of trauma or local infection, and degree of tenderness. Periorbital swelling associated with mucopurulent rhinorrhea, facial tenderness, and malodorous breath suggests periorbital cellulitis secondary to sinusitis. Ophthalmoplegia, proptosis, edema of the eyeball (chemosis), and abnormal visual acuity suggest orbital cellulitis. The presence of erythroderma with fever suggests infection or toxin (toxic shock, staphylococcal scalded skin syndrome, staphylococcal scarlet fever, leptosporosis) or Kawasaki's disease (p 114).

C. Hordeolum (stye) of the eyelid is caused by a staphylococcal infection of a hair follicle or sebaceous gland. A chalazion is a granulomatous inflammation of the meibomian glands.

D. Herpes simplex keratitis usually presents with marked irritation and eye pain. Fluorescein examination reveals branching dendritic etchings on the anterior part of the cornea. Symptoms may be exacerbated by the use of topical or systemic corticosteroids. Refer these patients to the ophthalmologist for confirmation and treatment with 0.5% idoxiuridine ophthalmic ointment or 0.1% solution or vidarabine or acyclovir. Reduce the patient's level of eye discomfort by instilling 5% homatropine and patching the eye.

E. Fluorescein examination of patients with phlyctenular keratoconjunctivitis reveals nodules located near the limbus with surrounding hyperemia. The lesions indicate a hypersensitivity reaction. Treat this disorder with topical steroids. Apply a PPD to rule out tuberculosis. The presence of hypertrophy of the dorsal conjunctiva with elevated greyish areas near the limbus is consistent with vernal conjunctivitis. Manage mild cases with topical steroids and refer more severe cases to the ophthalmologist.

REFERENCES

Ellis PP. Diseases of the conjunctiva. In: Kempe CH, Silver HK, O'Brien DO, eds. Current Pediatric Diagnosis and Treatment. Los Altos, California: Lange Medical Publications, 1982:213.

Poirier RH. Herpetic ocular infections of childhood. Arch Ophthalmol 1980; 98:704.

Teele DW. Management of the child with the red and swollen eye. Ped Infectious Disease 1983; 2:258.

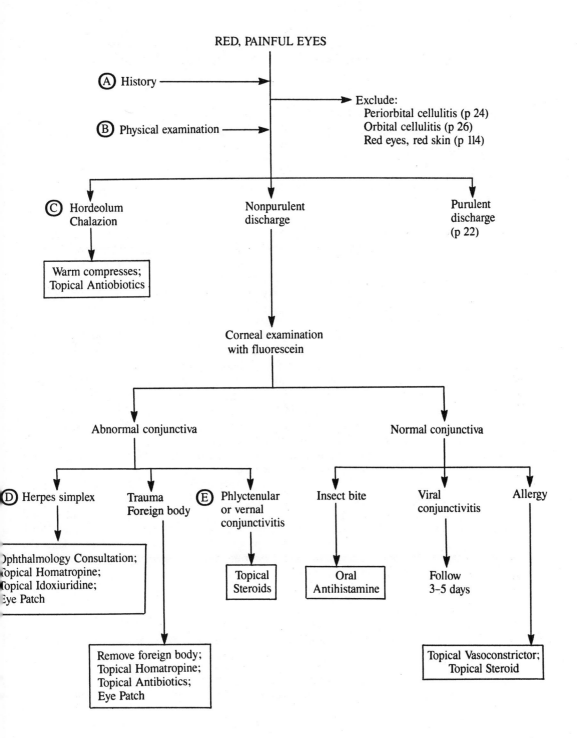

RED, PAINFUL EYES

(A) History

(B) Physical examination

Exclude:
  Periorbital cellulitis (p 24)
  Orbital cellulitis (p 26)
  Red eyes, red skin (p 114)

(C) Hordeolum
    Chalazion

Warm compresses;
Topical Antiobiotics

Nonpurulent
discharge

Purulent
discharge
(p 22)

Corneal examination
with fluorescein

Abnormal conjunctiva

Normal conjunctiva

(D) Herpes simplex

Trauma
Foreign body

(E) Phlyctenular
    or vernal
    conjunctivitis

Insect bite

Viral
conjunctivitis

Allergy

Ophthalmology Consultation;
Topical Homatropine;
Topical Idoxiuridine;
Eye Patch

Topical
Steroids

Oral
Antihistamine

Follow
3–5 days

Remove foreign body;
Topical Homatropine;
Topical Antibiotics;
Eye Patch

Topical Vasoconstrictor;
Topical Steroid

21

PURULENT CONJUNCTIVITIS

A. The use of silver nitrate as a method of prophylaxis against ophthalmic gonorrhea produces an excoriation of the superficial conjunctival layer and mild purulent discharge. The discharge appears within 24 hours of prophylaxis and resolves within 3 days.

B. The common organisms that cause neonatal conjunctivitis are *Chlamydia* followed by *S. aureus*, *S. pneumoniae*, *N. Gonorrhoeae*, *H. influenza* and gram-negative enteric organisms. Treat nongonococcal infections initially with topical antibiotic therapy (sulfonamide ophthalmic ointments). Failure to respond is an indication to switch topical antibiotics and consider oral erythromycin to cover *Chlamydia*. Chlamydia conjunctivitis develops in 20–44% of infants born vaginally to infected mothers. The incubation period varies from 5 to 15 days. Infants with Chlamydia conjunctivitis may become nasopharyngeal carriers and subsequently develop pneumonia. Oral erythromycin therapy decreases the risk of relapse or reinfection of conjunctivae and may eradicate the carrier state and prevent Chlamydia pneumonia.

C. Gonorrhea, which presents after a 1–3 day incubation period, is associated with a severe purulent discharge, edema of the eyelids, and occasional hemorrhage. Infection with gonorrhea can rapidly produce ulceration, perforation, and scarring. Start therapy with penicillin G 50,000 units/kg/day IV or IM when gram-negative diplococci are identified on Gram stain. Irrigate the purulent discharge with normal saline, and, in unilateral cases, cover the unaffected eye to prevent contamination. Topical erythromycin or penicillin antibiotics may also be of benefit.

D. Dacrocystitis presents as a purulent discharge with redness and swelling in the inferior/medial aspect of the eye. Stenosis of the lacrimal duct (dacrostenosis) predisposes to secondary bacterial infection of the lacrimal sac. After obtaining a culture, treat with amoxicillin and a topical antibiotic. Consider referral to an ophthalmologist when signs of dacrostenosis (excessive tearing with recurrent infections) persist beyond 7 months of age.

E. Infectious conjuctivitis occurring after the neonatal period can be bacterial or viral. The most common bacterial agents are *S. pneumoniae*, *H. influenzae*, and *S. aureus*. Less common agents are *N. gonorrhoea* and *N. meningitidis*. Initially treat purulent conjunctivitis with topical sulfacetamide ophthalmic ointment (10%) or solution (15%). In resistant cases, consider topical gentamicin, erythromycin, or neomycin which has more frequent allergic side effects. Viral agents causing conjunctivitis include echovirus, coxsackie virus, adenovirus, rubeola, and herpes simplex. Herpes infections often present with photophobia and pain, suggesting a keratitis. Fluorescein stain will reveal ulcerations and/or dendritic etchings. Refer suspected cases of herpes simplex infection to the ophthalmologist.

REFERENCES

Ellis PP. Diseases of the conjunctiva. In: Kempe CH, Silver HK, O'Brien DO, eds. Current Pediatric Diagnosis and Treatment. Los Altos, California: Lange Medical Publications 1982:213.

Hammerschlag MR. Conjunctivitis in infancy and childhood. Pediatr Rev 1984; 5:285.

Moore RA, Schmitt BD. Conjunctivitis in children. Clin Pediatrics 1979; 18:26.

Patamasucon P, Rettig PJ, Faust KL et al. Oral vs topical erythromycin therapies for chlamydial conjunctivitis. Am J Dis Child 1982; 136:817.

Teele DW. Management of the child with a red and swollen eye. Ped Infec Dis 1983; 2:258.

PURULENT CONJUNCTIVITIS

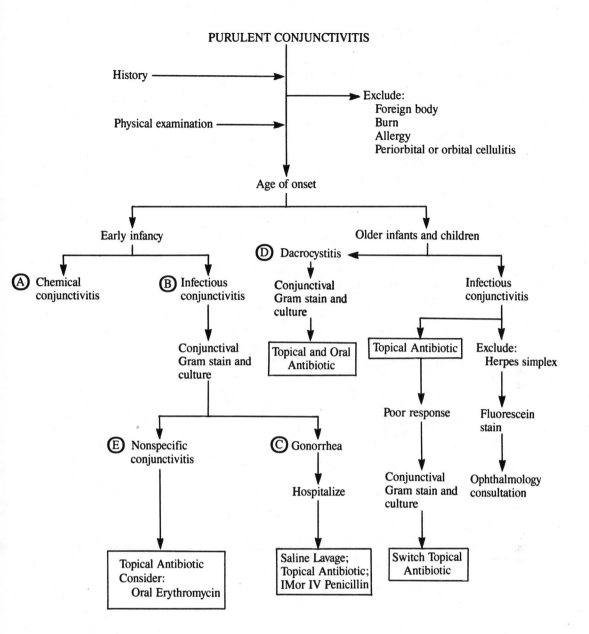

History ⟶

Physical examination ⟶

Exclude:
  Foreign body
  Burn
  Allergy
  Periorbital or orbital cellulitis

Age of onset

Early infancy

Older infants and children

Ⓐ Chemical conjunctivitis

Ⓑ Infectious conjunctivitis

Ⓓ Dacrocystitis

Conjunctival Gram stain and culture

Infectious conjunctivitis

Conjunctival Gram stain and culture

Topical and Oral Antibiotic

Topical Antibiotic

Exclude:
  Herpes simplex

Poor response

Fluorescein stain

Ⓔ Nonspecific conjunctivitis

Ⓒ Gonorrhea

Conjunctival Gram stain and culture

Ophthalmology consultation

Hospitalize

Switch Topical Antibiotic

Topical Antibiotic
Consider:
  Oral Erythromycin

Saline Lavage;
Topical Antibiotic;
IMor IV Penicillin

PERIORBITAL (PRESEPTAL) CELLULITIS

A. The swelling and redness of the eyelids of periorbital cellulitis can be caused by reactive preseptal edema (sinusitis) or cellulitis. Preseptal edema is often associated with sinusitis. Cellulitis can be related to local trauma, infection (conjunctivitis or impetigo), or bacteremia. Bacteremia with *H. influenzae* occurs in one-third of the children with periorbital cellulitis which is unrelated to local trauma or infection.

B. Assess the degree of illness. Severely ill patients appear toxic, with an altered mental status, high fever, or shock. Suspect CNS complication in these patients when they present with severe headache, seizures, focal neurologic findings, or meningeal signs. Moderately ill patients present with marked pain or headache or systemic signs of infection such as fever. Mildly ill patients are afebrile or have a low-grade fever without associated systemic symptoms.

C. Treat mildly ill patients in the outpatient setting with oral antibiotics. Use dicloxacillin, erythromycin/sulfamethoxazole, or a cephalosporin to treat periorbital cellulitis related to local trauma or infection since *S. aureus* and *S. pyogenes* are the most likely agents. Treat periorbital cellulitis that appears related to sinusitis (ethmoiditis) with amoxicillin or trimethoprim/sulfamethoxazole to cover *H. influenzae*, *S. pneumoniae*, and *B. catarrhalis*. Patients who do not respond to antibiotic therapy within 12–24 hours require hospitalization.

D. Admit moderate and severely ill children to the hospital and consider a septic workup (blood cultures, lumbar puncture, urine culture) to diagnose associated meningitis or sepsis. Obtain sinus films when paranasal sinusitis is suspected. Obtain a CT scan to exclude orbital cellulitis when ophthlmaplegia, proptosis, loss of vision, or edema of the eyeball is noted. Additional CNS complications such as brain abscess or cavernous sinus thrombosis, which present with severe headache, focal neurologic findings, seizures, or meningeal signs, will also be identified by CT scan. IV antibiotic therapy should include ampicillin with either moxolactam or chloramphenicol to cover ampicillin-resistant *H. influenzae* type B and a semisynthetic penicillin (oxacillin or nafcillin) to cover *S. aureus*.

REFERENCES

Barkin RM, Todd JK, Amer J. Periorbital cellulitis in children. Pediatrics 1978; 62:390.
Gellady AM, Shulman ST, Ayoub EM. Periorbital and orbital cellulitis in children. Pediatrics 1978; 61:272.
Teele DW. Management of the child with red and swollen eye. Ped Inf Dis 1983; 2:258.

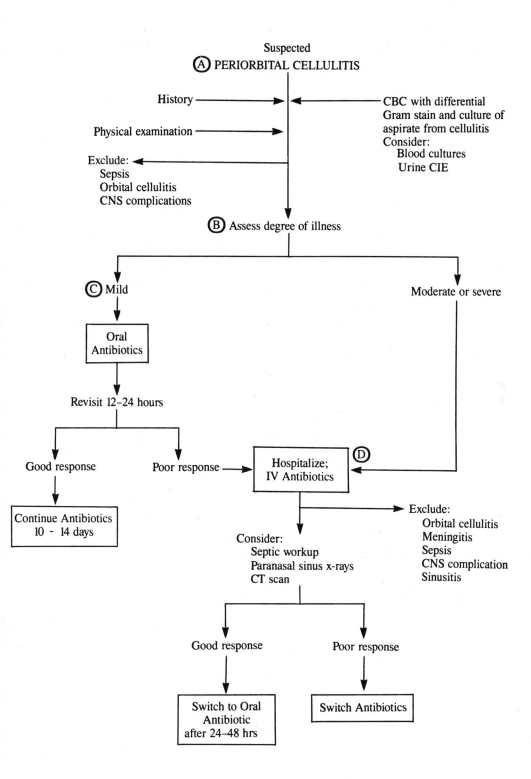

Suspected
Ⓐ PERIORBITAL CELLULITIS

History ⟶

⟵ CBC with differential
Gram stain and culture of
aspirate from cellulitis
Consider:
   Blood cultures
   Urine CIE

Physical examination ⟶

Exclude: ⟵
   Sepsis
   Orbital cellulitis
   CNS complications

Ⓑ Assess degree of illness

Ⓒ Mild

Moderate or severe

Oral
Antibiotics

Revisit 12–24 hours

Good response

Poor response ⟶

Ⓓ Hospitalize;
IV Antibiotics

Continue Antibiotics
10 - 14 days

Consider:
Septic workup
Paranasal sinus x-rays
CT scan

⟶ Exclude:
   Orbital cellulitis
   Meningitis
   Sepsis
   CNS complication
   Sinusitis

Good response

Poor response

Switch to Oral
Antibiotic
after 24–48 hrs

Switch Antibiotics

ORBITAL CELLULITIS OR ABSCESS

A. Orbital involvement is characterized by periorbital swelling, loss of vision, edema of the eyeball (chemosis), proptosis, and ophthalmoplegia.

B. Children with suspected orbital cellulitis should have a CT scan to determine the presence and extent of an abscess which requires surgical drainage. Perform a lumbar puncture because the risk of meningitis in children with orbital cellulitis is high, regardless of the presence of meningeal signs.

C. Orbital cellulitis is usually caused by *H. influenzae, S. pneumoniae, S. aureus,* or *S. pyogenes. S. aureus* and *S. pyogenes* are the most common organisms when local infection, impetigo, or trauma are predisposing factors. In children under 5 years of age without a predisposing condition, the most common organism is *H. influenzae.* Begin initial IV therapy with a semisynthetic penicillin (oxacillin or nafcillin 150–200 mg/kg/day), ampicillin 200–400 mg/kg/day and moxolactam 150 mg/kg/day or chloramphenicol 50 -75 mg/kg/day. Change antibiotics appropriately when culture and sensitivity results are available. Treat orbital infections for 10–21 days IV and then consider continuing therapy orally.

D. Altered mental status, severe headache, persistent high fever, persistent vomiting, seizures, paralysis, and focal neurologic signs suggest a CNS complication (meningitis, brain abscess, cavernous sinus thrombosis). Sudden loss of vision associated with pus in the anterior chamber of the eye (hypopyon) results from septic emboli in the posterior ciliary arteries.

REFERENCES

Gellady AM, Shulman ST, Ayoub EM. Periorbital and orbital cellulitis in children. Pediatrics 1978; 61:272.

Goldberg F, Berne AS, Oski FA. Differentiation of orbital cellulitis from preseptal cellulitis by computed tomography. Pediatrics 1978; 62:1000.

Gomez-Barreto J, Nahmias AJ. Hypopyon and orbital cellulitis associated with Haemophilus influenzae type B meningitis. Am J Dis Child 1977; 131:215.

Londer L, Nelson DL. Orbital cellulitis due to *Haemophilus influenzae.* Arch Opthalmol 1974; 91:89.

SUSPECTED ORBITAL ABSCESS OR CELLULITIS

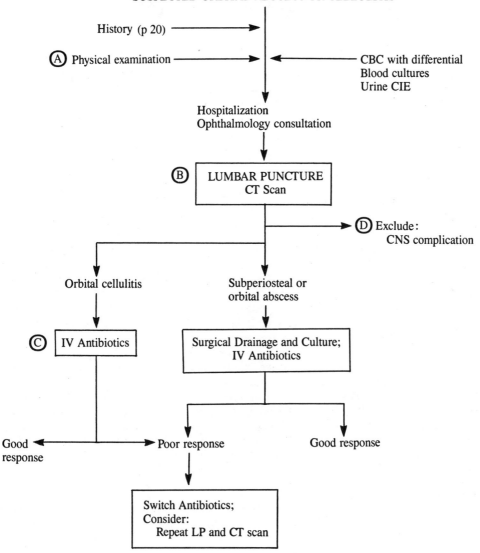

History (p 20)

Ⓐ Physical examination ← CBC with differential
Blood cultures
Urine CIE

Hospitalization
Ophthalmology consultation

Ⓑ LUMBAR PUNCTURE
CT Scan

Ⓓ Exclude:
CNS complication

Orbital cellulitis

Subperiosteal or
orbital abscess

Ⓒ IV Antibiotics

Surgical Drainage and Culture;
IV Antibiotics

Good
response ← Poor response

Good response

Switch Antibiotics;
Consider:
Repeat LP and CT scan

27

CYANOTIC HEART DISEASE

A. Cyanosis is produced by clinical conditions associated with one or more of the following physiologic abnormalities: alveolar hypoventilation, right to left shunt, ventilation-perfusion inequality, impairment of diffusion, and decreased affinity of hemoglobin for oxygen. Central cyanosis, related to the presence of 3 grams or more of reduced hemoglobin per 100 ml, is best detected by examining the lips, tongue, and mucous membranes. Peripheral cyanosis seen in the hands, feet, and circumoral areas may result from the slow blood flow with a large difference in arterial venous oxygen levels that may result from exposure to cold.

B. Document the onset and duration of cyanosis and the frequency of recurrent episodes. Note associated symptoms such as cough, dyspnea, orthopnea, poor feeding, sweating, fatigue, weight loss, and failure to thrive. Note precipitating factors such as eating, exercise, respiratory infections, seizures, or apnea. Identify predisposing conditions such as congenital heart disease, Kawasaki's disease, birth control pills, pulmonary disease, or hypercholesterolemia with a family history of early myocardial infarction.

C. Assess the circulatory status by evaluating blood pressure, heart rate, capillary refill, peripheral pulses, and skin color and temperature. Note signs of cardiac disease such as dysrhythmias, S3/S4 gallop, heart murmur, clicks, friction rub, or abnormal second heart sounds. Murmurs that disappear or change with position or are present with fever or anemia are often functional. Recognize signs of congestive heart failure such as tachypnea, tachycardia, gallop rhythm, rales, wheezes, retractions, peripheral edema, hepatomegaly, or ascites. Note signs of primary pulmonary disease. Assess mental status and evaluate for CNS disease (seizures, focal neurologic deficits, evidence of head trauma). Note signs of bacterial infections or sepsis.

D. The arterial blood gas (ABG) measures the partial pressure of dissolved oxygen in blood. The oxygen disassociation curve displays the relationship between the ABG and oxygen saturation. Perform an ABG shunt study by obtaining blood gases in both room air and 100% FIO_2. Suspect a fixed right-to-left shunt when the administration of 100% oxygen fails to increase the PAO_2 substantially. Echocardiography will usually detail structural abnormalities of the heart, specifically, great vessel relationships, function, and any major obstructions. Echocardiography also helps assess the presence of pulmonary hypertension.

REFERENCES

Guntheroth WG. Initial evaluation of child for heart disease. Pediatr Clin North Am 1978; 25:657.

Kawabori I. Cyanotic congenital heart defects with decreased pulmonary blood flow. Pediatr Clin North Am 1978; 25:759.

Kawabori I. Cyanotic congenital heart defects with increased pulmonary blood flow. Pediatr Clin North Am 1978; 25:777.

Kitterman JA. Cyanosis in the newborn infant. Pediatr Rev 1982; 4:13.

Shannon DC, Lasser M, Goldblatt A, et al. The cyanotic infant - heart disease or lung disease. New Engl J Med 1972; 287:951.

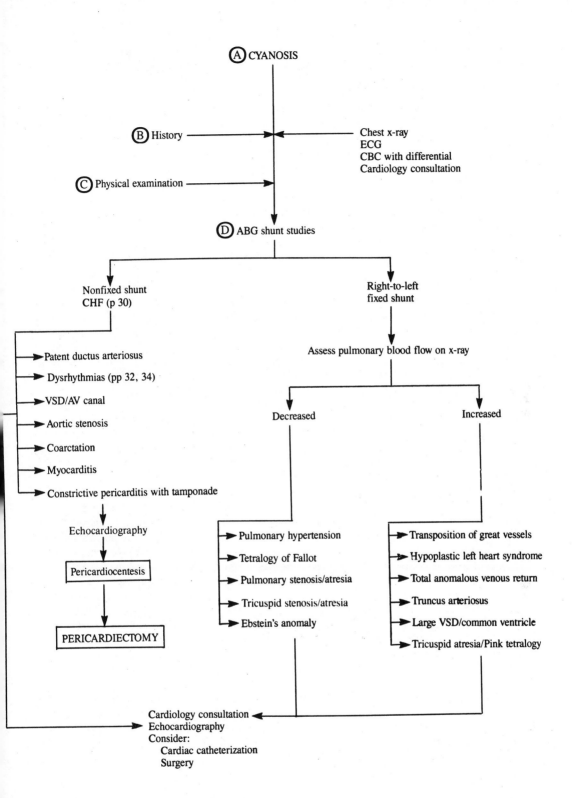

A CYANOSIS

B History — Chest x-ray
ECG
CBC with differential
Cardiology consultation

C Physical examination

D ABG shunt studies

Nonfixed shunt
CHF (p 30)

Right-to-left
fixed shunt

Assess pulmonary blood flow on x-ray

- Patent ductus arteriosus
- Dysrhythmias (pp 32, 34)
- VSD/AV canal
- Aortic stenosis
- Coarctation
- Myocarditis
- Constrictive pericarditis with tamponade

Echocardiography

Pericardiocentesis

PERICARDIECTOMY

Decreased

- Pulmonary hypertension
- Tetralogy of Fallot
- Pulmonary stenosis/atresia
- Tricuspid stenosis/atresia
- Ebstein's anomaly

Increased

- Transposition of great vessels
- Hypoplastic left heart syndrome
- Total anomalous venous return
- Truncus arteriosus
- Large VSD/common ventricle
- Tricuspid atresia/Pink tetralogy

Cardiology consultation
Echocardiography
Consider:
    Cardiac catheterization
    Surgery

CONGESTIVE HEART FAILURE

A. Congestive heart failure (CHF) results from pressure overload (left heart outflow or inflow obstructions), volume overload (left-to-right shunts, valvular regurgitation, severe anemia), depressed myocardial function (myocarditis, sepsis, ischemia, hypoglycemia, hypocalcemia, electrolyte abnormalities, cardiac toxins), and rhythm abnormalities.

B. Note symptoms of CHF such as feeding difficulties, sweating, cough, dyspnea, orthopnea, wheezing, and puffiness. Identify predisposing conditions such as congenital heart disease, acquired heart disease (rheumatic fever, cor pulmonale, endocarditis, storage diseases), medications and drugs, and hematologic disorders (thalassemia, sickle cell disease).

C. Assess the circulatory status; note signs of CHF and structural heart disease. These signs include tachycardia (>160 beats/min during infancy, >100 beats/min in older children), heart murmurs, clicks, S3 gallop, pulsus alterans (beat-to-beat variability in the strength of the pulse), jugular venous distention, hepatomegaly, and edema. Suspect pulmonary edema if cough, rales, wheezes, and retractions are present. Cool, mottled extremities suggest poor cardiac output and vasoconstriction. Chronic congestive heart failure results in failure to thrive and undernutrition.

D. On chest x-ray, note any cardiomegaly or pulmonary congestion. Cardiomegaly can be caused by ventricular dilatation secondary to volume overload, myocardial function abnormalities, or a pericardial effusion. On ECG note abnormal rhythms, cardiac ischemia, and ventricular hypertrophy. Consider myocarditis or a pericardial effusion if decreased voltage is noted across the precordial leads. An echocardiogram will identify a pericardial effusion and underlying structural heart disease and assess cardiac contractility and performance.

E. Treat arrhythmias related to digitalis toxicity with phenytoin (Dilantin). Perform a pericardiocentesis when a pericardial effusion produces tamponade. Correct electrolyte abnormalities that impair cardiac function such as hypochloremic alkalosis, hypokalemia, or hyponatremia. Correct a severe anemia with a packed red blood cell transfusion (consider a partial exchange). Treat underlying primary pulmonary disease such as pneumonia which contributes to CHF by causing hypoxia and pulmonary vasoconstriction.

F. Hospitalize in an ICU severely ill patients who present with shock, marked respiratory distress, or altered mental status. Monitor closely the arterial blood gas (ABG), central venous or pulmonary wedge pressure, and urine output. Supportive care should include humidified oxygen, temperature control, elevation of the head and shoulders, and correction of electrolyte and acid-base disturbances. Avoid sodium bicarbonate when respiratory failure is present. Consider morphine sulfate .05 to .1 mg/kg for hypoxic restlessness or air hunger. Treat the patient initially with Lasix 1–2 mg/kg IV. If a good urine flow is not established (>3 cc/kg/hour), repeat the dose after 1 hour.

G. Digitalize patients over 24 hours: give 1/2 total dosage initially, ¼ 8 hours later, and ¼ 16 hours later. Administer the dose IV when tissue perfusion is poor at 75% of the total oral dosage. The daily maintenance dose should be ¼ of the total digitalizing dosage given *bid*. Consider the possibility of either digitalis toxicity or inadequate levels of digitalis in patients who develop CHF. Avoid digitalis in patients with subvalvular stenosis or myocarditis.

H. Consider dopamine or isoproterenol for patients in shock or who have failed to respond to therapy. Dopamine has slightly less chronotropic cardiac effect and increases renal blood flow at infusion rates less than 10–15 μg/kg/per minute. Afterload-reducing agents such as hydralazine and nitroprusside have been used to produce vasodilatation and increase cardiac output. Use these agents with great caution.

REFERENCES

Driscoll DJ, Gillette PC, McNamara DG. The use of dopamine in children. J Pediatr 1978; 92:309.

Kaplan S, Gaum WE, Benzing G, et al. Therapeutic advances in pediatric cardiology. Pediatr Clin North Am 1978; 25:891.

Wolf RR. Cardiovascular diseases. In: Current Pediatric Diagnosis and Treatment. Kempe CH, Silver HK, O'Brien D, eds. Los Altos, California: Lange Medical Publications, 1983.

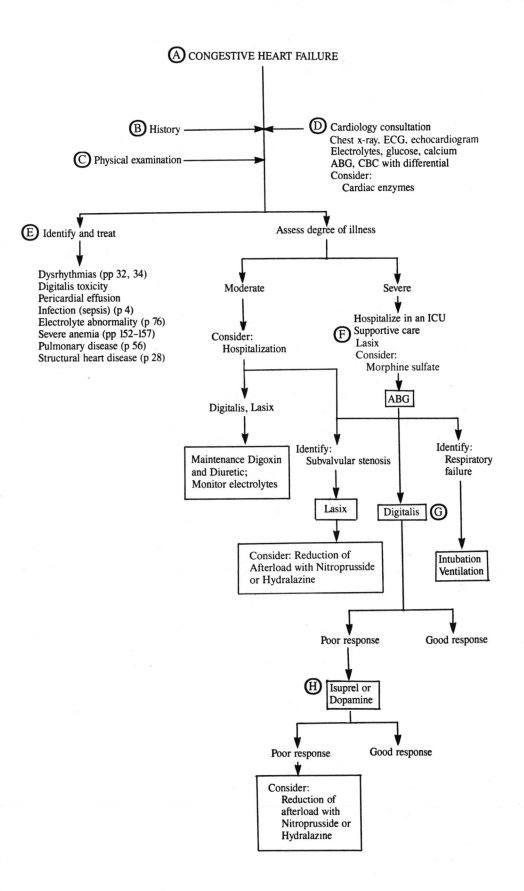

(A) CONGESTIVE HEART FAILURE

(B) History

(C) Physical examination

(D) Cardiology consultation
Chest x-ray, ECG, echocardiogram
Electrolytes, glucose, calcium
ABG, CBC with differential
Consider:
    Cardiac enzymes

(E) Identify and treat

Dysrhythmias (pp 32, 34)
Digitalis toxicity
Pericardial effusion
Infection (sepsis) (p 4)
Electrolyte abnormality (p 76)
Severe anemia (pp 152–157)
Pulmonary disease (p 56)
Structural heart disease (p 28)

Assess degree of illness

Moderate

Severe

Hospitalize in an ICU
(F) Supportive care
    Lasix
    Consider:
        Morphine sulfate

Consider:
Hospitalization

Digitalis, Lasix

ABG

Maintenance Digoxin
and Diuretic;
Monitor electrolytes

Identify:
Subvalvular stenosis

Identify:
Respiratory
failure

Lasix

Digitalis (G)

Intubation
Ventilation

Consider: Reduction of
Afterload with Nitroprusside
or Hydralazine

Poor response

Good response

(H) Isuprel or
Dopamine

Poor response

Good response

Consider:
    Reduction of
    afterload with
    Nitroprusside or
    Hydralazine

BRADYDYSRHYTHMIAS

A. Suspect a bradydysrhythmia when the resting awake heart rate is less than 100 beats per minute during the first 3 months of life, less than 80 for children under 2 years, less than 70 for children age 2 to 10 years, and less than 55 for adolescents. A sleeping heart rate is usually 10 to 20 beats per minute lower in infants and young children.

B. Determine the onset, duration, and severity of the slow heart rate. Note associated symptoms related to decreased cerebral flow such as syncope, dizziness, or confusion. Symptoms related to congestive heart failure include poor feeding, irritability, sweating, puffiness, cyanotic spells, and symptoms of respiratory distress. Chest pain and angina are symptoms which suggest decreased coronary artery blood flow. Identify predisposing conditons such as structural heart disease, prior cardiac surgery, medications or drug ingestions, collagen vascular diseases, hypothyroidism, CNS disorders, and recent viral illness.

C. Assess the cardiac status. Note signs of congestive heart failure and underlying structural heart disease (see pp 28, 30).

D. The ECG will identify most bradydysrhythmias as a complete or second-degree heart block, a sinus bradycardia, a slow junctional rhythm, a second-degree atrioventricular block or blocked premature atrial contractions (PACs). Suspect complete heart block when a ventricular rate of 40 to 80 is associated with an atrial rate greater than 100. A regular P-R interval is absent because conduction from the atria to the ventricles is disrupted. The presence of a normal and regular P-R interval and P waves preceding QRS complexes suggests a sinus bradycardia.

E. Complete heart block can be congenital or acquired. Causes of congenital heart block include structural heart disease (levo-transposition of the great vessels or asplenia-polysplenia syndrome) and maternal collagen vascular diseases. Most cases are idiopathic and may be first recognized only at the 2-week or 2-month well child visit. Acquired complete heart block has multiple etiologies including structural heart disease, cardiac surgery (transient or permanent), drugs (digoxin, propranolol), myocarditis or endocarditis with myocardial ischemia/infarction (Kawasaki's disease, coronary artery disease), collagen vascular diseases (rheumatic fever, lupus erythematosus,dermatomyositis),glycogen storage diseases (Pompe's disease), and cardiac tumors.

F. Causes of sinus bradycardia (sick sinus syndrome) include drugs (digoxin, propanolol), myocarditis or endocarditis, cardiac surgery, structural heart disease, hypothyroidism, and conditions associated with elevated intracranial pressure (meningoencephalitis, brain tumor).

G. Severely ill patients present with shock, congestive heart failure, or altered mental status. They require immediate supportive care and pharmacologic management; emergency transvenous pacing may be necessary. Moderately ill patients have a history of episodes that suggest decreased cerebral or coronary artery blood flow. Also, consider any infant with a ventricular rate persistently less than 50 with an atrial rate greater than 140 to be moderately ill because of an increased risk of sudden death during the first year of life. Additional criteria for moderate disease include a widened QRS complex or ventricular rate less than 45. Mildly ill patients are stable, appear asymptomatic, and have heart rates greater than 50 to 55.

H. Treat severely ill patients who have a complete AV block with an isoproterenol infusion of 0.2 to 0.4 μg/kg/min. If bradycardia persists, institute emergency transvenous pacemaking. Consider a trial of atropine (0.02–0.04 mg/kg) in patients with sinus bradycardia (avoid with blocked PACs). Close monitoring is essential since pharmacologic therapy may be complicated by a tachyarrhythmia.

I. Refer for a permanent pacemaker patients at high risk of developing a tachyarrhythmia, congestive heart failure, or episodes of decreased cerebral or coronary blood flow.

REFERENCES

Alpert MA, Flaker GC: Arrhythymias associated with sinus node dysfunction pathogenesis recognition and management. JAMA 1983; 250:2160.

Gewitz MH, Vetter VL. Cardiac emergencies. In: Fleisher G, Ludwig S, eds. Textbook of Pediatric Emergency Medicine. Baltimore: Williams & Wilkins, 1983.

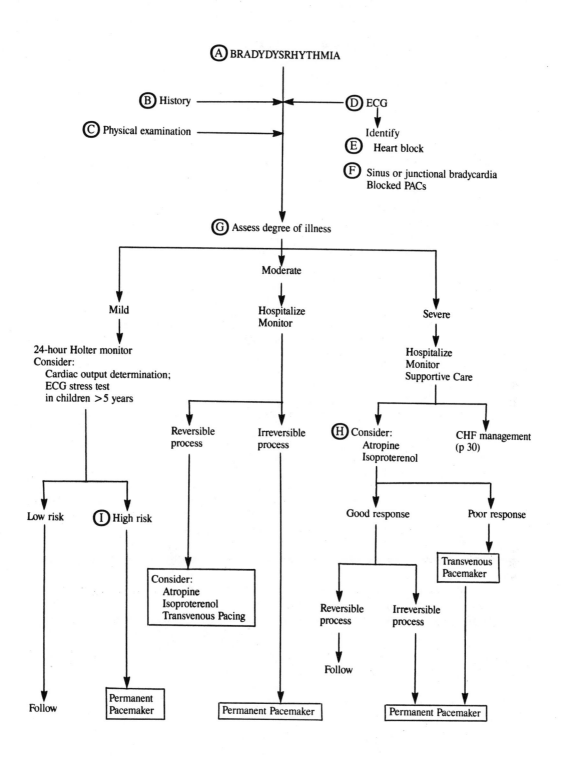

Gillette PC. Cardiac dysrhythmias in children. Peds in Rev 1981; 3:190.
Michaelson M, Engle MA: Congenital complete heart block: An international study of the natural history. Cardiovasc Circ 1972; 4:86.

ACUTE SUPRAVENTRICULAR TACHYCARDIAS

A. Supraventricular tachycardia (SVT) is most common during early infancy; the heart rate may be between 200 to 300 beats per minute. In older children, suspect an SVT when the heart rate is between 150 and 250. The SVT may originate in the atrial sinus node, the AV node, or the junctional conduction tissue.

B. Determine the onset, duration, severity, and frequency of recurrence of the rapid heart rate. Note palpitations and the presence of symptoms related to congestive heart failure (poor feeding, irritability, pallor, sweating, puffiness, cyanotic spells), respiratory distress (grunting, dyspnea, rapid breathing), and decreased coronary blood flow (chest pain or angina). Identify predisposing conditions or precipitating factors such as congenital heart disease, infection (myocarditis), fever, drugs (sympathomimetics, amphetamines), or Wolff-Parkinson-White syndrome.

C. Assess the cardiac status. Note signs of congestive heart failure and underlying structural heart disease (Ebstein's anomaly or transposition) (pp 28, 30).

D. Exclude a ventricular tachycardia which is suggested by wide QRS complexes. SVT usually presents with prolonged P-R intervals, abnormally shaped P waves, but narrow QRS complexes. Rarely, when an aberrant conduction pattern is present, SVT presents with widened QRS complexes. Suspect Wolff-Parkinson-White syndrome when a short P-R interval is associated with a widened QRS complex and slurred upstroke. This is caused by a bypass conduction tract which connects the atria and ventricles.

E. Assess the degree of illness. Severely ill patients present with hypotension, moderate or severe congestive heart failure, or altered mental status. Moderately ill patients have signs of mild congestive heart failure or a history of episodes which suggest decreased cerebral or coronary artery blood flow. Mildly ill patients appear asymptomatic.

F. Treat severely ill patients with direct current synchronized cardioversion. Synchronization of the discharge to the peak of the QRS complex is essential; it prevents discharge on the T wave and ventricular fibrillation. Use ¼ to ½ watts sec/lb. Since prior digitalization may increase the risk of ventricular fibrillation, digitalize the patient *after* cardioversion rather than before.

G. In older children and adolescents, attempt to disrupt the SVT with vagal maneuvers. Consider verapamil 0.05–0.1 mg/kg IV as an alternative to cardioversion or digitalization. Use propranolol rather than digoxin in patients with Wolff-Parkinson-White syndrome atrial flutter, or atrial fibrillation.

H. Treat infants after an initial episode and older children with recurrent SVT episodes with maintenance oral therapy. Possible oral regimens include digoxin, propranolol, dilantin, quinidine, and procainamide. Avoid the use of cold medicines that contain sympathomimetic amines.

REFERENCES

Garson A, Gillette PC, McNamara DG. Supraventricular tachycardia in children; Clinical features, response to treatment, and long-term followup in 217 patients. J Pediatr 1981; 98:875.

Gewitz MH, Vetter VL. Cardiac emergencies. In: Fleisher G, Ludwig S, eds. Textbook of Pediatric Emergency Medicine. Baltimore: Williams & Wilkins, 1983.

Gillette PC. Cardiac dysrhythmias in children. Peds in Rev 1981; 3:190.

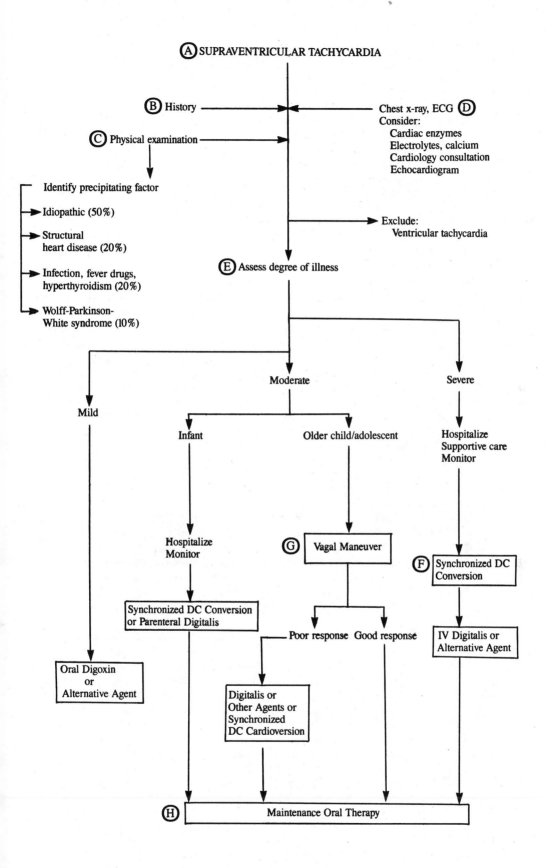

HYPOTENSION (SHOCK)

A. In shock, tissue oxygenation is impaired because of hypoperfusion related to poor cardiac function, hypovolemia, or loss of vascular tone (septic shock). Cardiac failure may be a primary and/or a secondary abnormality. Possible mechanisms adversely affecting cardiac function in shock include decreased coronary blood flow, marked acidosis, high levels of myocardial depressant factor, and increased peripheral vasoconstriction (afterload). Hypovolemia may be related to obvious events such as acute external hemorrhage, vomiting, diarrhea, diuresis, or extensive burns. Occult loss into the third space occurs with peritonitis, pulmonary edema, and intracranial or internal hemorrhage. Vasodilation produced by sepsis, spinal cord injuries, anaphylaxis, or drugs produces a relative hypovolemia without fluid loss from the vascular space.

B. Assess the circulatory status. Note the blood pressure, heart rate, respiratory rate, capillary refill, skin color, temperature and urine output. Evaluate the cardiac and pulmonary status (p 56). Evaluate the mental status and note signs of CNS disease (pp 132, 146).

C. The objective in the treatment of shock is the reestablishment of adequate tissue oxygenation. This requires monitoring of ventilation (PaO_2, PCO_2), cardiac function (arterial blood pressure), circulatory blood volume (central venous pressure, CVP), and oxygen-carrying capacity (hematocrit). A systemic arterial catheter allows continuous monitoring of systemic arterial pressure and access to the arterial circulation for blood sampling and blood gas determinations. Other venous lines should include a CVP line in the right atrium and large bore venous line for the infusion of fluids and drugs. Consider placing a balloon tip flow-directed quadralumen catheter to obtain a pulmonary artery wedge pressure; this allows measurement of right and left atrial pressures and enables determination of cardiac output by thermodilution. Place an ECG and heart rate monitor, and a catheter to document urine output.

D. After establishing adequate ventilation, stabilize the circulation with an isotonic fluid infusion of 10–20 cc/kg over 30 minutes and treat severe acidosis (pH <7.2) with an infusion of sodium bicarbonate; initially administer 1/2 of the dose calculated by the body weight (kg)×the base excess×0.4 (usually 2–3 mg/kg). Consider antibiotics and high dose steroids when septic shock is suspected.

E. Restore the circulatory blood volume using the CVP as a guide. In patients with a low hematocrit fluids should include either whole blood or packed red blood cells and fresh frozen plasma; use colloid (5% albumin or plasminate) for other patients. When the central venous pressure is less than 6 torr, administer at least 4 cc/kg of fluid over 10 minutes, and monitor the CVP. When the CVP changes by less than 2 torr, administer another 4 cc/kg bolus over 10 minutes. Continue administering boluses of fluid until the CVP rises to 5–10 torr indicating that circulatory blood volume has been restored and the patient becomes normotensive with good peripheral profusion.

F. Sympathomimetic amines increase cardiac output by improving myocardial contractility and increasing heart rate. Dopamine has slightly fewer chronotropic cardiac effects compared to isoproterenol and increases renal blood flow at infusion rates less than 15 μg/kg/min. Initiate therapy with dopamine at an infusion rate of 5 to 10 μg/kg/min. When 150 mg is added to 250 cc of D5W or normal saline 1 cc/kg/hr equals 10 μg/kg/min. Isoproterenol infusions can be started at 0.1 μg/kg/min and the infusion can be increased to 1 μg/kg/min if necessary but follow closely for the development of tachyarrhythmias or ischemia. Add 1.5 mg to 250 cc of D5W so that 1 cc/kg/hour equals 0.1 μg/kg/min.

G. The goal of vasodilator therapy is to reduce the resistance to left ventricular ejection (afterload). Consider using a short-acting vasodilator such as nitroprusside at a rate of 0.1 μg/kg/min. The maximum safe dosage of nitroprusside is 8 to 10 μg/kg/min as cyanide accumulates at higher infusion rates causing acidosis. An alternative is hydralazine 0.1 to 0.5 mg/kg IV every 3 to 6 hours.

REFERENCES
Perkin RM, Levin DL. Shock in the pediatric patient Part 1. J Pediatr 1982; 101:163.

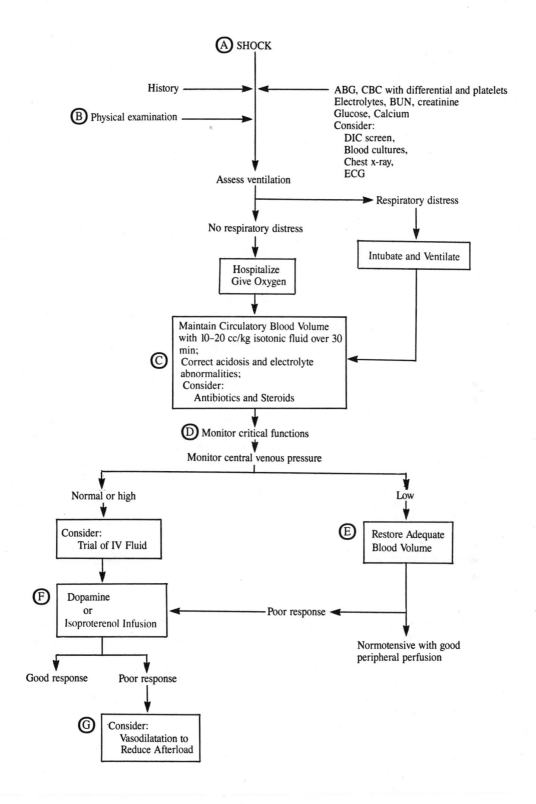

Ⓐ SHOCK

History

Ⓑ Physical examination

ABG, CBC with differential and platelets
Electrolytes, BUN, creatinine
Glucose, Calcium
Consider:
    DIC screen,
    Blood cultures,
    Chest x-ray,
    ECG

Assess ventilation

Respiratory distress

No respiratory distress

Intubate and Ventilate

Hospitalize
Give Oxygen

Ⓒ Maintain Circulatory Blood Volume
with 10–20 cc/kg isotonic fluid over 30 min;
Correct acidosis and electrolyte abnormalities;
Consider:
    Antibiotics and Steroids

Ⓓ Monitor critical functions

Monitor central venous pressure

Normal or high

Low

Consider:
    Trial of IV Fluid

Ⓔ Restore Adequate Blood Volume

Ⓕ Dopamine
or
Isoproterenol Infusion

Poor response

Normotensive with good peripheral perfusion

Good response

Poor response

Ⓖ Consider:
    Vasodilatation to Reduce Afterload

Perkin RM, Levin DL. Shock in the pediatric patient Part 2. J Pediatr 1982; 101:319.
Raphaely RC. Shock. In: Fleischer G, Ludwig S, eds. Pediatric Emergency Medicine. Baltimore: Williams & Wilkins, 1983:31.
Yabek SM. Management of Septic Shock. Pediatr Rev 1980; 2:83.

HYPERTENSION

A. Suspect hypertension when repeated supine blood pressures are > 100/70 mmHg in children under 2 years of age, > 110/74 mmHg in children 3 to 5 years, > 116/76 mmHg in children 6 to 9 years, and > 120/80 mmHg in children 10 to 13 years. In adolescents, repeated blood pressures > 135/85 mmHg in the seated position are abnormal. In taking blood pressure, use a cuff size such that the bladder width is ½ to ⅔ the length of the upper arm or the bladder width is equal to or greater than ½ the diameter of the upper arm. The bladder must entirely encircle the arm or leg. Use the muffling of the heart sound to indicate the diastolic pressure.

B. Note symptoms such as headache, abdominal pain, nausea, vomiting, recurrent nose bleeds, irritability, failure to thrive, visual disturbances, and deteriorating school performance.

C. Obtain both upper arm and lower extremity blood pressures. A systolic murmur, diminished femoral pulses, and a differential in blood pressure in the upper and lower extremities suggest coarctation of the aorta. Note signs of congestive heart failure. Examine the fundi for papilledema, arteriolar spasm, AV nicking, arterial tortuosity, and hemorrhage or exudates. Note signs of hypertensive encephalopathy such as seizures, stroke, focal neurologic deficits, decreased visual acuity, and altered mental status (confusion, stupor, coma). A continuous abdominal bruit suggests renal artery stenosis.

D. Evaluate preadolescents who present with hypertension and adolescents with elevations greater than 10 to 15 mmHg above the upper limits of normal to identify causes of secondary hypertension. Mild elevations in blood pressure in adolescents is usually essential and may be managed and followed without extensive workup.

E. Severely ill patients have signs of hypertensive encephalopathy or accelerated hypertension, defined as an acute rise in blood pressure superimposed on chronic moderate hypertension. Moderately ill patients have diastolic elevations greater than 10 to 15 mmHg above normal with significant symptoms. Mildly ill patients have minimal diastolic elevations with few if any symptoms.

F. Attempt a weight reduction program in obese adolescents and children, with reduction of salt intake. Avoid cigarette smoking and drugs such as sympathomimetics, amphetamines, steroids, contraceptive pills, and cold medications which elevate blood pressure. If possible, implement an endurance aerobic exercise program; avoid isometric exercises. Consider an ECG exercise stress test prior to implementing the exercise program.

G. Treat severely ill patients with diazoxide 3 to 5 mg/kg as a rapid IV push. Diazoxide may control blood pressure for 8 to 12 hours. Administer Lasix 1 to 2 mg/kg IV in patients who are normovolemic or volume overloaded; avoid Lasix in severely volume-contracted patients.

H. Treat moderate and severely ill patients with a diuretic, a beta-blocker (propranolol) 1 mg/kg PO *tid*, and a vasodilator (hydralazine) 0.1–0.2 mg/kg/dose *q 4–6 h*. Consider captopril, converting-enzyme inhibitor, in patients with resistant hypertension; avoid this drug in patients with renal artery stenosis because of adverse effects on renal function. Other antihypertensive agents include methyldopa, guanethedine, reserpine, and minoxidil. Follow patients for hypokalemia; consider potassium supplements or a potassium-sparing diuretic (spironolactone) when potassium levels fall below 3.2 mEq/L.

I. Consider the use of a nitroprusside infusion at 0.5 μg/kg/min for patients who do not respond to diazoxide and fursemide. Use nitroprusside with extreme caution because of the accumulation of cyanide.

REFERENCES

Balfe JW, Rentz CP: Recognition and management of hypertensive crises in childhood. Pediatr Clin North Am 1978; 25:159.

Goldring D, Hernandez A: Hypertension in children. Pediatr in Rev 1982; 3:235.

Robeson AM: Special diagnostic studies for the detection of renal and renovascular forms of hypertension. Pediatr Clin North Am 1978; 25:83.

Report of the Task Force on Blood Pressure Control in Children. Pediatr 1977; 59 (supplement):797.

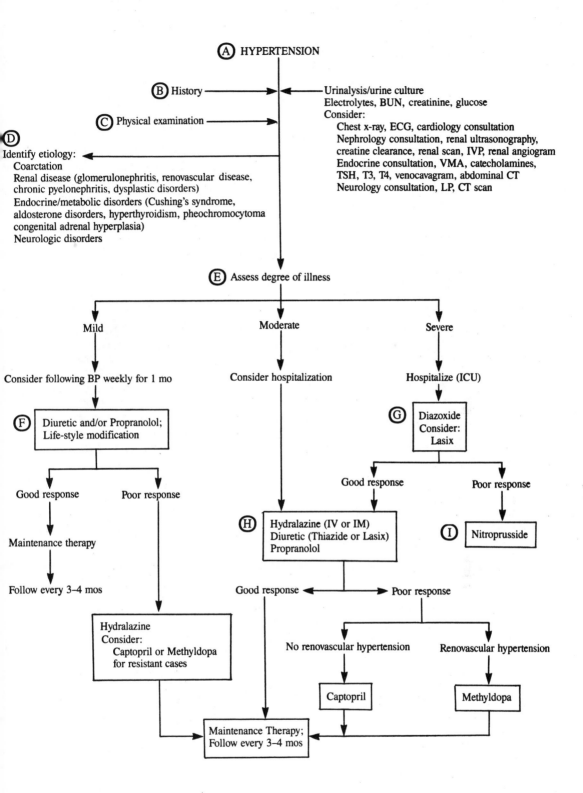

(A) HYPERTENSION

(B) History

(C) Physical examination

Urinalysis/urine culture
Electrolytes, BUN, creatinine, glucose
Consider:
    Chest x-ray, ECG, cardiology consultation
    Nephrology consultation, renal ultrasonography,
    creatine clearance, renal scan, IVP, renal angiogram
    Endocrine consultation, VMA, catecholamines,
    TSH, T3, T4, venocavagram, abdominal CT
    Neurology consultation, LP, CT scan

(D) Identify etiology:
    Coarctation
    Renal disease (glomerulonephritis, renovascular disease,
    chronic pyelonephritis, dysplastic disorders)
    Endocrine/metabolic disorders (Cushing's syndrome,
    aldosterone disorders, hyperthyroidism, pheochromocytoma
    congenital adrenal hyperplasia)
    Neurologic disorders

(E) Assess degree of illness

Mild

Moderate

Severe

Consider following BP weekly for 1 mo

Consider hospitalization

Hospitalize (ICU)

(F) Diuretic and/or Propranolol;
Life-style modification

(G) Diazoxide
Consider:
Lasix

Good response

Poor response

Good response

Poor response

Maintenance therapy

(H) Hydralazine (IV or IM)
Diuretic (Thiazide or Lasix)
Propranolol

(I) Nitroprusside

Follow every 3–4 mos

Good response ◄——————► Poor response

Hydralazine
Consider:
    Captopril or Methyldopa
    for resistant cases

No renovascular hypertension

Renovascular hypertension

Captopril

Methyldopa

Maintenance Therapy;
Follow every 3–4 mos

EVALUATION OF RESPIRATORY DISORDERS

A. Determine the presence, onset, duration, severity (associated dyspnea, inability to eat, vomiting, drooling, cyanosis, apnea) and pattern (relation to time of day, eating, position, exercise, season) of cough, stridor, or wheezing. Note associated upper respiratory symptoms such as rhinorrhea, nasal congestion, earache, conjunctivitis, sore throat, and hoarseness. Ask about systemic symptoms including fever, fatigue, malaise, vomiting, diarrhea, decreased oral intake, oliguria, weight loss, failure to thrive, and altered mental status. Document the current use of medications. Identify precipitating factors or predisposing conditions including environmental triggers (irritants, aspiration, allergens, drugs, exercise, infections, pets, birds), reactive airway disease, bronchopulmonary dysplasia, tracheomalacia, tracheoesophageal fistula, cystic fibrosis, cardiac disease, neuromuscular disease, or immunodeficiency states. Document adequate immunizations. Evaluate the family situation and note availability of a telephone and car, and the ability to properly manage a child at home.

B. On physical examination, note signs of upper respiratory tract involvement such as rhinorrhea (clear or mucopurulent). Identify upper respiratory tract infections such as otitis media, pharyngitis, and sinusitis. Hoarseness, drooling, suprasternal retractions, stridor, decreased air entry into the lungs, and cyanosis suggest an upper airway obstruction (croup, epiglottitis, foreign body). Signs of lower respiratory tract involvement include tachypnea, dyspnea, grunting respirations, intercostal and subcostal retractions, nasal flaring, decreased breath sounds or prolongation of the expiratory phase of respiration, wheezing, rales, and cyanosis. Tachypnea greater than 60 to 70, marked retractions, cyanosis, and agitation (air hunger, restlessness) suggest significant respiratory distress. Identify findings compatible with cardiac disease such as arrhythmias, abnormal heart sounds, clicks, friction rubs, heart murmur, and hepatomegaly.

REFERENCES

Brooks JG. Respiratory tract and mediastinum. In: Kempe CH, Silver HK, O'Brien D, eds. Current Pediatric Diagnosis and Treatment. 8th Ed. Los Altos, California: Lange Medical Publications, 1984:329.

EVALUATION OF RESPIRATORY DISORDERS

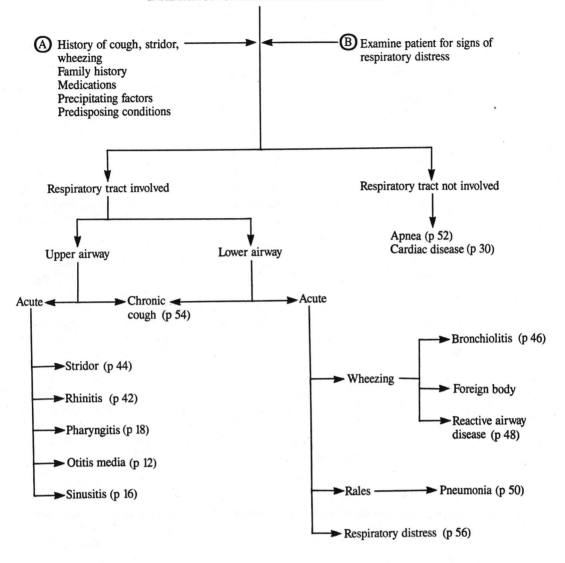

Ⓐ History of cough, stridor, ——————————→
wheezing
Family history
Medications
Precipitating factors
Predisposing conditions

Ⓑ Examine patient for signs of
respiratory distress

Respiratory tract involved

Respiratory tract not involved

Apnea (p 52)
Cardiac disease (p 30)

Upper airway

Lower airway

Acute ←——————→ Chronic ←——————→ Acute
cough (p 54)

→ Stridor (p 44)

→ Rhinitis (p 42)

→ Pharyngitis (p 18)

→ Otitis media (p 12)

→ Sinusitis (p 16)

→ Wheezing

→ Bronchiolitis (p 46)

→ Foreign body

→ Reactive airway
disease (p 48)

→ Rales ——————→ Pneumonia (p 50)

→ Respiratory distress (p 56)

RHINITIS

A. Determine the onset, severity, and pattern (season and time of day) of rhinitis. Note associated symptoms such as mucopurulent discharge (foreign body or sinusitis), or paroxysmal sneezing, nasal itching, burning of the eyes, and the allergic salute. Identify precipitating factors including current medications such as reserpine or beta–blockers, the overuse of nasal decongestants, pollen exposure, allergens, irritants, or climate changes. Identify atopic conditions such as eczema, asthma, or allergies in the patient or his family. Note predisposing endocrine–related conditions such as hypothyroidism, pregnancy, or menstruation.

B. Note the presence of a foreign body, mass or polyp. Check for choanal atresia or a deviated nasal septum. Mucopurulent nasal discharge associated with chronic cough and fetid breath suggests sinusitis. A clear nasal discharge with edematous, pale or bluish nasal mucosa suggests allergic rhinitis. Dark circles under the eyes related to venous congestion (allergic shiners) and a transverse nasal crease related to frequent allergic salutes also indicate allergic rhinitis.

C. Obtain a nasal smear for eosinophils by nose blowing or posterior nasopharyngeal swabbing. Stain the smear with Wright's stain and scan the slide for polymorphonuclear leukocytes, bacteria, and eosinophils. A percentage of eosinophils in relation to total leukocytes greater than 20% suggests allergic rhinitis.

D. The release of inflammatory mediators from sensitized mast cells in the nasal mucosa produces allergic rhinitis. Seasonal symptoms are usually related to pollen inhalation. Year–round symptoms (perennial) are usually related to indoor inhalent allergens such as dust, mold, dander, or feathers. Refer patients with allergic rhinitis for skin testing to identify specific allergens. Whenever possible, recommend limiting or avoiding exposure to known allergens.

E. Antihistamines decrease the release of mediators from the mast cell and block the binding of histamine to receptor sites. Commonly used classes of antihistamines include alkylamines (chlorpheneramine), ethanolamines (diphenhydramine), ethylenediamines (pyridiamine), and peparazine (hydroxyzine). Large doses are often necessary. Use the lowest dose sufficient to relieve symptoms without producing an unacceptable level of drowsiness. When one drug does not provide relief switch to a different class. Treat patients with seasonal rhinitis continuously during pollen season.

F. Add an oral decongestant such as pseudoephedrine if antihistamine therapy is inadequate. Oral sympathomimetics do not cause rebound congestion but are associated with side effects including headache, tachycardia, excitability, insomnia, tremor, and hypertension. Use nasal decongestants ≤ 5 days and only in patients with complete nasal obstruction secondary to congestion. Overuse of nasal decongestants results in rebound vasocongestion with dry, sore nasal mucosa (rhinitis medicamentosa).

G. In resistant cases of allergic rhinitis or rhinitis medicamentosa, try a short course (1–3 weeks) of a topical nasal steroid (1–2 sprays) such as beclomethasone (Vancenase or Beconase) or flunisolide (Nasalide). Side effects include nasal irritation, rhinorrhea, epistaxis, and sneezing. Adrenal suppression may occur with abuse.

H. Use cromolyn, available in a metered nasal spray, to treat severe seasonal rhinitis. Start 1 week prior to the usual onset of symptoms. This drug stabilizes mast cells and prevents allergen–induced release of inflammatory mediators. It has no sedative or stimulant effects.

REFERENCES

Bierman CW, Pierson WE, Donaldson JA. Diseases of the nose. In: Bierman CW, Perlman DS, eds. Allergic Diseases of Infancy, Childhood and Adolescence. Philadelphia: WB Saunders, 1980.

Miller RE, Paradise JL, Friday GA, et al. The nasal smear for eosinophils: its value in children with seasonal allergic rhinitis. Am J Dis Child 1982; 136:1009.

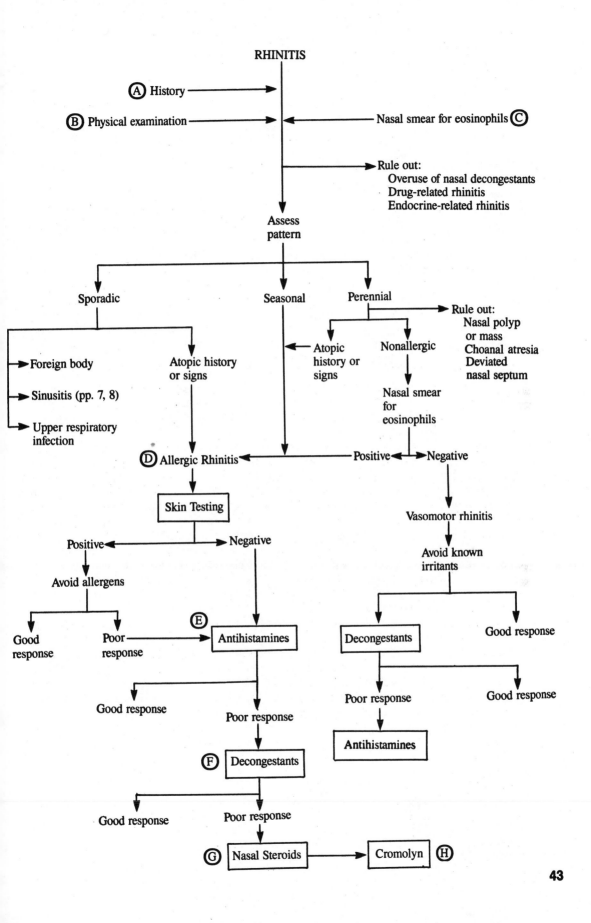

RHINITIS

(A) History

(B) Physical examination

Nasal smear for eosinophils (C)

Rule out:
Overuse of nasal decongestants
Drug-related rhinitis
Endocrine-related rhinitis

Assess
pattern

Sporadic   Seasonal   Perennial

Rule out:
Nasal polyp
or mass
Choanal atresia
Deviated
nasal septum

→ Foreign body

→ Sinusitis (pp. 7, 8)

→ Upper respiratory
infection

Atopic history
or signs

Atopic
history or
signs

Nonallergic

Nasal smear
for
eosinophils

(D) Allergic Rhinitis   Positive   Negative

Skin Testing

Vasomotor rhinitis

Positive   Negative

Avoid known
irritants

Avoid allergens

Good
response

Poor
response

(E)
Antihistamines

Decongestants   Good response

Good response

Poor response   Good response

Good response

Poor response

Antihistamines

(F) Decongestants

Good response

Poor response

(G) Nasal Steroids → Cromolyn (H)

STRIDOR

A. Signs of upper respiratory obstruction producing significant respiratory distress include audible stridor during quiet breathing, tachypnea, dyspnea, retractions, and decreased air entry into the lungs.

B. Suspect impending complete airway obstruction when the child presents with minimal air entry into the lungs, severe retractions, cyanosis, air hunger, or sudden increased restlessness related to hypoxia. The child must be closely monitored and constantly attended by someone trained in cardiopulmonary resuscitation. Disturb the child as little as possible, avoid all procedures, and have available a self-inflating bag and equipment necessary for emergency intubation. If possible, attempt intubation in a controlled setting, preferably in the operating room, with a surgeon available to perform an emergency tracheostomy. A self-inflating bag usually will ventilate an obstructed child, so long as the pressure release valve will not deter ventilating with extremely high pressures.

C. Causes of stridor identified by direct laryngoscopy include laryngomalacia, laryngeal web, laryngeal papilloma, redundant folds of mucus membrane in the glottic area, a floppy epiglottis, and supraglottic masses. Diagnoses associated with pharyngeal or retropharyngeal masses include enlarged adenoids, abscess or cellulitis, benign neoplasms such as cystic hygroma, hemangioma, goiter or neurofibroma, and malignancies such as neuroblastoma, lymphoma and histiocytoma.

D. Viral croup usually presents with several days of URI symptoms followed by the development of hoarseness, a barky cough, and low-grade fever. Viral croup usually occurs in children between 3 months and 3 years of age. Parainfluenza viruses, followed by RSV and influenza viruses account for most cases of viral croup. Children without stridor at rest may be managed at home. Avoid the use of racemic epinephrine in the emergency room if the child is to go home, because symptoms often reappear within 1 hour of therapy. The use of steroids in the outpatient managment of viral croup remains controversial. Treat children hospitalized with viral croup with a combination of mist and racemic epinephrine, given with nebulized air. If necessary, repeat this therapy hourly. Patients who fail to respond adequately should receiveDecadron0.3–0.4 mg/kg/dose q12h, in order to reduce the severity of the respiratory distress and shorten the hospital stay.

E. Suspect the development of bacterial tracheitis when croup is complicated by high fever, purulent tracheal secretions, and increasing respiratory distress. Infection with *S. aureus* has been implicated in many of these cases. If endotracheal intubation is necessary, maintain adequate pulmonary toilet; abundant purulent secretions increase the risk of plugging the endotracheal tube.

F. Acute epiglottitis may present initially with minimal respiratory distress. Signs which suggest this disease include the sudden onset of high fever, extreme sore throat with drooling and difficulty in swallowing, pain with movement of the neck, a muffled voice, and a confused and anxious affect. Acute epiglottitis is most often caused by infection with *H. influenza* type B. Intubate in a controlled situation; there is a high risk of acute airway obstruction and cardiac arrest associated with acute epiglottis. The endotracheal tube can be removed after 24–72 hours in most cases. Initiate antibiotic therapy with ampicillin 150–200 mg/kg/day and either chloramphenicol 50–100 mg/kg/day or moxolactam 150 mg/kg/day, pending the results of cultures. Blood cultures will be positive in over 50% of the cases with *H. influenza* type B. Identify extraepiglottic foci of infections such as pneumonia, septic arthritis, pericarditis or meningitis.

REFERENCES

Bates JR. Epiglottitis: diagnosis and treatment. Pediatr Rev 1979; 1:173.
Liston SL, Gehrz RC, Siegel LG et al. Bacterial tracheitis. Am J Dis Child 1983; 137:764.
Molteni RA. Epiglottitis- incidence of extraepiglottic infection. Pediatrics 1976; 58:526.
Tunnessen WW, Feinstein AR. The steroid croup controversy: an analytic review of methodologic problems. J Pediatr 1980; 96:751.

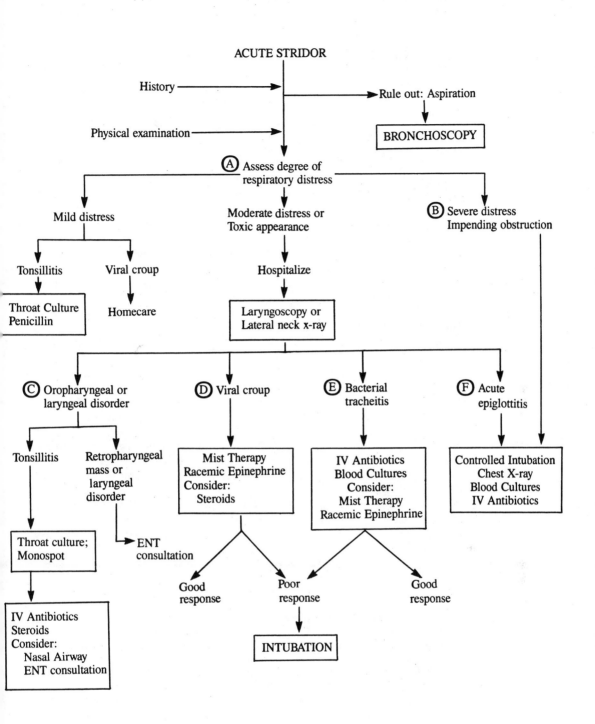

ACUTE STRIDOR

History → Rule out: Aspiration → BRONCHOSCOPY

Physical examination

Ⓐ Assess degree of respiratory distress

Mild distress

Moderate distress or Toxic appearance

Ⓑ Severe distress Impending obstruction

Tonsillitis — Throat Culture Penicillin

Viral croup → Homecare

Hospitalize → Laryngoscopy or Lateral neck x-ray

Ⓒ Oropharyngeal or laryngeal disorder

Ⓓ Viral croup

Ⓔ Bacterial tracheitis

Ⓕ Acute epiglottitis

Tonsillitis

Retropharyngeal mass or laryngeal disorder → ENT consultation

Mist Therapy
Racemic Epinephrine
Consider:
 Steroids

IV Antibiotics
Blood Cultures
Consider:
 Mist Therapy
Racemic Epinephrine

Controlled Intubation
Chest X-ray
Blood Cultures
IV Antibiotics

Throat culture; Monospot

IV Antibiotics
Steroids
Consider:
 Nasal Airway
 ENT consultation

Good response

Poor response → INTUBATION

Good response

Westley CR, Cotton EK, Brooks JG. Nebulized racemic epinephrine by IPPB for the treatment of croup. Am J Dis Child 1978; 132:484.

BRONCHIOLITIS

A. Bronchiolitis is a clinical syndrome characterized by inspiratory and expiratory wheezing. Inflammation of the small airways produces exudate, edema, necrosis, and bronchospasm and results in air trapping and emphysema. Respiratory syncytial virus most frequently causes this syndrome. Other agents include parainfluenza viruses, adenovirus, influenza virus, and *B. pertussis*.

B. Determine the onset, duration, severity, and pattern of respiratory symptoms. Note associated symptoms such as fever, earache, vomiting, oliguria, or alteration in mental status. Exclude the possibility of aspiration. Identify complicating conditions such as pulmonary disease (asthma, bronchopulmonary dysplasia, laryngomalacia, cystic fibrosis), cardiac disease, immune deficiency diseases, or prematurity.

C. Exclude noninfectious causes of wheezing such as foreign body, tracheoesophageal fistula, anomalies of the great vessels, gastroesophageal reflux, cystic fibrosis, alpha–1 antitrypsin deficiency, and anatomic malformations of the lung (sequestrations, bronchiogenic cysts, and teratomas).

D. Assess the degree of illness. Severely ill children appear toxic, dehydrated, or have hypotension or poor peripheral perfusion. They have marked respiratory distress with tachypnea > 70 respirations per minute, and retractions that may be associated with cyanosis or apnea. Moderately ill children have tachypnea with 50–70 respirations per minute, retractions, and often have a history of poor oral intake. Mildly ill children have good oral intake, appear well hydrated, and have minimal tachypnea and no retractions.

E. The radiologic findings of bronchiolitis include hyperexpansion with flattened diaphragm, peribronchial thickening, and patchy atelectasis with or without perihilar infiltrate.

F. Consider a trial of bronchodilator and steroid therapy in severe bronchiolitis. Maintain good supportive care with IV fluids and oxygen therapy. Monitor arterial blood gases. Indications of respiratory failure include inability to maintain a PaO_2 > 55 torr on 100% oxygen, a PCO_2 < 50 torr or a PCO_2 rising more than 5 torr per hour. Intubate and ventilate children with progressive respiratory failure or severe apnea.

G. Apnea complicates 20–25% of the cases of RSV bronchiolitis. Infants < 3 months of age who were born prematurely are at the greatest risk of becoming apneic. The mechanism of apnea is unclear; however, it appears to correlate with the degree of hypoxemia. Recurrent or prolonged apnea requires intubation and assisted ventilation for 24–48 hours.

REFERENCES

Bruhn FW, Mokrohisky ST, McIntosh K. Apnea associated with respiratory syncytial virus infection in young infants. J Pediatr 1977; 129:777.

Hall CB, Hall WJ, Speers DM. Clinical and physiological manifestations of bronchiolitis and pneumonia. Am J Dis Child 1979; 133:7908.

Henderson FW, Clyde WA, Collier AM et al. The etiologic and epidemiologic spectrum of bronchiolitis in pediatric practice. J Pediatr 1979; 95:183.

Tal A, Bavilski C, Yohai D et al. Dexamethasone and salbutamol in the treatment of acute wheezing in infants. Pediatrics 1983; 71:13.

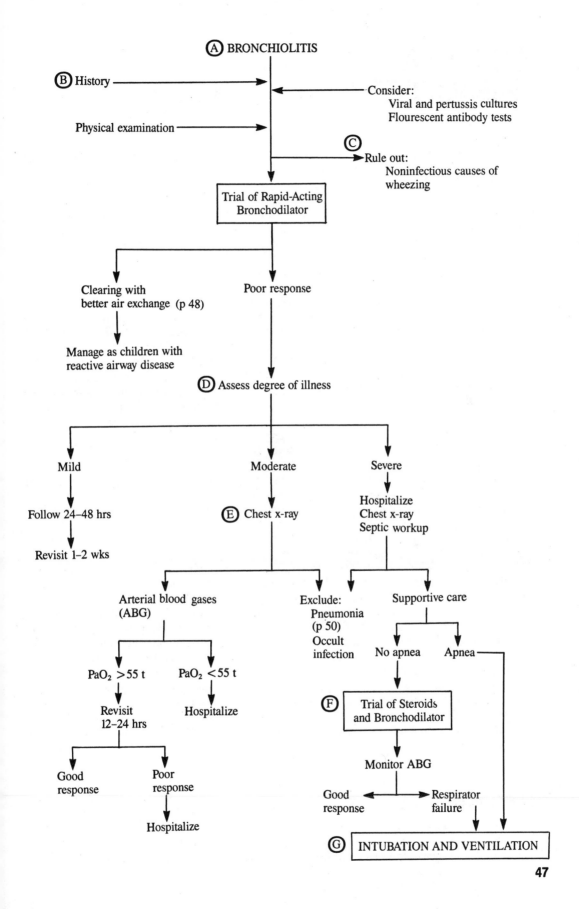

Ⓐ BRONCHIOLITIS

Ⓑ History

Consider:
Viral and pertussis cultures
Flourescent antibody tests

Physical examination

Ⓒ Rule out:
Noninfectious causes of
wheezing

Trial of Rapid-Acting
Bronchodilator

Clearing with
better air exchange (p 48)

Poor response

Manage as children with
reactive airway disease

Ⓓ Assess degree of illness

Mild

Moderate

Severe

Follow 24–48 hrs

Ⓔ Chest x-ray

Hospitalize
Chest x-ray
Septic workup

Revisit 1–2 wks

Arterial blood gases
(ABG)

Exclude:
Pneumonia
(p 50)
Occult
infection

Supportive care

No apnea

Apnea

$PaO_2 > 55$ t

$PaO_2 < 55$ t

Revisit
12–24 hrs

Hospitalize

Ⓕ Trial of Steroids
and Bronchodilator

Good
response

Poor
response

Monitor ABG

Hospitalize

Good
response

Respirator
failure

Ⓖ INTUBATION AND VENTILATION

ASTHMA
(REACTIVE AIRWAY DISEASE)

A. Determine the onset, duration, and therapy of the current episode. Note the course and outcomes of recent previous episodes. Identify precipitating factors such as infection, allergens, drugs, or exercise. Note changes in mental status, oral intake, vomiting, diarrhea, and frequency of urination. Assess parental attitude and the ability of the family to care for the child at home. Accurate knowledge of the type and timing of any prior theophylline is necessary in order to determine a safe loading dose without knowledge of theophylline blood levels.

B. Note signs of respiratory distress including tachypnea, dyspnea, nasal flaring, retractions, use of accessory muscles, ability to talk, wheezing, prolongation of the expiratory phase, and decreased breath sounds. Do spirometry if the facilities are available. Signs of severe respiratory distress include markedly decreased or absent breath sounds, cyanosis, and an increased pulsus paradoxsus (exaggeration of the normal variation of cardiac output with the respiratory cycle). An altered mental status with restlessness, disorientation, and air hunger indicates severe hypoxia.

C. Treat the patient initially with a rapid-acting bronchodilator subcutaneously or by nebulization. Injectable preparations include epinephrine (adrenalin) 1:1000; 0.01 ml/kg/dose (maximum 0.5 cc) or terbutaline sulfate (Brethine, Bricanyl) 1 mg/ml; 0.01 mg/kg/dose. Nebulized agents include isoetharine (Bronchosol) 1%; 0.25–0.5 ml diluted in 2 ml water or metaproterenol (Alupent) 5%; 0.1–0.3 ml diluted in 2 ml water. Use an initial loading dose of theophylline (6–9 mg/kg) to achieve a therapeutic blood level of 10–20 μg/ml. Knowledge of the current blood level is necessary to determine the loading dose in patients already taking theophylline (Loading dose=0.5×weight in kg×desired change in level). Treat mildly ill patients with an oral preparation or rectal solution, and moderate-to-severely ill patients with IV theophylline. Never use theophylline suppositories because of their erratic absorption.

D. The maintenance dose of oral theophylline in children under 12 years of age (excluding infants under 6 months) is approximately 20 mg/kg/day and in children 12–18 years of age approximately 18 mg/kg/day. Other adrenergic agents are metaproterenol (Alupent) 10 mg *q6h* for children under 60 pounds and 20 mg *q6h* for children over 60 pounds or an Alupent metered–dose inhaler 2–3 inhalations *q3–4h*; terbutaline (Brethine, Bricanyl) 2.5–5 mg *q6h*; or salbutamol (Proventil, Ventolin) 1–2 inhalations (metered dose 0.90 mg) *q4h*.

E. Admit patients with moderate–to–severe respiratory distress who fail to respond to a trial of rapid-acting bronchodilators. Administer IV aminophylline (85% theophylline) as a loading dose; follow with a continuous infusion at an initial rate of 0.85–1.1 mg/kg/hour. Calculate the loading dose to raise the theophylline level to 15–20 μg/ml. Monitor theophylline levels 2, 6, and 24 hours after starting the constant infusion. Increase the infusion by 0.1 mg/kg/hour every 6 hours until an adequate blood level is achieved. In the absence of adequate monitoring equipment, nursing care, and ability to determine serum theophylline levels; administer theophylline as a bolus 4–5 mg/kg over 20 minutes *q4h*.

F. Suspect respiratory failure when the patient has poor air exchange, persistent cyanosis, or a depressed level of consciousness. Check arterial blood gases; if the PCO_2 rises by 5 mmHg per hour, or if the PCO_2 level reaches 50–60 mmHg, admit patient to an intensive care unit and treat for acute respiratory failure. Consider an isoproterenol drip prior to intubation and mechanical ventilation.

REFERENCES

Easton J et al. Management of asthma. Pediatrics 1981; 68:874.
Lefert F. The management of acute severe asthma. J Pediatr 1980; 96:1.
Rachelefsky GS. Pharmacologic management of childhood asthma. Pediatr Rev 1980; 1:301.

ASTHMA (REACTIVE AIRWAY DISEASE)

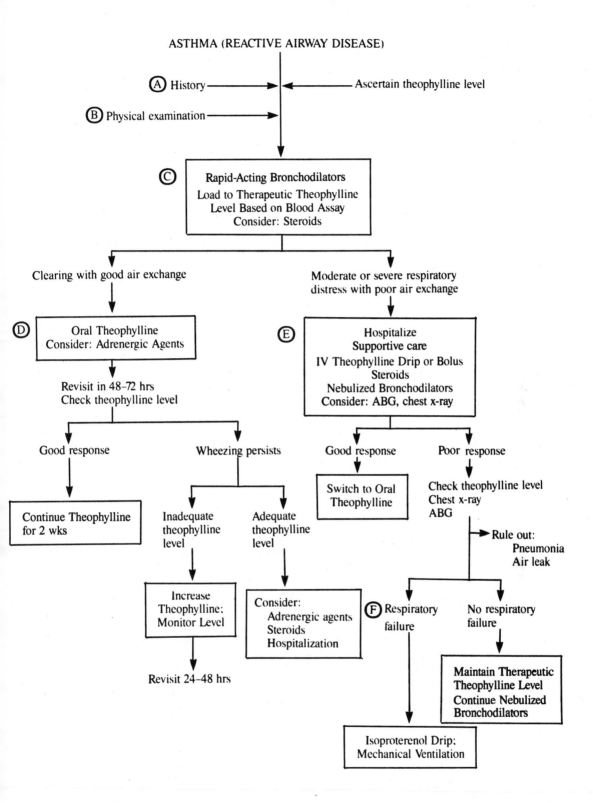

(A) History ────── Ascertain theophylline level

(B) Physical examination ──────

(C) **Rapid-Acting Bronchodilators**
Load to Therapeutic Theophylline
Level Based on Blood Assay
Consider: Steroids

Clearing with good air exchange

Moderate or severe respiratory
distress with poor air exchange

(D) Oral Theophylline
Consider: Adrenergic Agents

(E) Hospitalize
Supportive care
IV Theophylline Drip or Bolus
Steroids
Nebulized Bronchodilators
Consider: ABG, chest x-ray

Revisit in 48–72 hrs
Check theophylline level

Good response

Wheezing persists

Good response

Poor response

Continue Theophylline
for 2 wks

Inadequate
theophylline
level

Adequate
theophylline
level

Switch to Oral
Theophylline

Check theophylline level
Chest x-ray
ABG

Rule out:
Pneumonia
Air leak

Increase
Theophylline;
Monitor Level

Consider:
Adrenergic agents
Steroids
Hospitalization

(F) Respiratory
failure

No respiratory
failure

Revisit 24–48 hrs

**Maintain Therapeutic
Theophylline Level
Continue Nebulized
Bronchodilators**

Isoproterenol Drip;
Mechanical Ventilation

Silver RB, Ginsburg CM. Early prediction of the need for hospitalization in children with acute asthma. Clin
Pediatrics 1984; 23:81.
Weinberger M, Hendeles L. Slow-release theophylline: rationale and basis for product selection. New Engl J
Med 1983; 308:760.

PNEUMONIA

A. Determine the onset, duration, severity and pattern of respiratory symptoms. Note associated symptoms such as fever, earache, vomiting, oliguria, and altered mental status. Identify underlying conditions including pulmonary disease (asthma, bronchopulmonary dysplasia, cystic fibrosis), cardiac disease, malnutrition, or immune deficiency disorders.

B. Assess the degree of illness. Severely ill children present with tachypnea >70 respirations/min, severe retractions, cyanosis, dehydration, hypotension, or a "toxic" appearance. Moderately ill children have tachypnea (50–70 respirations/min) with retractions, poor fluid intake, or a fever ≥39°C. Consider children moderately ill when the CBC with differential suggests a bacterial process. Mildly ill children appear well hydrated with minimal signs of respiratory distress and temperature <39°C. Consider all infants under 6 months of age with suspected pneumonia to be either moderately or severely ill.

C. Obtain a chest x-ray in all children under 6 months of age with suspected pneumonia and in older children who appear moderately or severely ill. Hyperexpansion with perihilar or diffuse infiltrate are most frequently caused by viruses, *Chlamydia* (in infants <6 months of age), or *M. pneumoniae* (children >3 years of age). Lobar or segmental infiltrates and empyema are frequently associated with bacterial infections. Patchy infiltrates (bronchopneumonia) are associated with viral or bacterial disease.

D. In patients under 6 months of age, organisms associated with pneumonia include *Chlamydia, S. aureus, S. pneumoniae, H. influenzae, group A* and *B streptococcus*, and *Klebsiella. Chlamydia* is the most common agent causing pneumonia in this age period. Clinical features include respiratory symptoms for more than one week (80%), conjunctivitis (50%), and eosinophilia (70%). Treat suspected cases with erythromycin 40 mg/kg/day in 4 divided doses. In older infants and children, *S. pneumoniae*, and *H. influenzae* are the most frequent bacterial agents causing pneumonia. Treat with amoxicillin 50–75 mg/kg/day in 3 divided doses. Consider giving one dose of ampicillin or penicillin IM when compliance is questionable or vomiting is present. Failure to improve after 24–48 hours of therapy suggests a viral infection, or infection with a resistant organism. Consider a change in antibiotics to cover resistant *H. influenzae*, a repeat chest x-ray, and hospitalization.

E. Treat hospitalized severely ill children with IV antibiotic therapy. When pneumonia with *S. aureus* is suspected, use a semisynthetic penicillin (oxacillin or nafcillin) and gentamicin. Use ampicillin and either chloramphenicol or moxolactam for severe pneumonia associated with sepsis or meningitis and infections with *H. influenzae*. Use an aminoglycoside antibiotic for possible gram-negative enteric infections. Treat patients with cystic fibrosis with carbenicillin and gentamicin since Pseudomonas infections are common. Consider gram-negative enteric organisms and pneumocystis in immunocompromised children at any age. Empyema is associated with many bacterial infections including *S. pneumoniae, S. aureus, H. influenzae, group A streptococcus*, and gram-negative enteric organisms. Obtain a repeat chest x-ray if the clinical status deteriorates after 48–72 hours of therapy in order to identify air leaks, effusions, or empyema, or resistant infection.

REFERENCES

Eichenwald HF. Pneumonia syndromes in children. Hosp Prac 1976; May:89.
Jacobs NM, Harris VJ. Acute haemophilus pneumonia in childhood. Am J Dis Child 1979; 133:603.
Marks MI. Pediatric pneumonia: viral or bacterial. J Resp Dis 1982; March:108.
McLaughlin FJ, Goldman DA, Rosenbaum DM. Empyema in children: clinical course and long-term follow-up. Pediatrics 1984; 73:587.

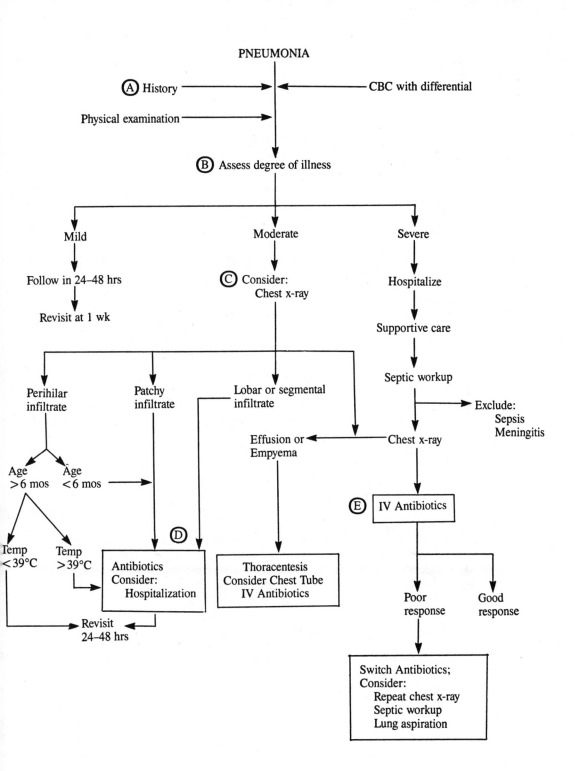

PNEUMONIA

(A) History ⟶ ⟵ CBC with differential

Physical examination ⟶

(B) Assess degree of illness

Mild — Moderate — Severe

Mild:
Follow in 24–48 hrs
Revisit at 1 wk

Moderate:
(C) Consider:
Chest x-ray

Severe:
Hospitalize
Supportive care
Septic workup

Perihilar infiltrate — Patchy infiltrate — Lobar or segmental infiltrate

Exclude:
Sepsis
Meningitis

Effusion or Empyema ⟵ Chest x-ray

Age >6 mos   Age <6 mos ⟶

(E) IV Antibiotics

Temp <39°C   Temp >39°C

(D)
Antibiotics
Consider:
Hospitalization

Thoracentesis
Consider Chest Tube
IV Antibiotics

Poor response   Good response

Revisit 24–48 hrs

Switch Antibiotics;
Consider:
    Repeat chest x-ray
    Septic workup
    Lung aspiration

APNEA

A. Apnea is defined as a failure to breathe spontaneously for 20 seconds or an episode without breathing associated with cyanosis, pallor, bradycardia ($<$ 80 beats/min), or loss of muscle tone.

B. Determine onset, duration, frequency, pattern (relationship to feeding, crying, sleep), severity (type of resuscitation required and degree of cyanosis, pallor, or hypotonia) of the apnea. Note associated symptoms suggestive of seizures such as muscle jerks, eye rolling, tongue thrusting, a postictal state, and frequent recurrences. Suspect breathholding spells when the episode occurs while the child is awake, is precipitated by crying, sudden pain or fear, and is associated with stiffening and/or clonus. With breathholding, cyanosis and hypotonia precede any abnormal movements and there is no postictal state. Identify precipitating factors such as respiratory infection, possible drug ingestion, head trauma, and predisposing conditions including prematurity, heart disease, pulmonary disease (bronchopulmonary dysplasia, asthma), CNS disorders, mucopolysaccharidosis, hypothyroidism, congenital syndrome (Prader–Willi, Pierre Robin), or hematologic diseases causing severe anemia.

C. Assess the degree of illness. Severely ill infants appear toxic and have an altered mental status or signs of significant cardiac or pulmonary compromise. Moderately ill infants have symptoms such as fever, lethargy, and poor feeding, or findings of respiratory or cardiac disease. Mildly ill infants are vigorous and asymptomatic.

D. In obstructive apnea, the infant or child makes inspiratory efforts but fails to inspire adequate air to the lungs. When no inspiratory efforts are associated with a cessation of breathing, apnea is called central or nonobstructive.

E. Diagnoses of upper airway obstruction include macroglossia (mucopolysaccharide syndromes, hypothyroidism), enlarged tonsils and/or adenoids, pharyngeal/retropharyngeal masses, Pierre Robin syndrome, choanal stenosis or atresia, epiglottitis, and supraglottic mass.

F. A barium swallow identifies gastric reflux, a vascular ring, or tracheoesophageal fistula. The role of gastric reflux as a cause of apnea of infancy is unclear, since gastroesophageal reflux in early infancy is a common finding in children without apnea. Rarely, gastric reflux may result in laryngospasm. Refluxed gastric contents may stimulate upper airway or laryngeal receptors, producing apnea and bradycardia.

G. In sudden infant death syndrome (SIDS), the cause of death cannot be explained by either the history or autopsy. Risk factors include a family history of either SIDS or apnea of infancy (recurrence risk for nextborn sibling is 5.6/1000), recurrent apnea requiring intervention, a severe apneic episode (near SIDS), and prematurity. These infants should have home monitoring until at least 6 months of age. After 6 months of age, discontinue monitoring if the infant has not experienced a significant apneic spell requiring intervention during the preceding 2 months. Document the infant's ability to handle the stress of immunizations and URIs prior to discontinuation of home monitoring.

H. Hypoxia and respiratory distress secondary to infection, pulmonary disease, or cardiac disease can cause apnea. The risk of apnea associated with infection is highest in infants under 3 months of age who were born prematurely. Apnea is associated with 20–25% of cases of RSV lower respiratory infections.

REFERENCES

Aras N, Boettrich C, Hall CB et al. The association of apnea and respiratory syncytial virus infection in infants. J Pediatr 1982; 101:65.

Berger D. Child abuse simulating "near miss" sudden infant death syndrome. J Pediatr 1979; 95:554.

Brooks JG. Apnea of infancy and sudden infant death syndrome. Am J Dis Child 1982; 136:1012.

Irgens LM, Skjaeruen R, Peterson DR. Prospective assessment of recurrence risk in sudden infant death syndrome siblings. J Pediatr 1984; 104:349.

McBride JT. Infantile apnea. Pediatr Rev 1984; 5:275.

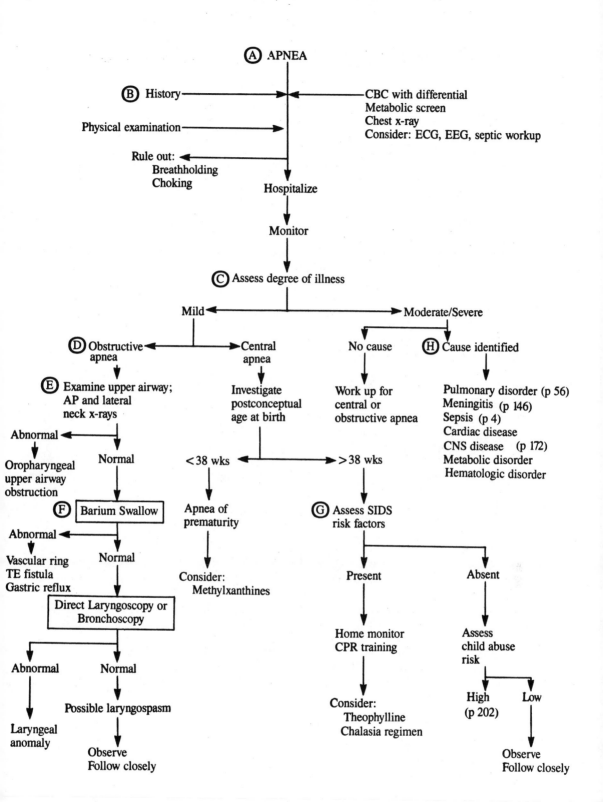

Ⓐ APNEA

Ⓑ History — CBC with differential
Metabolic screen
Chest x-ray
Consider: ECG, EEG, septic workup

Physical examination —

Rule out:
Breathholding
Choking

Hospitalize

Monitor

Ⓒ Assess degree of illness

Mild — Moderate/Severe

Ⓓ Obstructive apnea — Central apnea

No cause — Ⓗ Cause identified

Ⓔ Examine upper airway; AP and lateral neck x-rays

Investigate postconceptual age at birth

Work up for central or obstructive apnea

Pulmonary disorder (p 56)
Meningitis (p 146)
Sepsis (p 4)
Cardiac disease
CNS disease (p 172)
Metabolic disorder
Hematologic disorder

Abnormal —

Oropharyngeal upper airway obstruction

Normal

< 38 wks — > 38 wks

Ⓕ Barium Swallow

Apnea of prematurity

Ⓖ Assess SIDS risk factors

Abnormal —

Vascular ring
TE fistula
Gastric reflux

Normal

Consider:
Methylxanthines

Present — Absent

Direct Laryngoscopy or Bronchoscopy

Home monitor
CPR training

Assess child abuse risk

Abnormal — Normal

Possible laryngospasm

Consider:
Theophylline
Chalasia regimen

High (p 202) — Low

Laryngeal anomaly

Observe
Follow closely

Observe
Follow closely

Brooks JG. Apnea of infancy and sudden infant death syndrome. Am J Dis Child 1982; 136:1012.
Irgens LM, Skjaeruen R, Peterson DR. Prospective assessment of recurrence risk in sudden infant death syndrome siblings. J Pediatr 1984; 104:349.
McBride JT. Infantile apnea. Pediatr Rev 1984; 5:275.

CHRONIC COUGH

A. Children with a history of persistent cough longer than 4 weeks in duration need a thorough evaluation. The type of cough often suggests the etiology: productive (reactive air way disease, infection), brassy (habit cough, tracheitis), barky (croup), paroxysmal (foreign body, pertussis, cystic fibrosis). The pattern of cough can be helpful: nocturnal (sinusitis, reactive air way disease), early morning (cystic fibrosis, bronchiectasis), exercise-induced (reactive air way disease, cystic fibrosis, bronchiectasis), absent during sleep (habit cough).

B. Institute a trial of bronchodilator therapy in patients without an upper respiratory tract disorder who have a normal chest x-ray. Reactive airway disease which causes chronic cough without wheezing is often exercise-induced. Patients who fail to respond to this therapy and who are moderately ill or have associated systemic symptoms such as failure to thrive, recurrent infections, recurrent fever, stridor, or wheezing should be given a workup with sinus x-rays and/or a barium swallow.

C. Work up chest x-ray findings of tracheal deviation, localized infiltrate, or localized hyperexpansion with additional studies to diagnose a foreign body, infection, or mass lesion obstructing the air way (intrinsic or extrinsic obstruction). Consider bronchoscopy when a foreign body or obstructing mass is suspected. Manage patients with suspected localized infection with a trial of antibiotic therapy combined with postural drainage.

D. The workup for mediastinal masses includes a CT scan, possibly tomograms, and a surgical consultation for thoracotomy or mediastinoscopy. The most comon masses (and their usual location in the mediastinum) are neurogenic tumors (33%, posterior), lymphoma (14%, anterior or middle), teratoma (10%, anterior), thymic lesion (9%, anterior), bronchiogenic cyst (7.5%, middle), angioma (7%, anterior), duplication cyst (7%, posterior), and lymph node infection (4%, middle).

E. Causes of pulmonary mass include pulmonary sequestration, bronchiogenic cysts, eventration of the diaphragm, cystic adenematoid malformation, lung abscess, massive atelectasis, and tumor. Work up a pulmonary mass with tomograms, CT scan, and fluoroscopy. Consider skin tests, bronchoscopy, and angiography.

F. Investigate diffuse pulmonary infiltrates for an infectious etiology with skin tests; rapid diagnostic tests; and cultures for bacterial disease (tuberculosis, pertussis, mycoplasma pneumonia, and chlamydia), fungal disease (monilia, histoplasmosis coccidiomycosis), parasitic disease (pneumocystis echinococcus); and viral infections (RSV, CMV, adenovirus, influenza, parainfluenza). Obtain a pulmonary consultation for pulmonary function testing in order to diagnose restrictive lung disease. Consider a brush biopsy or open lung biopsy to diagnose noninfectious etiologies such as hypersensitivity pneumonitis (exposure to organic antigens), pulmonary hemosiderosis, pulmonary alveolar proteinoses, fibrosing alveolitis, and Goodpasture's syndrome.

G. Causes of bronchiectasis include cystic fibrosis, immunodeficiency syndrome, Kartagener's syndrome, and chronic infection. When sweat chlorides are normal, obtain immunoglobulins and a nasal mucosa biopsy for cilia studies.

REFERENCES

Cloutier MM, Loughlin GM. Chronic cough in children; a manifestation of airway hyperactivity. Pediatrics 1981; 67:6.

Eigen H. The clinical evaluation of chronic cough. Pediatr Clin North Am 1982; 29:67.

Feller RM, Simpson JS, Ein SH. Mediastinal masses in infants and children. Pediatr Clin North Am 1979; 26:677.

Mellis CM. Evaluation and treatment of chronic cough in children. Pediatr Clin North Am 1979; 26:553.

CHRONIC COUGH

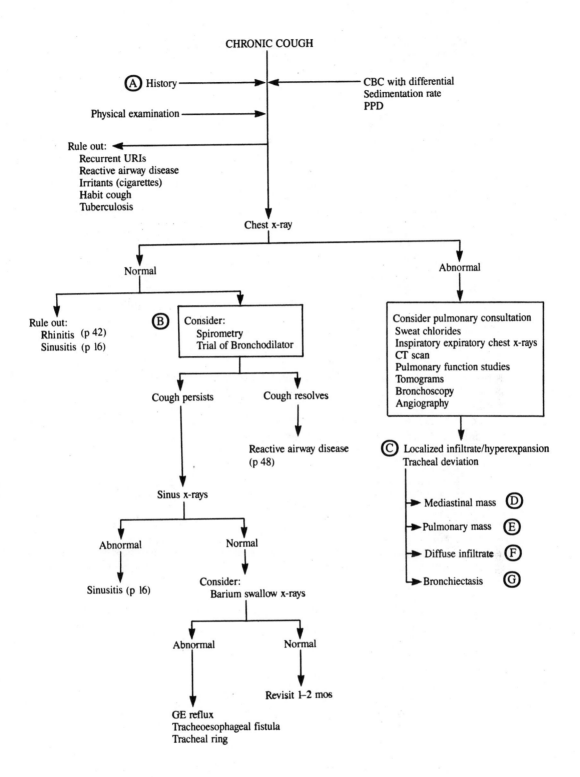

A History

CBC with differential
Sedimentation rate
PPD

Physical examination

Rule out:
  Recurrent URIs
  Reactive airway disease
  Irritants (cigarettes)
  Habit cough
  Tuberculosis

Chest x-ray

Normal

Abnormal

Rule out:
  Rhinitis (p 42)
  Sinusitis (p 16)

B Consider:
  Spirometry
  Trial of Bronchodilator

Consider pulmonary consultation
Sweat chlorides
Inspiratory expiratory chest x-rays
CT scan
Pulmonary function studies
Tomograms
Bronchoscopy
Angiography

Cough persists

Cough resolves

Reactive airway disease
(p 48)

C Localized infiltrate/hyperexpansion
Tracheal deviation

Sinus x-rays

Mediastinal mass D

Pulmonary mass E

Diffuse infiltrate F

Bronchiectasis G

Abnormal

Normal

Sinusitis (p 16)

Consider:
  Barium swallow x-rays

Abnormal

Normal

Revisit 1–2 mos

GE reflux
Tracheoesophageal fistula
Tracheal ring

55

RESPIRATORY DISTRESS

A. Cyanosis related to pulmonary disease can be produced by alveolar hypoventilation, ventilation profusion inequality, and impairment of oxygen diffusion. Cyanosis is related to the presence of 3 grams or more of reduced hemoglobin per 100 mls. It is best detected by examining the lips, tongue, and mucous membranes. Peripheral cyanosis related to slow blood flow and large differences in arteriovenous oxygen is often present in the hands, feet, and circumoral areas.

B. The arterial blood gas (ABG) measures the partial pressure of dissolved oxygen in blood. The relationship between the ABG and O_2 saturation is displayed in the oxygen dissociation curve. Pulmonary disease is suggested when the administration of 100% oxygen results in a substantial increase in the PaO_2 compared to a gas obtained in room air. The shunt study is useful in identifying fixed right to left shunts which suggest cardiac disease or marked pulmonary hypertension. A PaO_2 less than 55 torr on 80 to 100% oxygen or a PCO_2 over 50 torr suggests respiratory failure. Intubate and ventilate these children. Consider the use of sedation/paralysis when the patient is fighting the ventilator.

C. Adult respiratory distress syndrome results when severe damage to the capillary endothelial cells decreases surfactant levels causing massive atelectasis. Use assisted ventilation with positive end expiratory pressure to maintain adequate oxygenation.

D. Pulmonary edema results from circulatory overload, decreased oncotic pressure (hypoproteinemia) or capillary damage and leak. Capillary damage can result from a direct pulmonary insult such as a toxic inhalation or near drowning, or a systemic process such as shock, anoxia, or overwhelming sepsis. CNS disorders such as meningitis or encephalitis, mass lesions (hematoma, tumor or intracranial hemorrhage) can also produce pulmonary edema. Circulatory overload secondary to renal failure, the syndrome of inappropriate ADH, or water intoxication can cause pulmonary edema. High-altitude pulmonary edema (HAPE) occurs in children and adolescents who live at low altitude and travel above 8500 feet, in residents of high-altitude areas who return home from low altitudes, and in residents of high-altitude areas who develop a viral URI. Clinical signs include dyspnea, cough, periodic breathing, and frothy sputum. Pulmonary edema on x-ray may be only right-sided with basilar involvement. Manage cases with oxygen and return to lower altitude.

E. Space-occupying pulmonary lesions with air leak include pneumothorax, pneumomediastinum, pneumopericardium, and pulmonary interstitial emphysema. Space-occupying lesions without air leaks include diaphragmatic hernia, congenital lobar emphysema, cystic adenomatoid malformation, bronchiogenic cysts, eventration of the diaphragm, lung abscess, and tumor. Work up a pulmonary mass with tomograms and a CT scan. Consider fluoroscopy, bronchoscopy, and angiography.

F. Obstructive lesions of the upper airway include choanal atresia, Pierre Robin syndrome, vocal cord paralysis, stenosis of the trachea, vascular rings, foreign body or congenital webs or cysts.

REFERENCES

Kitterman JA. Cyanosis in the newborn infant. Pediatr in Rev 1982; 4:13.
Newth CJL. Recognition and management of respiratory failure. Pediatr Clin North Am 1979; 26:617.
Pagtakhan RD, Chernick V. Respiratory failure in the pediatric patient. Pediatr in Rev 1982; 3:247.
Shannon DC, Lasser M, Goldblatt A, et al. The cyanotic infant-heart disease or lung disease. N Engl J Med 1972; 287:951.

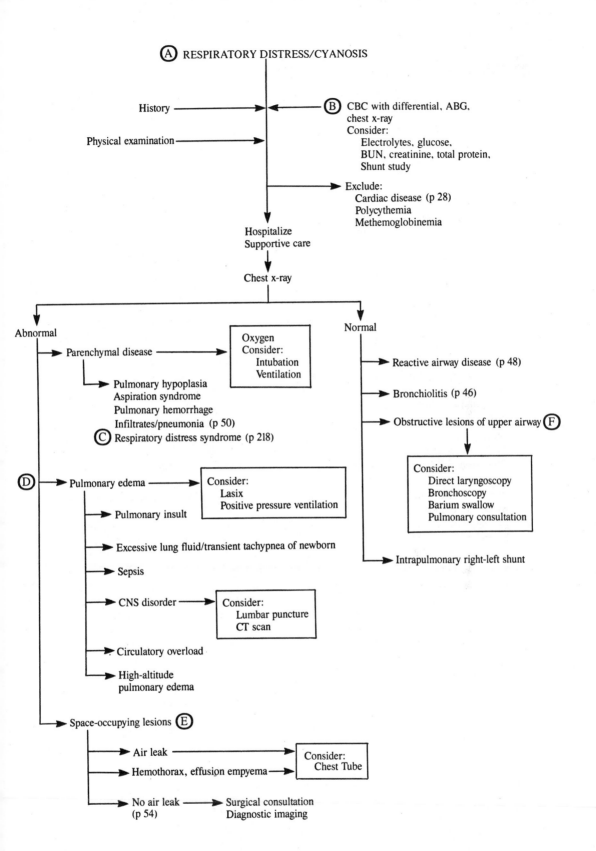

(A) RESPIRATORY DISTRESS/CYANOSIS

History

Physical examination

(B) CBC with differential, ABG,
chest x-ray
Consider:
Electrolytes, glucose,
BUN, creatinine, total protein,
Shunt study

Exclude:
Cardiac disease (p 28)
Polycythemia
Methemoglobinemia

Hospitalize
Supportive care

Chest x-ray

Abnormal

Parenchymal disease

Oxygen
Consider:
Intubation
Ventilation

Pulmonary hypoplasia
Aspiration syndrome
Pulmonary hemorrhage
Infiltrates/pneumonia (p 50)
(C) Respiratory distress syndrome (p 218)

(D) Pulmonary edema

Consider:
Lasix
Positive pressure ventilation

Pulmonary insult

Excessive lung fluid/transient tachypnea of newborn

Sepsis

CNS disorder

Consider:
Lumbar puncture
CT scan

Circulatory overload

High-altitude
pulmonary edema

Space-occupying lesions (E)

Air leak

Hemothorax, effusion empyema

Consider:
Chest Tube

No air leak
(p 54)

Surgical consultation
Diagnostic imaging

Normal

Reactive airway disease (p 48)

Bronchiolitis (p 46)

Obstructive lesions of upper airway (F)

Consider:
Direct laryngoscopy
Bronchoscopy
Barium swallow
Pulmonary consultation

Intrapulmonary right-left shunt

57

SHORT STATURE

Michael S. Kappy, M.D., Ph.D.

A. Ask about the heights of parents and siblings (familial short stature) and whether the mother had a history of delayed menarche or father a delayed adolescent growth spurt (constitutional short stature). Obtain an appropriate nutritional and psychosocial data base. Identify predisposing conditions such as congenital infections, small for gestational age at birth (primordial short stature), congenital syndromes, and chronic illness involving any organ system (especially the GI tract and the cardiac, pulmonary, and renal systems).

B. Document the accurate height of the child and calculate the height:weight ratio. Note the presence of congenital abnormalities and assess carefully the gastrointestinal, cardiovascular, and pulmonary systems. Note the presence or absence of a goiter. Evaluate the child's pubertal development. Assess the child's dentition.

C. Consider the diagnosis of Turner's syndrome in girls. Approximately 60% of cases do not have the classical syndrome stigmata (web neck, widely spaced nipples, and delayed sexual maturation). After 9 to 10 years of age, FSH and LH measurements will identify ovarian failure, which is common with Turner's syndrome. Karyotyping confirms the diagnosis.

D. Document the child's growth rate from one year of age through preadolescence. The lower limit of normal growth is approximately 5 cm per year. A short child with a normal growth rate is unlikely to have significant illness or endocrinopathy.

E. Rule out thyroid or growth hormone deficiency in children with a significantly delayed bone age who are growing less than 4 cms a year. In primary hypothyroidism, a low free T4 or total T4 is associated with an elevated TSH.

F. The bone age (single AP view of the left hand) is useful in correlating the degree of physical maturation with chronologic age. Causes of delayed bone age include constitutional delay, emotional deprivation, chronic illness, malnutrition, growth hormone deficiency, and thyroid hormone deficiency.

G. In constitutional delay, the child's rate of physical maturation is delayed compared to that of his/her peers. The bone age is usually equal to the height age. Pubertal maturation is correspondingly delayed. The ultimate height of these children is usually normal since the pubertal growth spurt often occurs between 15 and 17 years, and growth continues until 18 to 20 years of age.

H. Children with familial short stature have a normal physical examination, growth rate of greater than 4 cm a year, and a bone age appropriate for chronologic age. Patients with primordial short stature were small for gestational age at birth or may have in addition a congenital syndrome (e.g., Russell-Silver syndrome).

I. Rule out growth hormone deficiency in children with normal thyroid function, delayed bone age, and growth rate less than 4 cms per year.

J. A low T4 not accompanied by an elevated TSH suggests thyroid binding protein deficiency, secondary (pituitary) disorders, or tertiary (hypothalamic) disorders. Refer these patients with suspected pituitary or hypothalamic disorders for further evaluation.

REFERENCES

Fisher DA. Hypothyroidism in childhood. Pediatr Rev 1980; 2:67.

Frasier SD. Short stature in children. Pediatr Rev 1981; 3:171.

Horner JM et al. Growth deceleration in children with constitutional short stature. Pediatrics 1978, 62:529.

Rimoin DL, Horton WA. Short stature. J Pediatr 1978; 92:523-697.

Schaff-Blass E, Burstein S, Rosenfield RL. Advances in diagnosis and treatment of short stature with special reference to the note of growth hormone. J Pediatrics 1984; 104:81.

Schaff-Blass E et al. Advances in diagnosis and therapy of short stature with special reference to the role of GH. J Pediatr 1984; 104:801.

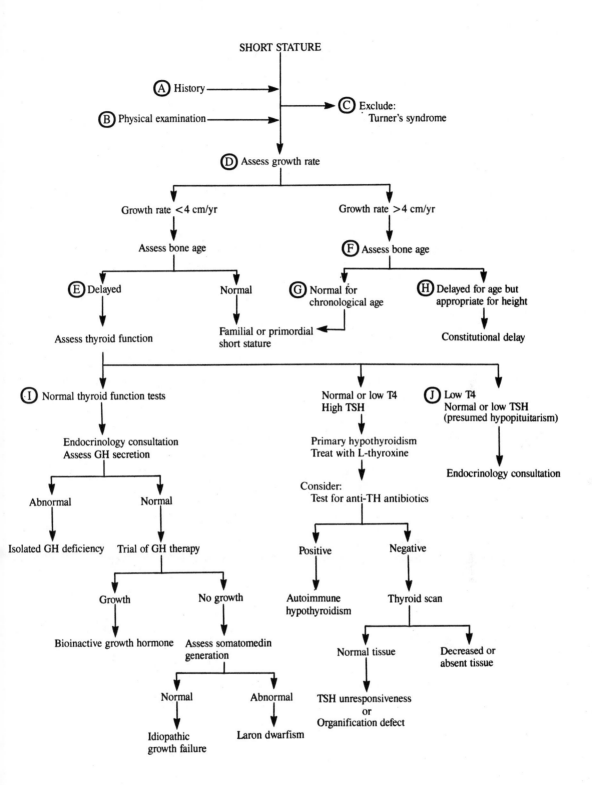

SHORT STATURE

(A) History

(B) Physical examination

(C) Exclude:
Turner's syndrome

(D) Assess growth rate

Growth rate <4 cm/yr

Assess bone age

(E) Delayed

Normal

Assess thyroid function

Familial or primordial
short stature

Growth rate >4 cm/yr

(F) Assess bone age

(G) Normal for
chronological age

(H) Delayed for age but
appropriate for height

Constitutional delay

(I) Normal thyroid function tests

Endocrinology consultation
Assess GH secretion

Abnormal

Normal

Isolated GH deficiency   Trial of GH therapy

Growth

No growth

Bioinactive growth hormone   Assess somatomedin
generation

Normal

Abnormal

Idiopathic
growth failure

Laron dwarfism

Normal or low T4
High TSH

Primary hypothyroidism
Treat with L-thyroxine

Consider:
Test for anti-TH antibiotics

Positive

Negative

Autoimmune
hypothyroidism

Thyroid scan

Normal tissue

Decreased or
absent tissue

TSH unresponsiveness
or
Organification defect

(J) Low T4
Normal or low TSH
(presumed hypopituitarism)

Endocrinology consultation

AMBIGUOUS GENITALIA
Michael S. Kappy, M.D., Ph.D.

A. Note predisposing factors or conditions such as birth control pills during pregnancy, a positive family history for ambiguous genitalia, congenital adrenal hyperplasia, or infant deaths, or the presence of maternal virilization.

B. Accurately describe the infant's phallus as well as the relationship of the urethral opening to the glans. The absence of palpable testes in the scrotal, labial, or inguinal region implies that the child is female with salt-losing congenital adrenal hyperplasia. The presence of associated abnormalities suggests a dysmorphic syndrome as opposed to an inherited metabolic disorder.

C. The results of the karyotyping separate cases into genetic males (XY) with incomplete virilization, genetic females (XX) with excessive virilization, and chromosomal aberrations.

D. Evaluate genetic males for defects in the biosynthetic pathway of androgens (testosterone and dihydrotestosterone), the major virilizing factors during intrauterine development. Some conditions may be associated with electrolyte abnormalities related to mineralocorticoid deficiencies. Consider an exploratory laparotomy and gonadal biopsy when the metabolic workup is negative. Examine internal structures including the gonads and the Wolffian derivatives (seminal vesicles, prostatic urethra, epididymis and vas deferens) to identify XY gonadal dysgenesis, true hermaphroditism, and idiopathic ambiguity. Normal testicular tissue with reduced or absent Wolffian structures associated with normal circulating testosterone and dihydrotestosterone indicates a receptor defect termed partial androgen insensitivity (testicular feminization syndrome).

E. The absence of maternal virilization or elevated androgens suggests idiopathic ambiguity (dysmorphia) or true hermaphroditism. Consider an exploratory laparotomy and gonadal biopsy to diagnose these conditions. Karyotyping of gonadal cells may show a mixed XX and XY despite a peripheral XX karyotype.

F. Treat patients with 21-hydroxylase deficiency with mineralocorticoid and glucocorticoid replacement. The usual mineralocorticoid is Florinef (.05–0.15 mg daily). For glucocorticoid replacement, use the lowest possible dose of hydrocortisone that suppresses adrenal androgen secretion and allows for normal growth and development. The full replacement dose (25 mg/m²/day in 3 divided doses) may inhibit normal growth.

G. The management of ambiguous genitalia may involve surgery. Assignment of gender to the infants should be made soon after birth, with consultations of both surgical and endocrine subspecialists. Even in cases where the karyotype indicates a genetic male, incomplete virilization that significantly compromises the size of the phallus often necessitates raising the child as a female.

REFERENCES

Hung W, August GP, Glasgow AM. Pediatric Endocrinology. New York: Medical Exam Publ, 1983.
Sainger P. Abnormal sex differentiation. J Pediatr 1984; 104:1.

Figure 1 Steroid Hormone Biosynthesis

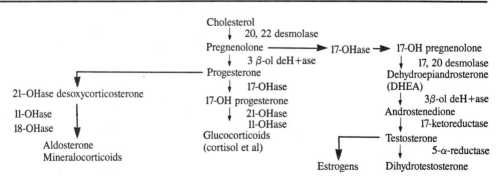

AMBIGUOUS GENITALIA

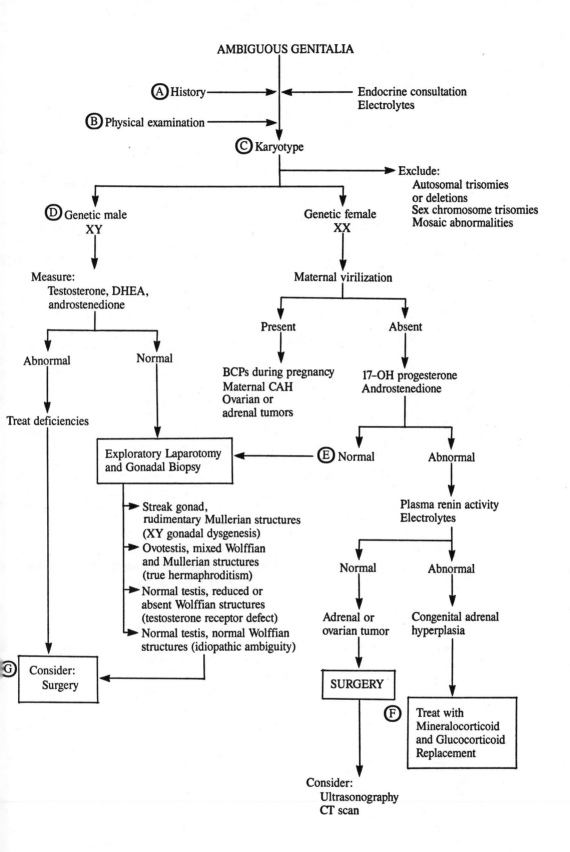

Ⓐ History

Endocrine consultation
Electrolytes

Ⓑ Physical examination

Ⓒ Karyotype

Exclude:
Autosomal trisomies
or deletions
Sex chromosome trisomies
Mosaic abnormalities

Ⓓ Genetic male
XY

Genetic female
XX

Measure:
Testosterone, DHEA,
androstenedione

Maternal virilization

Abnormal   Normal

Present   Absent

Treat deficiencies

BCPs during pregnancy
Maternal CAH
Ovarian or
adrenal tumors

17-OH progesterone
Androstenedione

Exploratory Laparotomy
and Gonadal Biopsy

Ⓔ Normal   Abnormal

→ Streak gonad,
rudimentary Mullerian structures
(XY gonadal dysgenesis)
→ Ovotestis, mixed Wolffian
and Mullerian structures
(true hermaphroditism)
→ Normal testis, reduced or
absent Wolffian structures
(testosterone receptor defect)
→ Normal testis, normal Wolffian
structures (idiopathic ambiguity)

Plasma renin activity
Electrolytes

Normal   Abnormal

Adrenal or
ovarian tumor

Congenital adrenal
hyperplasia

Ⓖ Consider:
Surgery

SURGERY

Ⓕ Treat with
Mineralocorticoid
and Glucocorticoid
Replacement

Consider:
Ultrasonography
CT scan

PRECOCIOUS PUBERTY IN THE MALE

Michael S. Kappy, M.D., Ph.D.

A. Note the age of onset of sexual development and recent increase in growth velocity. Identify predisposing CNS conditions such as tumor, head injury, and meningitis. Obtain a family history for similar conditions. The normal onset of pubertal development (mean/range) in the male is genitals (11¾ years/9½–14 years); pubic hair (12½ years/10¾–14 years); gynecomastia (12½ years/10¾–14 years); peak height velocity (13¾ years/11¾–16 years); axillary hair (14 years/12–16 years).

B. Carefully plot heights and weights. Assess the genitalia, and note the presence or absence of acne and pubic hair. Obtain accurate measurements of both testes and penis. In pseudo (end-organ) precocity, testosterone or other androgens are secreted without gonadotropin stimulation. Thus, the penis is enlarged, but the testes are not (unless tumor is present). This suggests a disorder in the testes or adrenal glands rather than the central nervous system. In central, or true precocious puberty, increased gonadotropin secretion stimulates testosterone prior to the normal pubertal age, and penile and testicular enlargement are present. Note skeletal abnormalities (commonly in the lower extremities) and rough-bordered café-au-lait spots which suggest McCune-Albright's syndrome. Signs of androgen excess with moon face, central adiposity, and striae suggest Cushing's syndrome. Premature adrenarche or the development of acne, pubic and axillary hair associated with normal or slightly increased levels of hormones and a normal growth velocity is benign.

C. Congenital adrenal hyperplasia accounts for 70–80% of cases with precocious puberty. An elevated 17-OHP suggests this diagnosis. Measure the gonadotropins (FSH and LH) and testosterone to determine whether or not gonadotropin secretion has stimulated testosterone. Consider luteinizing releasing hormone (LRH) testing to determine maturity of the pituitary response.

D. A low serum testosterone concentration in the absence of elevated FSH and LH (prepubertal level) suggests abnormal secretion of other androgens, most commonly of adrenal origin. Measure either the urinary excretion products of androgens (17-ketosteroids) or the hormones directly (17-hydroxyprogesterone, androstenedione, dehydroepiandrosterone [DHEA]).

E. In patients with congenital adrenal hyperplasia and Cushing's disease, dexamethasone will suppress endogenous production of cortisol by inhibiting ACTH secretion. In patients whose virilization results from an autonomously functioning adrenal tissue (an adrenal tumor) or an ACTH-producing tumor, dexamethasone will not suppress cortisol secretion.

REFERENCES

Lee PA. Normal ages of pubertal events among American males and females. J Adolescent Health Care 1980; 1:26.
Hung W, August GP, Glasgow AM. Pediatric Endocrinology. New York: Medical Exam Publ, 1983.
Parks JS. Endocrine disorders of childhood. Hosp Pract 1977; 12:93.
Rosenfeld RG. Evaluation of growth and maturation in adolescence. Pediatr Rev 1982; 4:175.

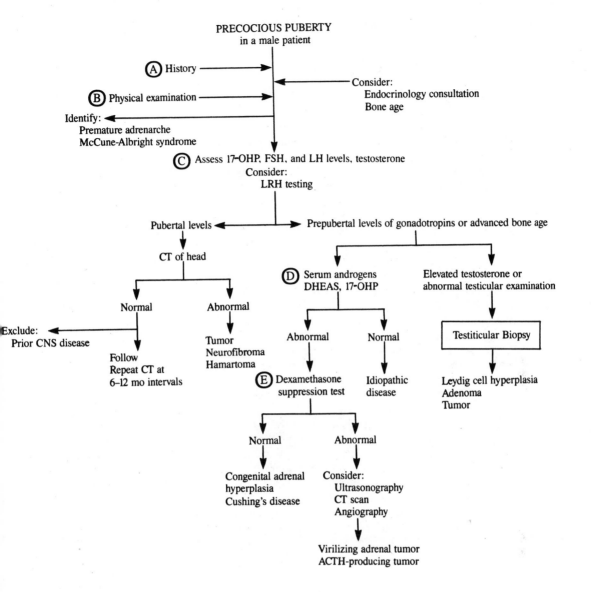

PRECOCIOUS PUBERTY
in a male patient

(A) History

Consider:
    Endocrinology consultation
    Bone age

(B) Physical examination

Identify:
    Premature adrenarche
    McCune-Albright syndrome

(C) Assess 17-OHP, FSH, and LH levels, testosterone
    Consider:
        LRH testing

Pubertal levels → ← Prepubertal levels of gonadotropins or advanced bone age

CT of head

Normal   Abnormal

Exclude:
    Prior CNS disease

Follow   Tumor
Repeat CT at   Neurofibroma
6–12 mo intervals   Hamartoma

(D) Serum androgens
    DHEAS, 17-OHP

Abnormal   Normal

(E) Dexamethasone   Idiopathic
    suppression test   disease

Elevated testosterone or
abnormal testicular examination

Testicular Biopsy

Leydig cell hyperplasia
Adenoma
Tumor

Normal   Abnormal

Congenital adrenal   Consider:
hyperplasia   Ultrasonography
Cushing's disease   CT scan
                              Angiography

Virilizing adrenal tumor
ACTH-producing tumor

63

PRECOCIOUS PUBERTY IN THE FEMALE

Michael S. Kappy, M.D., Ph.D.

A. Note the age of onset of signs of puberty and recent increase in growth velocity. The normal onset of pubertal development (mean/range) is breast development (11 ¼ years/8–15 years), pubic hair (12 years/9–15 years), menarche (13 ¼ years/10½–16 years), peak height velocity (12 ½ years/9½–15 years), and axillary hair (13 ¼ years/11 ½–14 ½ years). Identify exogenous sources of hormones. Note family history of early sexual development.

B. Note signs of central nervous system abnormalities. Rough-bordered, unilateral café-au-lait spots or skeletal abnormalities suggest McCune-Albright syndrome. Document the presence or absence of the adrenal aspects of puberty (acne, pubic hair). Their absence implies that estrogen excess produces the pubertal changes. Virilization or heterosexual precocity without signs of estrogen effect (breast development or lightening of the color of the vaginal mucosa) suggests an excess of circulating testosterone or adrenal androgens. Perform a careful abdominal, rectal-abdominal, or vaginal-abdominal examination (depending on the age of the patient) to rule out an ovarian mass or uterine enlargement. Consider an abdominal ultrasound in place of rectal-abdominal or vaginal-abdominal examinations.

C. Premature thelarche (early breast development) has normal or slight elevations in circulating gonadotropins or estrogen and is an innocent nonpathologic finding. Premature adrenarche (the early development of pubic or axillary hair without other signs of virilization such as clitoral enlargement or facial hair) has normal or slight elevations in circulating androgens. It is also an innocent nonpathologic finding. Follow these patients at regular intervals to monitor their growth rate and the progress of pubertal development.

D. Measure serum FSH/LH and estradiol in girls with isosexual precocity. In pseudoprecocity, hormones are secreted without gonadotropin stimulation. The presence of elevated gonadotropins is necessary for the diagnosis of central (true) precocity. Elevation of serum estradiol without concomitant elevation of gonadotropin (pseudoprecocity) suggests an autonomous source of estrogen secretion (functioning ovarian tumor).

E. Excessive or abnormal changes or virilization in the female (pubic/axillary or facial hair, acne, clitoromegaly) warrants the measurement of testosterone and of adrenal androgens as estimated by a 24-hour urinary ketosteroids test or by direct measurement of dehydroepiandrosterone (DHEA) and androstenedione in the serum.

F. Low serum testosterone concentration in the absence of elevated FSH and LH suggests the abnormal secretion of other androgens, most commonly those of adrenal origin. Measure the urinary excretion products of androgens (17–ketosteroids) or the hormones directly (17-hydroxyprogesterone, androstenedione, DHEA).

G. In patients with congenital adrenal hyperplasia and Cushing's disease, dexamethasone will suppress endogenous production of cortisol by inhibiting ACTH secretion. In patients whose virilization results from autonomously functioning adrenal tissue (an adrenal tumor or an ACTH-producing tumor), a dose of dexamethasone will not suppress cortisol secretion.

H. In a virilized female who has elevated serum testosterone concentration, abdominal ultrasonography is necessary to help rule out ovarian neoplasms such as arrhenoblastomas. If ultrasonography is abnormal, a laparoscopy or laporotomy is indicated for both diagnostic and therapeutic purposes.

REFERENCES

Hung W, August GP, Glasgow AM. Pediatric Endocrinology. New York: Medical Exam Publ, 1983.

Lee PA. Normal ages of pubertal events among American males and females. J Adolescent Health Care 1980; 1:26.

Parks JS. Endocrine disorders of childhood. Hosp Pract 1977; 12:93.

Rosenfeld RG. Evaluation of growth and maturation in adolescence. Pediatr Rev 1982; 4:175.

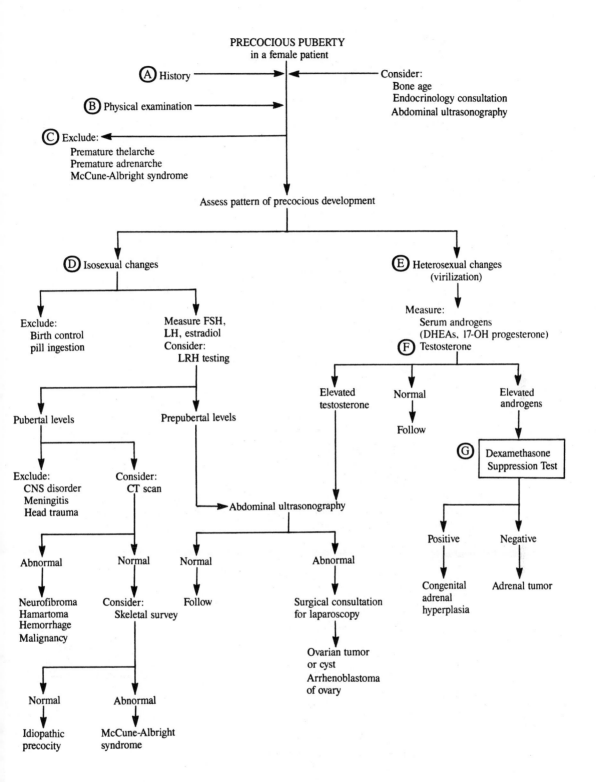

PRECOCIOUS PUBERTY
in a female patient

Ⓐ History

Ⓑ Physical examination

Consider:
　Bone age
　Endocrinology consultation
　Abdominal ultrasonography

Ⓒ Exclude:
　Premature thelarche
　Premature adrenarche
　McCune-Albright syndrome

Assess pattern of precocious development

Ⓓ Isosexual changes

Ⓔ Heterosexual changes
(virilization)

Exclude:
　Birth control
　pill ingestion

Measure FSH,
LH, estradiol
Consider:
　LRH testing

Measure:
　Serum androgens
　(DHEAs, 17-OH progesterone)
Ⓕ Testosterone

Pubertal levels

Prepubertal levels

Elevated
testosterone

Normal

Follow

Elevated
androgens

Exclude:
　CNS disorder
　Meningitis
　Head trauma

Consider:
　CT scan

Abdominal ultrasonography

Ⓖ Dexamethasone
Suppression Test

Abnormal

Normal

Normal

Abnormal

Positive

Negative

Neurofibroma
Hamartoma
Hemorrhage
Malignancy

Consider:
　Skeletal survey

Follow

Surgical consultation
for laparoscopy

Congenital
adrenal
hyperplasia

Adrenal tumor

Normal

Abnormal

Ovarian tumor
or cyst
Arrhenoblastoma
of ovary

Idiopathic
precocity

McCune-Albright
syndrome

HYPERGLYCEMIA

Michael S. Kappy, M.D., Ph.D.

A. Note symptoms that suggest diabetes, such as polyuria, polydipsia, and weight loss. Identify predisposing conditions or factors such as known diabetes mellitus, steroid medications, recent head injury, and excessive oral or IV glucose administration. This is especially pertinent in premature infants, whose ability to metabolize an infused glucose load is less than that of full-term infants or older children. In patients with insulin dependent diabetes note symptoms of infection.

B. Assess vital signs, circulatory status, and hydration. Note alterations in mental status and abnormal or focal neurologic signs. Assess growth and development.

C. The management of diabetic ketoacidosis includes the correction of dehydration, restoration of adequate circulation and renal function, replacement of electrolyte losses (potassium and phosphorus), correction of metabolic acidosis, lowering of hyperglycemia without causing hypoglycemia or cerebral edema, and stopping ketogenesis. Initiate therapy during the first hour with 20 cc/kg of normal saline or Ringer's lactate solution. When the initial venous pH is less than 7.0 or the patient experiences cardiac or pulmonary depression resulting from acidosis, consider giving 2 to 3 mEq of bicarbonate per kg as a 1:6 dilution during the first 2 hours of IV therapy. Discontinue bicarbonate after the venous pH is more than 7.1. Begin an IV insulin infusion with an IV push of 0.1 units/kg of regular insulin (maximum 2–3 units) followed by 0.1 units/kg/hour (maximum 3 units/hr). Monitor blood glucose concentrations hourly. The blood glucose concentration should fall approximately 75 mg/dl/hr. Add 5% glucose to the IV fluids when the plasma glucose reaches 250 to 300 mg/dl to prevent hypoglycemia. Intravenous fluid should include a potassium concentration of 40 mEq/L. This is given as 20 mEq of KCl and 20 mEq of potassium phosphate per liter. When the venous plasma CO_2 content or calculated bicarbonate is more than 15 mEq/L, consider beginning subcutaneous regular insulin 0.2 to 0.25 units/kg/dose. repeat the dose every 4 to 6 hours as determined by monitoring the blood glucose with Chemstrips.

D. Nonketotic hyperosmolar syndrome occurs when changes in sensorium are associated with blood sugar greater than 800 mg/dl in the absence of significant metabolic acidosis. Hospitalize the patient and begin a regular insulin infusion 0.1 units/kg/hr to slowly lower blood sugar. Replace calculated fluid deficits slowly over 36 to 48 hours to prevent cerebral edema. Monitor the blood sugar closely with hourly determinations.

E. Institute insulin therapy for a new diabetic as an outpatient when ketoacidosis is not present. Use a short-acting (regular) insulin 0.2 to 0.25 units/kg given every 6 hours for 2 or 3 days to determine the child's insulin requirements. Have the patient or parents monitor the blood glucose concentration with a reagent strip such as Chemstrip which can be read directly or with an electronic metering device. Adjust the insulin dose on the basis of these blood measurements. After determining the child's insulin requirements, give approximately three-quarters of the total dose as intermediate-acting insulin (NPH) and supplement with short-acting (regular) insulin as necessary. In addition to insulin therapy, implement a complete educational program covering diet, exercise, the techniques of glucose monitoring, insulin administration, and a review of the complications of diabetes.

REFERENCES

Costells S. Juvenile diabetes. Pediatr Clin North Am 1984; 31.
Olefsky J. Insulin resistance and insulin action. Diabetes 1981; 30:148.

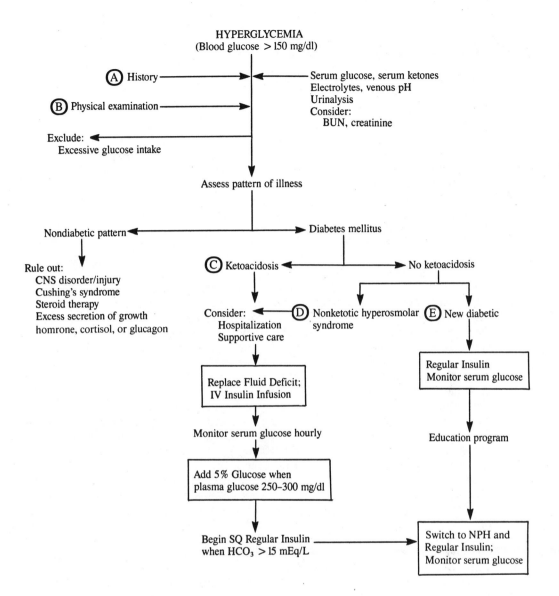

HYPERGLYCEMIA
(Blood glucose > 150 mg/dl)

(A) History

(B) Physical examination

Serum glucose, serum ketones
Electrolytes, venous pH
Urinalysis
Consider:
    BUN, creatinine

Exclude:
    Excessive glucose intake

Assess pattern of illness

Nondiabetic pattern

Diabetes mellitus

Rule out:
    CNS disorder/injury
    Cushing's syndrome
    Steroid therapy
    Excess secretion of growth
    homrone, cortisol, or glucagon

(C) Ketoacidosis

No ketoacidosis

Consider:
Hospitalization
Supportive care

(D) Nonketotic hyperosmolar
    syndrome

(E) New diabetic

Replace Fluid Deficit;
IV Insulin Infusion

Regular Insulin
Monitor serum glucose

Monitor serum glucose hourly

Add 5% Glucose when
plasma glucose 250–300 mg/dl

Education program

Begin SQ Regular Insulin
when HCO₃ > 15 mEq/L

Switch to NPH and
Regular Insulin;
Monitor serum glucose

HYPOGLYCEMIA

Michael S. Kappy, M.D., Ph.D.

A. Note symptoms of hypoglycemia such as pallor, sweating, dizziness, tachycardia, tremor, altered mental status, and seizures. Assess the pattern of symptoms and their relationship to meals or specific foods. Note episodes of febrile illness. Identify precipitating factors or predisposing conditions such as drug or toxin ingestion (aspirin or ethanol) and insulin use (diabetes mellitus). Note any family history of hypoglycemia, especially in the newborn period.

B. Assess the vital signs and neurologic status (mental status, weakness, and seizures). Note pallor, tachycardia, tachypnea, and increased sweating. Consider galactosemia, liver failure, glycogen storage disease, or α-1-antitrypsin when jaundice and/or hepatomegaly are present. Cataracts suggest galactosemia. Congenital adrenal hyperplasia in the female presents with ambiguous genitalia. Micropenis in the hypoglycemic male newborn suggests panhypopituitarism since gonadotropin secretion is necessary for normal phallic size at birth. Darkening of the skin, especially in fold creases, is present with Addison's disease.

C. Functional fasting (ketotic) hypoglycemia, the most common form of hypoglycemia, usually occurs in children between 1 and 5 years of age during periods of decreased food intake (e.g., during acute febrile illnesses). When glucose production is inadequate, the breakdown of fat stores for energy causes the excretion of ketones in the urine. Ketonuria usually precedes hypoglycemia; therefore, the parents can test the child's urine for ketones at home, especially during an illness, and help prevent hypoglycemia by instituting frequent small feedings of foods containing carbohydrate if ketonemia is present.

D. Treat acute hypoglycemia with 2 to 4 ml of 25% glucose per kg (0.5–1.0 g/kg), followed by a glucose infusion of 6 to 8 mg/kg/min as a 10–15% glucose solution. Except in cases of endogenous insulin excess, it is rarely necessary to use rates of glucose administration >10 mg/kg/min. Consider a dose of glucagon 0.03 mg/kg IV (a maximum of 1 mg). Prolonged difficulty in maintaining normal blood glucose concentrations may be alleviated by giving hydrocortisone 10 mg/kg IV followed by the same daily dosage in 3 or 4 divided oral doses if necessary.

E. The diagnosis of hyperinsulinism depends on documenting an inappropriately high insulin level (insulin:glucose ratio during hypoglycemia >0.4) for the observed blood glucose concentration. Consider medical therapy with diazoxide prior to subtotal or total pancreatectomy.

F. The ACTH test assesses adrenal cortex function. Low serum cortisol before and after stimulation suggest primary adrenal insufficiency; high serum cortisol suggests that the patient has a deficiency in pituitary secretion of ACTH.

G. In the fasting state, normal blood glucose levels are maintained initially by the breakdown of glycogen and subsequently by the synthesis of glucose from protein (gluconeogenesis). There are at least 4 major types of glycogen breakdown disorders (glycogen storage diseases) with many subtypes now being described. Many present with hepatomegaly and failure to thrive. Disorders of gluconeogenesis (fructal 1,6 diphosphate deficiency, galactosemia, fructose intolerance) are associated with absent, defective, or blocked enzymes.

REFERENCES

Cornblath M, Schwartz R. Disorders of Carbohydrate Metabolism in Infancy. Philadelphia: WB Saunders, 1976.
Fisher GW et al. Neonatal islet cell adenoma. Pediatrics 1974; 3:75.
Sexson WR. Incidence of neonatal hypoglycemia: a matter of definition. J Pediatr 1984; 105:149.

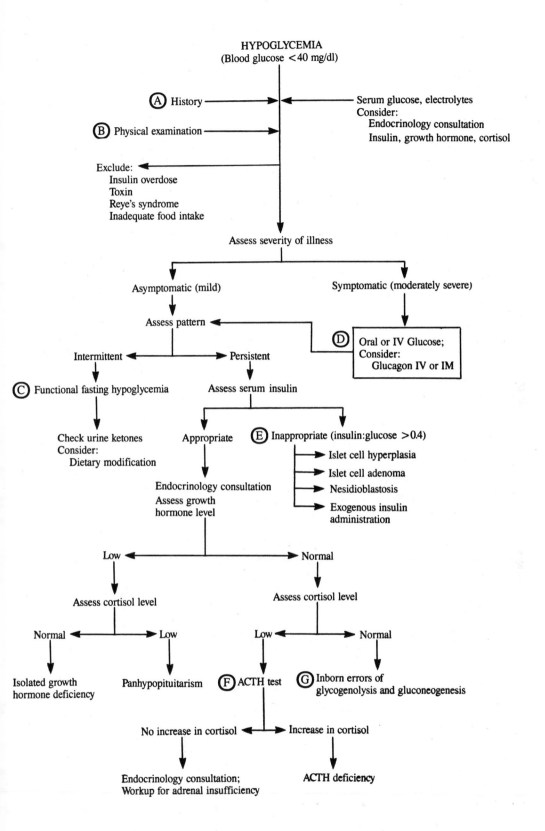

HYPOGLYCEMIA
(Blood glucose <40 mg/dl)

Ⓐ History

Ⓑ Physical examination

Serum glucose, electrolytes
Consider:
    Endocrinology consultation
    Insulin, growth hormone, cortisol

Exclude:
    Insulin overdose
    Toxin
    Reye's syndrome
    Inadequate food intake

Assess severity of illness

Asymptomatic (mild)

Symptomatic (moderately severe)

Assess pattern

Ⓓ Oral or IV Glucose;
Consider:
    Glucagon IV or IM

Intermittent

Persistent

Ⓒ Functional fasting hypoglycemia

Assess serum insulin

Check urine ketones
Consider:
    Dietary modification

Appropriate

Ⓔ Inappropriate (insulin:glucose >0.4)

Islet cell hyperplasia

Islet cell adenoma

Nesidioblastosis

Exogenous insulin
administration

Endocrinology consultation
Assess growth
hormone level

Low

Normal

Assess cortisol level

Assess cortisol level

Normal

Low

Low

Normal

Isolated growth
hormone deficiency

Panhypopituitarism

Ⓕ ACTH test

Ⓖ Inborn errors of
glycogenolysis and gluconeogenesis

No increase in cortisol

Increase in cortisol

Endocrinology consultation;
Workup for adrenal insufficiency

ACTH deficiency

HYPERKALEMIA

Michael S. Kappy, M.D., Ph.D.

A. Note symptoms of hyperkalemia such as anorexia, nausea, vomiting, and weakness. Identify predisposing factors such as renal disease, metabolic acidosis (diabetic ketoacidosis or aspirin intoxication), acute hemolysis, or acute rhabdomyolysis. Consider excessive intravenous administration of potassium in patients receiving intravenous fluids.

B. Note vital signs, and assess the circulatory status (skin color, capillary refill). Suspect congenital adrenal hyperplasia in infants with ambiguous genitalia. Addison's disease is associated with a characteristic slate-grey skin color. Note the signs of diabetic ketoacidosis (dehydration, Kussmaul respirations, acetone breath).

C. Electrocardiographic findings in hyperkalemia include peaked T waves which may progress to widening of the QRS complex, decreased P-wave amplitude, and increased P-R interval. Serum potassium concentrations above 8 mEq/L may produce bradycardia, dysrhythmias, and cardiac arrest.

D. Since potassium is the major intracellular cation, any significant cellular damage (acute hemolysis, or acute rhabdomyolysis) may elevate serum potassium levels. Consider the possibility that hemolysis of red blood cells during blood sampling is responsible for a false elevation of serum potassium. Metabolic acidosis elevates serum potassium as a result of displacement of potassium from within the cell by hydrogen ions.

E. When serum potassium levels are more than 7 mEq/L and ECG changes are present, administer: sodium bicarbonate, 1 to 2 mEq/kg IV over 10 to 15 minutes; calcium gluconate, 50 to 100 mg/kg by slow IV drip over 5 to 10 minutes with a maximum single dose of 1 gram; and/or glucose D25, 2 cc/kg with insulin 0.2 units/kg IV over 10 to 15 minutes. Treat less urgent situations with D5 or D10 isotonic solution, 20 cc/kg/hr, and consider Lasix. When adrenal disorders are suspected, give hydrocortisone (Solucortef), 10 mg/kg IV stat, and the same dosage on a daily basis divided into 4 equal doses to be given each 6 hours. At the same time, give DOCA, 1.0 mg IM. In addition, lower potassium with a potassium-binding resin, Kayexalate 1.0 g/kg by rectum as an enema. Serum potassium may be expected to decrease by 0.5 to 2.0 mEq/L with each enema. This may be repeated 2 or 3 times per day. In life-threatening situations, consider peritoneal dialysis and/or hemodialysis.

F. Defects in mineralocorticoid secretion or action may result in excessive sodium excretion and potassium retention. Causes of a deficiency of mineralocorticoid (desoxycorticosterone or aldosterone) include deficiencies in enzymes (20, 22 desmolase, 3 β–OL deH$^+$ase, 21-OHase, 18-OHase). A defect in the 20–22 desmolase enzyme results in an accumulation of cholesterol in the adrenal gland (lipoid hyperplasia) which is usually fatal in early infancy. Defects in 3 β–OL deH$^+$ase and 21-OHase produce adrenal hyperplasia due to the excessive ACTH secretion that accompanies decreased cortisol production. A defect in enzyme 11-OHase decreases aldosterone production but does not result in hyperkalemia since desoxycorticosterone has significant mineralocorticoid effect. Adrenal failure (Addison's disease) caused by adrenal injury or autoantibodies presents with mineralocorticoid and glucocorticoid deficiencies. Additional causes of hyperkalemia include end-organ unresponsiveness to aldosterone and congenital adrenal hypoplasia, a rare embryological deficiency of the adrenal gland.

REFERENCES

Wallach J. Interpretation of Pediatric Tests. Boston: Little, Brown, 1983; 389.
Winters RW. Principles of Pediatric Fluid Therapy. 2nd ed. Boston: Little, Brown, 1982.

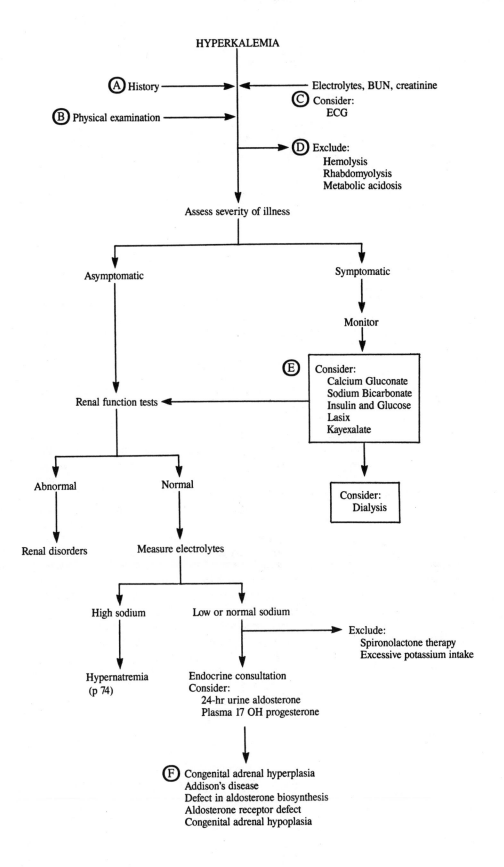

HYPERKALEMIA

(A) History

(B) Physical examination

Electrolytes, BUN, creatinine

(C) Consider:
ECG

(D) Exclude:
Hemolysis
Rhabdomyolysis
Metabolic acidosis

Assess severity of illness

Asymptomatic

Symptomatic

Monitor

(E) Consider:
Calcium Gluconate
Sodium Bicarbonate
Insulin and Glucose
Lasix
Kayexalate

Renal function tests

Consider:
Dialysis

Abnormal

Normal

Renal disorders

Measure electrolytes

High sodium

Low or normal sodium

Exclude:
Spironolactone therapy
Excessive potassium intake

Hypernatremia
(p 74)

Endocrine consultation
Consider:
24-hr urine aldosterone
Plasma 17 OH progesterone

(F) Congenital adrenal hyperplasia
Addison's disease
Defect in aldosterone biosynthesis
Aldosterone receptor defect
Congenital adrenal hypoplasia

HYPOKALEMIA

Michael S. Kappy, M.D., Ph.D.

A. Note symptoms of weakness, lethargy, and vomiting. Identify predisposing factors or conditions such as diuretic therapy, steroid therapy, persistent vomiting (pyloric stenosis), and renal disorders. Treatment of diabetic ketoacidosis may lead to hypokalemia because of bicarbonate therapy and loss of potassium secondary to an osmotic diuresis. An inadequate potassium concentration in IV fluids also produces hypokalemia.

B. Note vital signs, especially blood pressure. The presence of a moon face, purplish striae, and central adiposity suggests Cushing's syndrome or prolonged steroid therapy.

C. ECG findings of hypokalemia include flattened T-waves, depressed ST segments, and a prominent U-wave.

D. When plasma renin activity is suppressed with primary mineralocorticoid excess (adrenal hyperactivity), obtain a 24-hour urine collection and test for aldosterone (serum aldosterone levels fluctuate widely during the day). Clinical conditions characterized by suppressed renin activity without an elevation in daily aldosterone production include inborn errors of metabolism within the adrenal gland such as 11- or 17-hydroxylase deficiency. These inborn errors and Cushing's syndrome result in increased levels of mineralocorticoids and cortisol which are responsible for producing hypokalemia.

E. Plasma renin activity is high in renal disorders. A defect in chloride absorption (Bartter's syndrome) produces a hypokalemic metabolic alkalosis that is associated with a normal serum sodium and blood pressure. Elevated plasma renin activity, hypokalemia, and hypertension are characteristic of renal vascular disease and tumors of the juxtaglomerular cells. The workup for these disorders includes renal scan and digital subtraction angiography.

F. Congenital adrenal hyperplasia due to either 11- or 17-hydroxylase deficiency differs from 21-hydroxylase deficiency in that mineralocorticoid synthesis is not impaired. Treat with glucocorticoid replacement. Boys and girls with this disorder require testosterone or estrogen replacement respectively, during the pubertal and postpubertal periods because the 17-hydroxylase enzyme is necessary for the synthesis of androgen and estrogens.

G. Clinical signs of adrenal excess (Cushing's syndrome) have different etiologies. Bilateral adrenal hyperplasia caused by inappropriate secretion of ACTH by the pituitary is Cushing's disease. Possible treatments of Cushing's disease include pituitary irradiation, transsphenoidal hypophysectomy, and the use of an antipituitary drug (cyproheptadine) or, alternatively, drugs that act on the adrenal gland. Other causes of Cushing's syndrome include excessive ingestion of steroid hormones, ectopic production of ACTH by tumors such as pheochromocytoma, neuroblastoma, islet cell tumors and Wilm's tumors, and tumors of the adrenal gland (carcinomas or adenomas). Consider total adrenalectomy when Cushing's syndrome is caused by an adrenal carcinoma or adenoma or when more conservative treatments are ineffective.

H. Treat Bartter's syndrome with a sodium-wasting/potassium-retaining diuretic such as spironolactone and the supplemental use of potassium and magnesium as their respective chloride salts. This regimen blocks endogenous aldosterone action and restores electrolyte balances in potassium, magnesium, and chloride. Success has been reported recently with the use of a prostaglandin synthesis-inhibitor, indomethacin.

REFERENCES

Bacchus H. Metabolic and Endocrine Emergencies. Baltimore: University Park Press, 1977:131.
Hung W, August GP, Glasgow AM. Pediatric Endocrinology. New York: Medical Exam Publ, 1983:232.

HYPOKALEMIA

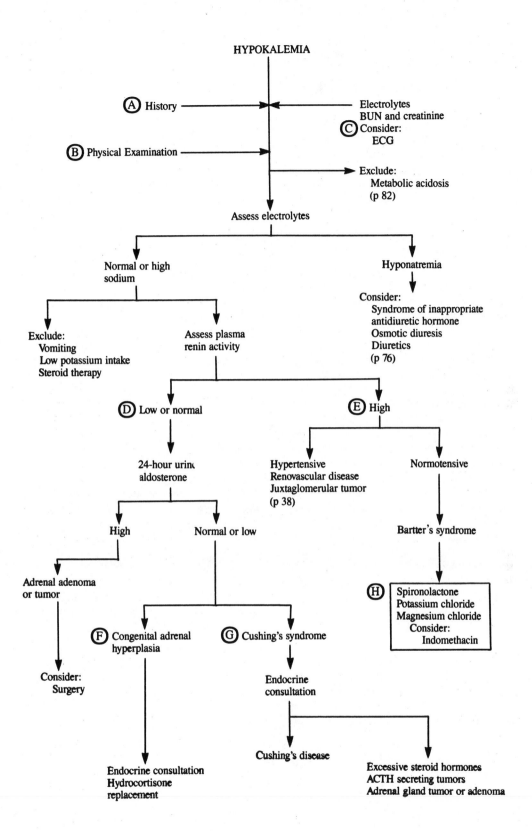

(A) History ← → Electrolytes
BUN and creatinine
(C) Consider:
ECG

(B) Physical Examination →

→ Exclude:
Metabolic acidosis
(p 82)

Assess electrolytes

Normal or high
sodium

Hyponatremia

Consider:
Syndrome of inappropriate
antidiuretic hormone
Osmotic diuresis
Diuretics
(p 76)

Exclude:
Vomiting
Low potassium intake
Steroid therapy

Assess plasma
renin activity

(D) Low or normal

(E) High

24-hour urine
aldosterone

Hypertensive
Renovascular disease
Juxtaglomerular tumor
(p 38)

Normotensive

Bartter's syndrome

High

Normal or low

Adrenal adenoma
or tumor

(H) Spironolactone
Potassium chloride
Magnesium chloride
Consider:
Indomethacin

(F) Congenital adrenal
hyperplasia

(G) Cushing's syndrome

Consider:
Surgery

Endocrine
consultation

Endocrine consultation
Hydrocortisone
replacement

Cushing's disease

Excessive steroid hormones
ACTH secreting tumors
Adrenal gland tumor or adenoma

HYPERNATREMIA

Michael S. Kappy, M.D., Ph.D.

A. Note the presence of polyuria (central or nephrogenic diabetes insipidus). Identify children receiving steroid therapy or excessive sodium in oral or IV fluids. Identify predisposing central nervous system (CNS) disorders such as head injuries, brain tumor, or meningitis.

B. Assess the patient's vital signs and hydration status. Note alterations in mental status and abnormal neurologic signs. Recognize cushingoid features (moon face, purplish striae, and central adiposity).

C. Suspect hypertonic dehydration when patients with gastroenteritis have been managed at home with high-sodium fluids such as boiled skim milk. Treat hypernatremic dehydration by replacing the fluid deficits and lowering the serum sodium at an acceptable rate (0.5 to 1 mEq of sodium per hour). This can be accomplished by administering a ⅔ normal IV solution which contains small amounts of free water to correct fluid deficits without rapidly lowering serum sodium. When dehydration is not significant, administer the fluid deficit replacement together with maintenance fluids over 48 hours as ¼ normal saline with 40 mEq KCl per liter.

D. When the hydration status is normal, exclude a history of excessive sodium intake (salt intoxication). The presence of hypertension suggests the possibility of primary renal disease or a mineralocorticoid excess. The plasma renin activity should be high in primary renal disease (renovascular disorders or juxtaglomerular cell tumors) and low primary mineralocorticoid excess.

E. Hypernatremia associated with a low urine specific gravity or osmolality suggests either an inability to secrete antidiuretic hormone or an impairment of end-organ responsiveness to the hormone. A trial of antidiuretic hormone (ADH) distinguishes a primary deficiency from end-organ unresponsiveness. Patients with central diabetes insipidus (failure of ADH secretion) respond within 20 to 30 minutes to a trial of 0.1 units per kg of aqueous pitressin (maximum of 5 units) IM by decreasing urine output and increasing urine specific gravity. Patients with nephrogenic diabetes insipidus (end-organ insensitivity to ADH) fail to respond to pitressin. Causes of central diabetes insipidus include tumors of the hypothalamus or pituitary, histiocytosis X, trauma, toxins, and infections of the CNS. A sudden appearance of central diabetes insipidus in a patient with underlying CNS pathology is a poor prognostic sign frequently associated with brain death. A familial form of central diabetes insipidus due to an inherited decrease in the number of cells in the supraoptic or paraventricular nuclei in the hypothalamus is a rare cause of diabetes insipidus. Nephrogenic diabetes insipidus is an unusual condition that may be related to the failure of the distal tubular cells to generate cyclic AMP in response to ADH End-organ unresponsiveness may also occur when serum concentrations of potassium or calcium are low.

REFERENCES

Hung W, August GP, Glasgow AM. Pediatric Endocrinology. New York: Medical Exam Publ, 1983.
Levy M. The pathophysiology of sodium balance. Hosp Pract 1978; 13:95.
Winters RW. Principles of Pediatric Fluid Therapy. 2nd ed. Boston: Little, Brown, 1982.

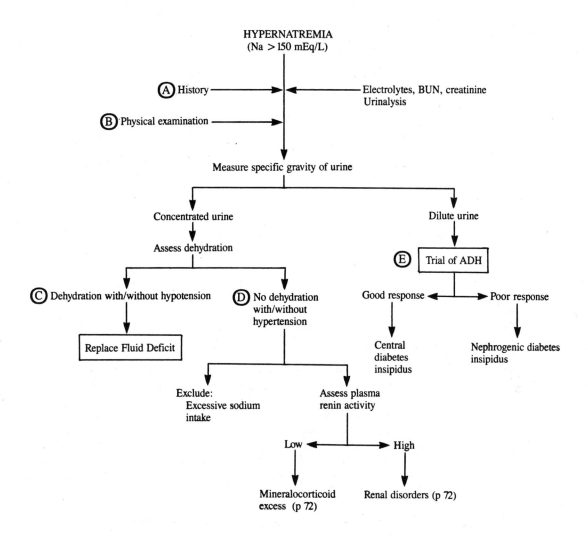

HYPERNATREMIA
(Na > 150 mEq/L)

Ⓐ History

Electrolytes, BUN, creatinine
Urinalysis

Ⓑ Physical examination

Measure specific gravity of urine

Concentrated urine

Assess dehydration

Dilute urine

Ⓔ Trial of ADH

Ⓒ Dehydration with/without hypotension

Ⓓ No dehydration
with/without
hypertension

Good response

Poor response

Replace Fluid Deficit

Central
diabetes
insipidus

Nephrogenic diabetes
insipidus

Exclude:
Excessive sodium
intake

Assess plasma
renin activity

Low

High

Mineralocorticoid
excess (p 72)

Renal disorders (p 72)

HYPONATREMIA
Michael S. Kappy, M.D., Ph.D.

A. Identify predisposing factors such as diabetes mellitus, cystic fibrosis, central nervous system (CNS) disorders, gastroenteritis, excessive water intake, diuretics, renal disease, exposure to heavy metals, pneumonia, and liver disease with ascites.

B. Assess vital signs, circulatory status, and hydration status. Note signs of circulatory overload such as congestive heart failure with pulmonary edema, gallop, and hepatomegaly. Note signs of CNS disorder (altered mental status, abnormal or focal neurologic signs), respiratory distress (pneumonia, cystic fibrosis), liver disease (ascites, hepatomegaly, jaundice, portal hypertension), and renal disease. Suspect the syndrome of inappropriate antidiuretic hormone secretion (SIADH) in well-hydrated patients, especially those with associated CNS pathology.

C. Identify patients whose plasma osmolality is increased due to substances other than sodium. In hyperglycemia, total body sodium may not be decreased since movement of water from intracellular to vascular space causes an osmotic dilution of sodium. In hyperlipidemia, the sodium measurement is falsely low since the volume of lipid reduces the volume of serum in the centrifuged specimen of blood.

D. A low urinary sodium suggests insufficient sodium intake or excessive nonrenal sodium loss. Excessive sodium may be lost in sweat (cystic fibrosis) or from the GI tract (vomiting or diarrhea). Prolonged treatment with clear fluids of low sodium content may produce hyponatremia.

E. When the urine osmolality exceeds the plasma osmolality, suspect SIADH. The hypothalamus produces ADH inappropriately without physiologic cause. Patients with SIADH usually do not appear dehydrated and have a concentrated urine in the face of hyponatremia and lowered plasma osmolality. Consider CNS disorders such as head injury, meningitis, encephalitis, and brain tumor. Bronchopneumonia and chronic liver disease with ascites may also stimulate (appropriate) secretion of ADH because of reduced blood flow to the left atrium and baroreceptor activation. Manage patients with SIADH by restricting the intake of free water. Consider replacing only insensible loss plus urine output. When SIADH results in severe hyponatremia (< 120 mEq/L) with associated seizures, consider using a hypertonic saline infusion and Lasix to quickly increase serum sodium.

F. Diuretics (thiazides and furosemide) inhibit renal tubular reabsorption of sodium and potassium. An important exception is spironolactone, which inhibits aldosterone action on the tubule resulting in a selective loss of sodium with retention of potassium. Osmotic diuresis (hyperglycemia, mannitol, glycerol) also results in excessive urinary losses of sodium and potassium. In hyponatremia secondary to osmotic diuresis or diuretic therapy, the urine osmolality remains less than or equal to that of the serum.

G. In Fanconi's syndrome, multiple transport functions of the tubule are disturbed, including impaired tubular reabsorption of glucose, amino acids, phosphate, bicarbonate, and electrolytes. These disorders may be secondary to tubular injury from exogenous toxic agents (heavy metals, outdated tetracyclines) or from toxic products of metabolic disorders such as cystinosis, tyrosinosis, and fructose intolerance. In chronic renal insufficiency, urinary sodium excretion is high because the kidney fails to reabsorb normal amounts of sodium. In Bartter's syndrome (a primary disorder of chloride transport), the loss of potassium and chloride may be accompanied by hyponatremia during periods of low sodium intake.

REFERENCES

Harrison HE, Harrison HC. Disorders of calcium and potassium metabolism in childhood and adolescence. Philadelphia: WB Saunders, 1979.

Kelsch RC, Oliver WJ. Hyponatremia in children. Pediatr Rev 1980; 2:187.

Levy M. The pathophysiology of sodium balance. Hosp Pract 1978.

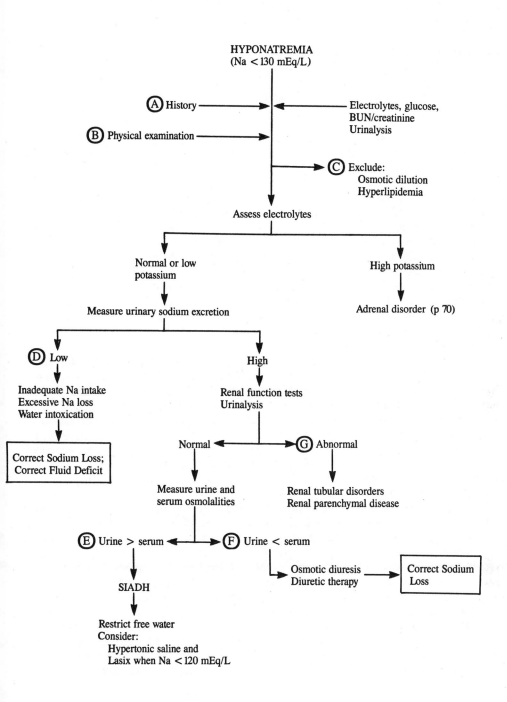

HYPONATREMIA
(Na < 130 mEq/L)

Ⓐ History

Electrolytes, glucose,
BUN/creatinine
Urinalysis

Ⓑ Physical examination

Ⓒ Exclude:
Osmotic dilution
Hyperlipidemia

Assess electrolytes

Normal or low
potassium

High potassium

Measure urinary sodium excretion

Adrenal disorder (p 70)

Ⓓ Low

Inadequate Na intake
Excessive Na loss
Water intoxication

Correct Sodium Loss;
Correct Fluid Deficit

High

Renal function tests
Urinalysis

Normal

Ⓖ Abnormal

Renal tubular disorders
Renal parenchymal disease

Measure urine and
serum osmolalities

Ⓔ Urine > serum

Ⓕ Urine < serum

Osmotic diuresis
Diuretic therapy

Correct Sodium
Loss

SIADH

Restrict free water
Consider:
Hypertonic saline and
Lasix when Na < 120 mEq/L

Wallach J. Interpretation of Pediatric tests. Boston: Little, Brown, 1983.
Winters RW. Principles of Pediatric Fluid Therapy. 2nd ed. Boston: Little, Brown, 1982.

HYPERCALCEMIA

Michael S. Kappy, M.D., Ph.D.

A. Note symptoms such as anorexia, weakness, constipation, polyuria, behavioral changes, and headache. Identify predisposing factors including a history of treated renal disease, hyperparathyroidism, dietary excess of vitamin D or A (fish oil), the use of thiazide diuretics, or immobilization of a major limb.

B. Note the presence of abnormal deep tendon reflexes, bone pain, hypertension, failure to thrive, or developmental delay. A characteristic elf-like face with hypertelorism and large, low set ears, with or without craniostenosis suggests Williams syndrome. Note cardiac findings associated with this syndrome such as supravalvular aortic stenosis or pulmonary artery stenosis.

C. Williams syndrome is characterized by poor feeding, failure to thrive, elfin face, heart defects (e.g., supravalvular aortic stenosis), and hypercalcemia with a normal IPTH level. Hypercalcemia may result from excessive maternal intake of vitamin D or unusual sensitivity to vitamin D; treatment consists of decreasing the intake of vitamin D and calcium. Familial benign hypercalcemia, an autosomal dominant disorder, results in mildly elevated calcium concentrations (12–13 mg/dl with normal IPTH levels). Urinary calcium excretion is low, and treatment is unnecessary.

D. Elevation of immunoreactive parathyroid hormone (IPTH) identifies cases of hyperparathyroidism which are usually due to generalized hyperplasia of the chief cells of the parathyroid glands. Other causes of primary hyperparathyroidism include parathyroid adenoma and two forms of autosomal dominant multiple endocrine neoplasia (MEN). In MEN type I, hyperparathyroidism is associated with a nonfunctioning chromophobe adenoma, insulinoma, and peptic ulceration due to a gastrin-secreting tumor of the pancreas. In MEN type II, hyperparathyroidism is associated with medullary carcinoma of the thyroid, pheochromocytoma, and mucosal neuromas. Hyperparathyroidism may also be associated with renal disease since defective renal excretion of phosphate leads to hypophosphatemia and decreased serum calcium levels. The hypocalcemia stimulates parathormone secretion secondarily so that a normal serum calcium is maintained. This secondary hyperparathyroidism may persist even after the renal disease has been treated by dialysis or transplantation, and hypercalcemia with variable serum phosphorus levels ensues. This autonomous hyperfunctioning of the parathyroid glands has been termed tertiary hyperparathyroidism and is treatable by removal of one or more of the parathyroid glands.

E. Hypercalcemia is seen in a variety of conditions, including sarcoidosis and hyper- and hypothyroidism, and a variety of tumors, in particular, leukemias. Some of these tumors secrete hormones that are immunologically similar to parathormone; in other tumors, prostaglandins or unknown factors are thought to be responsible for the hypercalcemia.

F. When hypercalcemia requires emergency therapy, administer a diuretic (furosemide) with generous amounts of IV normal saline with 40 mEq of potassium chloride per liter. Consider oral phosphorus supplements as well as corticosteroids. In some patients with renal disease, the use of salmon calcitonin with or without peritoneal dialysis may be necessary.

REFERENCES

Harrison HE, Harrison HC. Disorders of calcium and potassium metabolism in childhood and adolescence. Philadelphia: WB Saunders, 1979.

Hung W, August GP, Glasgow AM. Pediatric Endocrinology. New York: Medical Exam Publ, 1983.

Tsang RC, Noguche A, Steichen JJ. Pediatric parathyroid disorders. Pediatr Clin North Am 1979; 26:223.

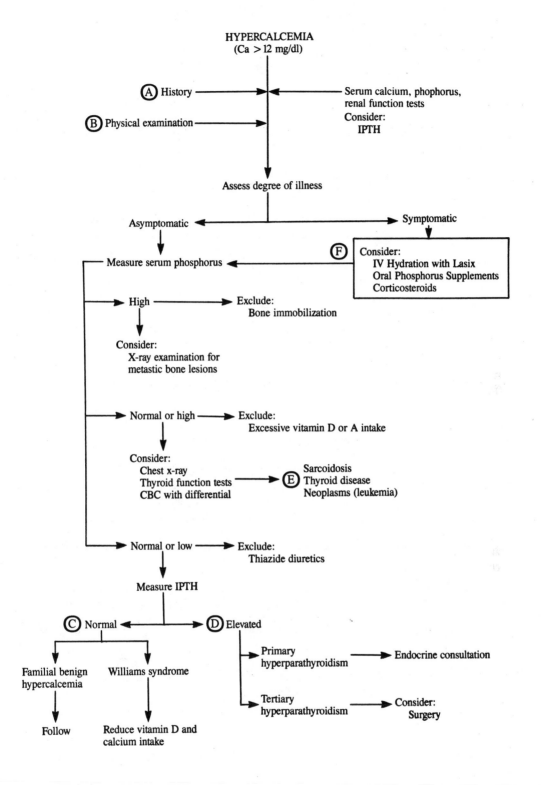

HYPERCALCEMIA
(Ca > 12 mg/dl)

Ⓐ History

Serum calcium, phophorus,
renal function tests
Consider:
  IPTH

Ⓑ Physical examination

Assess degree of illness

Asymptomatic   Symptomatic

Ⓕ Consider:
  IV Hydration with Lasix
  Oral Phosphorus Supplements
  Corticosteroids

Measure serum phosphorus

High ——————→ Exclude:
                 Bone immobilization

Consider:
  X-ray examination for
  metastic bone lesions

Normal or high ——→ Exclude:
                      Excessive vitamin D or A intake

Consider:
  Chest x-ray   Sarcoidosis
  Thyroid function tests ——→ Ⓔ Thyroid disease
  CBC with differential   Neoplasms (leukemia)

Normal or low ——→ Exclude:
                    Thiazide diuretics

Measure IPTH

Ⓒ Normal ←——————→ Ⓓ Elevated

Familial benign   Williams syndrome
hypercalcemia

                                    Primary
                                    hyperparathyroidism ——→ Endocrine consultation

Follow   Reduce vitamin D and
                calcium intake

                                    Tertiary
                                    hyperparathyroidism ——→ Consider:
                                                             Surgery

79

HYPOCALCEMIA
Michael S. Kappy, M.D., Ph.D.

A. Note symptoms such as lethargy, poor feeding, vomiting, diarrhea, photophobia, and tetany. Identify predisposing factors such as thyroid surgery (inadvertent removal of the parathyroid glands), renal disease, liver disease, nutritional deficiencies of calcium or vitamin D, and chronic ingestion of medications (phenytoin, steroids) that interfere with the normal metabolism of vitamin D. Note family history of hypocalcemic disorders.

B. Treat acute hypocalcemia with intravenous administration of 10% calcium gluconate (9 mg of elemental calcium per ml), 1 to 2 ml/kg over 10–15 min *q6h*. Monitor heart rate to identify dysrhythmias that may be produced by the too rapid infusion of calcium. Treat coexisting magnesium deficiencies with magnesium chloride, citrate, or lactate, (elemental magnesium 24–48 mg/kg/day in divided doses) up to a maximum of 1 gram of elemental magnesium per day.

C. When urinary phosphorus is low or normal, consider nutritional deficiencies of calcium and phosphorus (especially common in premature infants) or vitamin D. Nutritional deficiencies may be caused by excessive loss through malabsorption (GI or liver disease). Abnormalities in vitamin D metabolism decrease the formation of active vitamin D (1,25-dihydroxy D3). These conditions are not usually accompanied by severe hypocalcemia since elevated secretion of parathyroid hormone (PTH) tends to keep the serum calcium concentrations from falling. Hypocalcemia may occur if the PTH effect is inadequate, particularly when serum vitamin D concentrations are very low.

D. In patients with high urinary phosphorus excretion, suspect renal tubular diseases such as Fanconi's syndrome, renal tubular acidosis (distal RTA), and x- linked dominant familial hypophosphatemic rickets. In these conditions, hypophosphatemia is the more commonly seen abnormality; however, hypocalcemia may occur as well.

E. A decrease in the amount of parathyroid tissue or diminished secretion of PTH results in a low level of immunoreactive parathyroid hormone (IPTH). Causes of decreased tissue include DiGeorge syndrome (hypoplasia of the parathyroid glands, absence of the thymus, and coarctation of the aorta) and removal of parathyroid tissue during thyroid surgery. Decreased secretion related to autoimmune parathyroid insufficiency is produced either alone or as part of an autoimmune polyendocrinopathy (thyroid, adrenal, pernicious anemia, moniliasis, vitiligo, and insulin-dependent diabetes mellitus).

F. Increased secretion of PTH occurs as a result of end-organ unresponsiveness to the hormone. In pseudohypoparathyroidism, unresponsiveness is related to disorders beyond the PTH receptors in the bone and/or kidney. Additional causes of unresponsiveness to PTH include hypomagnesemia, hypernatremia, hypokalemia, and infections.

G. Renal parenchaymal disease reduces excretion of phosphorus. Elevated serum phosphorus levels lower serum calcium by forming insoluble calcium phosphate salts that are then deposited in various tissues including the kidney. The low serum calcium may be partially corrected by increased levels of PTH. Another cause for hypocalcemia is the relative inability of an abnormal kidney to convert vitamin D3 to its active metabolite 1,25-dihydroxy D3. The rate-limiting enzyme is deficient in the failing kidney and may result in a deficiency in active vitamin D and hypocalcemia despite secondary hyperparathyroidism.

REFERENCES

Cholst IN et al. The influence of hypermagnesemia on serum calcium and PTH levels in human subjects. N Engl J Med 1984; 310:1221.

Donckerwolcke RA. Diagnosis and treatment of renal tubular disorders in children. Pediatr Clin North Am 1982; 29:895.

Harrison HE, Harrison HC. Disorders of calcium and potassium metabolism in childhood and adolescence. Philadelphia: WB Saunders, 1979.

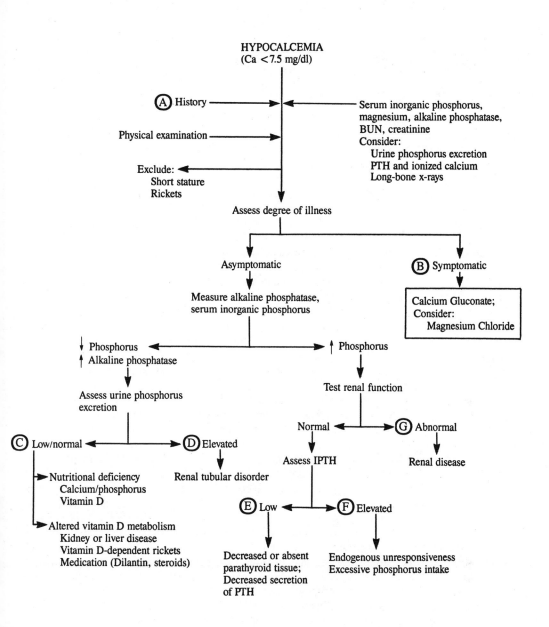

HYPOCALCEMIA
(Ca <7.5 mg/dl)

Ⓐ History — Serum inorganic phosphorus, magnesium, alkaline phosphatase, BUN, creatinine

Physical examination

Consider:
  Urine phosphorus excretion
  PTH and ionized calcium
  Long-bone x-rays

Exclude:
  Short stature
  Rickets

Assess degree of illness

Asymptomatic

Ⓑ Symptomatic

Measure alkaline phosphatase, serum inorganic phosphorus

Calcium Gluconate;
Consider:
  Magnesium Chloride

↓ Phosphorus
↑ Alkaline phosphatase

↑ Phosphorus

Assess urine phosphorus excretion

Test renal function

Normal

Ⓖ Abnormal

Ⓒ Low/normal

Ⓓ Elevated

Assess IPTH

Renal disease

Nutritional deficiency
  Calcium/phosphorus
  Vitamin D

Renal tubular disorder

Ⓔ Low

Ⓕ Elevated

Altered vitamin D metabolism
  Kidney or liver disease
  Vitamin D-dependent rickets
  Medication (Dilantin, steroids)

Decreased or absent
parathyroid tissue;
Decreased secretion
of PTH

Endogenous unresponsiveness
Excessive phosphorus intake

Rienhoff HY. Pseudohypoparathyroidism. Johns Hopkins Med J 1982; 151:137.
Tsang RC, Noguchi A, Steichen JJ. Pediatric parathyroid disorders. Pediatr Clin North Am 1979; 26:223.

METABOLIC ACIDOSIS
Michael S. Kappy, M.D., Ph.D.

A. Metabolic acidosis results in a decrease in the buffering capacity (sodium bicarbonate) of the blood; this decrease is produced either by an abnormal increase in circulating acid (endogenous or exogenous) or by loss of bicarbonate from the gastrointestinal tract or kidneys. The kidneys are the major site for the regulation of buffer capacity. The lungs also alter pH by determining the clearance of carbon dioxide, an end product of normal metabolism. Acidosis associated with the diminished clearance of carbon dioxide from the lungs is called respiratory acidosis.

B. Note the presence of vomiting, diarrhea, failure to thrive, polyuria, fever, or altered neurologic status (seizures). Identify predisposing factors such as renal disease, diabetes mellitus, diarrhea and vomiting, hypothermia, toxin ingestion, known hypoglycemic syndrome, or inborn errors of metabolism. Ask about family history of neonatal death or metabolic disorders.

C. Note the patient's vital signs; assess the circulatory status. Note signs consistent with respiratory distress, sepsis, or a CNS disorder.

D. Calculate the anion gap by determining the difference between the serum sodium concentration and the sum of the serum chloride and bicarbonate concentration. Since the sums of all serum anions and cations are equal because of the electroneutrality of the body, the anion gap represents the difference between the unmeasured serum anions (anions except chloride and bicarbonate) and unmeasured serum cations (cations except sodium). The normal value is usually 12 mEq/L ± 4.

E. Hypoglycemia, positive urinary ketones, and an elevated anion gap suggest a disorder of glycogenolysis or gluconeogenesis. Excessive ketone production is due to the utilization of fat stores to provide energy in the absence of glucose. Type 1 of glycogen storage disease produce elevated lactic and uric acid levels that contribute to the metabolic acidosis. Premature infants may develop metabolic acidosis when they receive an acid load that exceeds the renal capacity (excessive phosphate or protein from cow's milk).

F. Inborn errors of metabolism that can produce a lactic acidosis include deficiencies in pyruvate dehydrogenase enzyme complex and enzyme defects between pyruvate and phosphylenol pyruvate. Lactic acidosis may also be a nonspecific finding related to long periods of hypoxia.

G. Abnormal renal function produces metabolic acidosis because of impaired acid excretion and/or inability to retain sodium bicarbonate. Renal tubular disease results in acidosis due to the failure to reabsorb sodium bicarbonate in normal amounts. Renal tubular disorders include Fanconi's syndrome and proximal and distal renal tubular acidoses. In proximal renal tubular acidosis there is a lowered threshold for the reabsorption of bicarbonate; patients can acidify their urine only when plasma bicarbonate falls below the renal threshold (approximately 15 mEq/L). While the exact mode of inheritance is unknown, it appears to have a genetic component. In distal renal tubular acidosis, the kidney is unable to excrete an acid urine at any plasma bicarbonate concentration. Impaired distal tubular hydrogen ion excretion results in excessive urinary loss of both potassium and phosphorus. This leads to hypokalemic acidosis. Distal renal tubular acidosis also may result in mild to moderate antidiuretic hormone unresponsiveness at the renal tubule; the subsequent polyuria accentuates both hypokalemia and hypophosphatemia.

REFERENCES

Kappy MS, Morrow G. A diagnostic approach to metabolic acidosis in children. Pediatrics 1980; 65:351.
Winters RW. Principles of Pediatric Fluid Therapy. 2nd ed. Boston: Little, Brown, 1982.

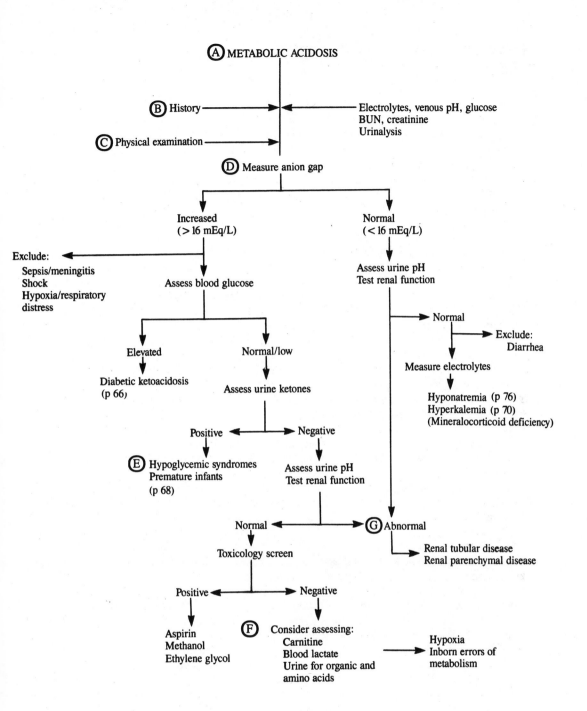

Ⓐ METABOLIC ACIDOSIS

Ⓑ History ———————→ ┃ ←——————— Electrolytes, venous pH, glucose
                    ┃   BUN, creatinine
Ⓒ Physical examination ———→ ┃   Urinalysis

Ⓓ Measure anion gap

Increased   Normal
(> 16 mEq/L)   (< 16 mEq/L)

Exclude: ←   Assess urine pH
  Sepsis/meningitis   Test renal function
  Shock
  Hypoxia/respiratory
  distress
                                                      Normal
          Assess blood glucose
                                                           → Exclude:
                                                              Diarrhea
                                          Measure electrolytes
  Elevated   Normal/low
                                          Hyponatremia (p 76)
Diabetic ketoacidosis Assess urine ketones   Hyperkalemia (p 70)
(p 66)   (Mineralocorticoid deficiency)

            Positive ←   → Negative

Ⓔ Hypoglycemic syndromes   Assess urine pH
  Premature infants   Test renal function
  (p 68)

                Normal ←   → Ⓖ Abnormal

              Toxicology screen   Renal tubular disease
                                             Renal parenchymal disease
     Positive ←   → Negative

Aspirin   Ⓕ Consider assessing: Hypoxia
Methanol   Carnitine   → Inborn errors of
Ethylene glycol   Blood lactate   metabolism
                        Urine for organic and
                        amino acids

VULVOVAGINITIS

A. Note the onset, duration, quantity, color, and odor of the vaginal discharge. Identify associated symptoms such as abdominal pain, pruritis, dysuria, and fever. Identify precipitating factors such as poor perinanal hygiene (wiping from back to front), trauma, masturbation, recent antibiotics, possible foreign body, bubble baths, harsh soaps, and nylon tights. In the preadolescent, explore the possibility of sexual abuse. In the adolescent, determine sexual activity and menstrual history.

B. Inspect the external genitalia for redness or excoriation of labia majora, labia minora, clitoris, and introitus. Note any signs of trauma (bruising, hematoma, tear). Examine the prepubertal child in the knee-chest position in order to best visualize the vagina and cervix. In the adolescent, perform an appropriate pelvic examination which includes a speculum examination of the vagina, a bimanual rectovaginal abdominal palpation and a wet prep, Gram stain, and GC culture of cervical discharge. In the prepubertal child, obtain specimens with a moistened (nonbacteriostatic saline) cotton-tipped applicator. Culture the specimens on Thayer-Martin agar, blood agar, MacConkey agar, and chocolate agar. Inflammation of the vulva with fissures or excoriations suggests a monilial infection. Herpes simplex infections cause a vesicular eruption. Note the presence of cervical erosion, ectropion, or discharge. The presence of adnexal tenderness suggests pelvic inflammatory disease/salpingitis. When *Candida* is suspected, consider a fungal culture. When vulvar or anal pruritis is present in a prepubertal child, consider a morning scotch tape specimen to identify pin worms.

C. Trichomonas infections are identified when flagellated, motile organisms are seen on wet prep. Budding hypha seen with a KOH prep indicates monilia infection. Clue cells or epithelial cells coated with refractile bacteria on wet prep are consistent with Gardinella (H. vaginalis) infections. Sheets of epithelial cells seen on wet prep indicate leukorrhea which is a normal variant. The presence of > 10 polymorphonuclear cells per hpF in the discharge of a sexually active adolescent suggests gonorrhea and/or chlamydia.

D. Most cases of prepubertal vulvovaginitis are related to poor perianal hygiene. Normal vaginal flora include *E. coli, S. epidermidis, alpha streptococci,* and *lactobacillus*. Manage cases with nonspecific vaginitis with sitz baths and improved perianal hygiene (cotton underpants, front to back wiping, avoid nylon tights and tight fitting pants). Consider a trial of zinc oxide cream *tid* before topical antibiotic creams such as sultrin, vagitrol, and AVC cream. Failure to respond is an indication for an oral antibiotic such as ampicillin or a cephalosporin.

E. Recommended antibiotic therapy for gonorrheal disease includes the following possibilities: procaine penicillin G 4.8 million units IM plus 1 g oral probenecid; ampicillin 3.5 g orally (amoxicillin 3.0 g) plus 1 gram oral probenecid PO; and tetracycline 500 mg orally 4 times a day for 5 days in adolescents. Treat *Chlamydia* with tetracycline 500 mg *qid* for 10 days or oral erythromycin 500 mg *aid* for 10 days.

F. Treat cases of *Trichomonas vaginalis* with metronidazole (Flagyl 1.5 or 2 grams PO in a single dose). Infection with *Candida* is infrequent in the prepubertal child. When present, it is usually associated with recent antibiotic therapy or diabetes mellitus. Treat cases of *Candida vaginalis* with nystatin suppositories 1 twice a day for 14 days, or myconazole 2% (Monostat) or clotrimazole 1% (Gyne Lotrimin) creams at night for 7 days. Consider the use of 1% hydrocortisone cream if inflammation is severe. Treat infections with *H. vaginalis* (*Gardinella vaginalis*) with oral ampicillin 500 mg 4 times a day for 10 days or metronidazole 250 mg *bid* for 7 days (not approved yet for this indication).

G. When a sexually transmitted agent is identified, perform a thorough evaluation for possible sexual abuse. All contacts (extended family, babysitter, parents) should be interviewed. The patient should have repeated interviews, with trained personnel utilizing play therapy when appropriate. Consider hospitalization in order to carry out the evaluation.

VULVOVAGINITIS

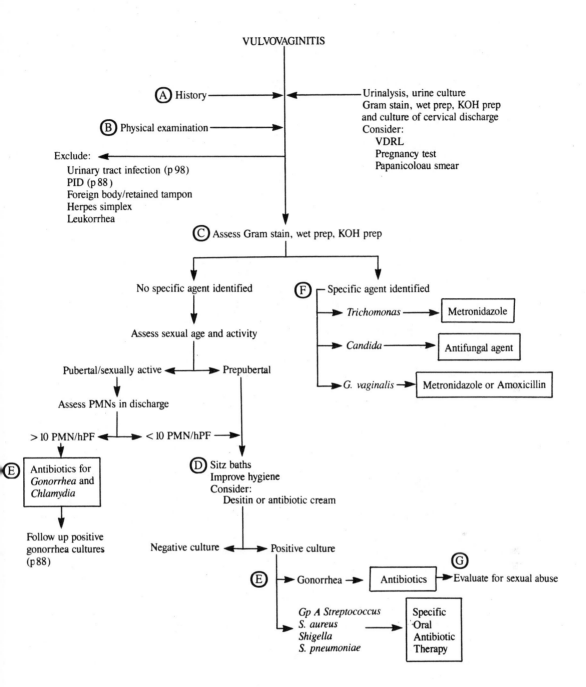

REFERENCES

Brunham RC, Paavonen J, Steven CE, et al. Mucopurulent cervicitis: the ignored counter-part in women of urethritis in men. N Engl J Med 1984; 311:1.

Emans SJ. Vulvovaginitis in children and adolescents. Pediatr Rev 1981; 2:319.

Paradise JE, Campos JM, et al. Vulvovaginitis in premenarcheal girls: clinical features and diagnostic evaluation. Pediatrics 1982; 70:193.

Treatment of sexually transmitted disease. Medical Letter 1984; 26:5.

PELVIC PAIN IN THE ADOLESCENT FEMALE

A. Determine the onset, frequency, severity, pattern, and location of pain. Note associated symptoms such as fever, nausea, vomiting, rash, jaundice, arthritis, organomegaly, change in bowel pattern, and weight loss. Inquire as to symptoms of urinary tract infection such as dysuria, urgency, or frequency and gynecologic symptoms such as dysmenorrhea and vaginal discharge. Document the timing and duration of the last menstrual period, recent sexual relations, possible exposure to venereal disease, or a history of prior abdominal surgery. Obtain a psychosocial history to identify presence of stress in the patient's life and level of anxiety (family and school) (p 191).

B. Perform an appropriate pelvic examination which includes a speculum examination of the vagina, a bimanual rectovaginal abdominal palpation and a wet prep, Gram stain, and GC culture of cervical discharge. Consider any discharge other than a normal thin, clear to partially opaque fluid as abnormal and indicative of infection. The presence of adnexal tenderness with or without a cervical discharge suggests pelvic inflammatory disease, salpingitis, or tubal pregnancy.

C. Dysmenorrhea results from prostaglandin F_2 alpha and E_2 activity on the myometrium. Treat with ibuprofen (Motrin) 200–400 mg every 4–6 hours or naproxen sodium, 550 mg orally at the start of menses, followed by 275 mg every 6–8 hours for the first day. Consider adding a combination oral contraceptive if pain persists despite prostaglandin inhibitor therapy. Failure of the pain to respond to therapy requires a gynecology consultation for laparoscopy to rule out pelvic pathology such as endometriosis.

REFERENCES

Barr RG. Abdominal pain in the female adolescent. Pediatr Rev 1983; 4:281.

Emans SJ. Pelvic examination of the adolescent patient. Pediatr Rev 1983; 4:307.

Emans SJ, Goldstein DP. Pediatric and adolescent gynecology. 2nd ed. Boston: Little, Brown, 1982.

Goldstein DP, de Cholnoky C, Emans SJ, et al. Laparoscopy in the diagnosis and management of pelvic pain in adolescents. J Reprod Med 1980; 24:251.

Litt IF. Menstrual problems during adolescence. Pediatr Rev 1983; 4:203.

PELVIC PAIN IN THE ADOLESCENT FEMALE

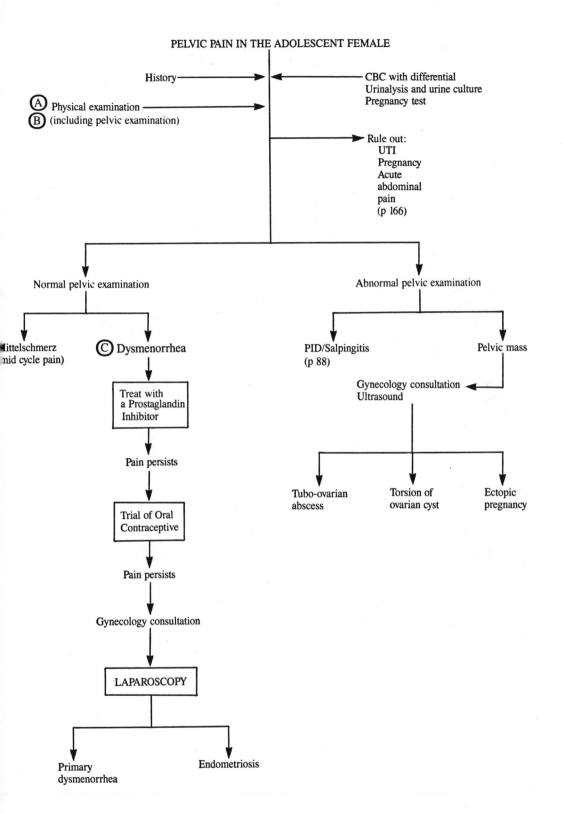

History

CBC with differential
Urinalysis and urine culture
Pregnancy test

Ⓐ Physical examination
Ⓑ (including pelvic examination)

Rule out:
UTI
Pregnancy
Acute
abdominal
pain
(p 166)

Normal pelvic examination

Abnormal pelvic examination

Mittelschmerz
(mid cycle pain)

Ⓒ Dysmenorrhea

PID/Salpingitis
(p 88)

Pelvic mass

Treat with
a Prostaglandin
Inhibitor

Gynecology consultation
Ultrasound

Pain persists

Trial of Oral
Contraceptive

Tubo-ovarian
abscess

Torsion of
ovarian cyst

Ectopic
pregnancy

Pain persists

Gynecology consultation

LAPAROSCOPY

Primary
dysmenorrhea

Endometriosis

PELVIC INFLAMMATORY DISEASE

A. Hospitalize moderate or severely ill adolescents who present with fever, pain which interferes with normal walking, or marked pain on abdominal palpation. Adequate follow-up of adolescents with PID is necessary to assess response to therapy, to identify persistent cases, and to reduce sequelae; however, a study has shown that approximately ⅔ of adolescents with PID fail to return for follow-up appointments.

B. Pathogens which can cause PID include gonorrhea, *Chlamydia*, urea plasma/urealyticum, mycoplasma hominis, gram-negative bacilli, and anaerobic bacteria. Recommended outpatient therapy includes coverage for both chlamydia and gonorrhea. Oral tetracycline 500 mg *qid* for 10 days or erythromycin 500 mg *qid* for 15 days will treat both. An alternative is to use tetracycline or trimethoprim/sulfamethoxazole (9 tablets as a single dose for 3 days) plus recommended therapy for gonorrheal disease. Possibilities include: procaine penicillin G, 4.8 million units IM plus probenecid, 1 g orally; ampicillin, 3.5 g orally (amoxicillin 3 g), plus probenecid, 1 g orally; tetracycline, 500 mg orally *qid* for 5 days; or cefoxitin, 2 g IM, plus probenecid, 1 g orally followed by doxycycline 100 mg orally *bid* for 10 days. Patients allergic to penicillin can be treated with oral tetracycline, 500 mg *qid* for 15 days, or oral erythromycin, 500 mg *qid* for 15 days.

C. Treat hospitalized patients with cefoxitin, 2 g IV *qid*, plus doxycycline, 100 mg IV *bid* until an adequate response is achieved; then switch to oral doxycycline to complete a 10-day course of therapy. Remove an IUD. When symptoms do not improve, consider adding clindamycin, an aminoglycoside, or metronidazole. Simultaneous infection with multiple agents is likely in patients with an IUD and in those who have severe infection such as a tubo-ovarian abscess or septic abortion.

D. Reasons for treatment failure include reinfection by a sexual partner, poor compliance, and resistant organisms. Resistant penicillinase producing gonorrhea can be treated with spectinomycin, 2 g IM, or cefoxitin, 2 g IM, plus probenecid, 1 g orally.

REFERENCES

Centers for Disease Control Recommended Treatment Schedules 1982. US Dept. of Health and Human Services.

Emans SJ, Goldstein DP. Pediatric and Adolescent Gynecology. 2nd ed. Boston: Little, Brown, 1982.

Fraser J, Reitig PJ, Kaplan DW. Prevalence of cervical trachomatis and *Neisseria gonorrhoeae* in female adolescents. Pediatrics 1983; 71:333.

Murphy M, Shubow J, Wise PH. Pelvic inflammatory disease: Is hospitalization necessary to ensure therapeutic compliance? Abstract Am J Dis Child 1983; 137:540.

Treatment of Sexually Transmitted Disease. Medical Letter 1984; 26:5.

PELVIC INFLAMMATORY DISEASE

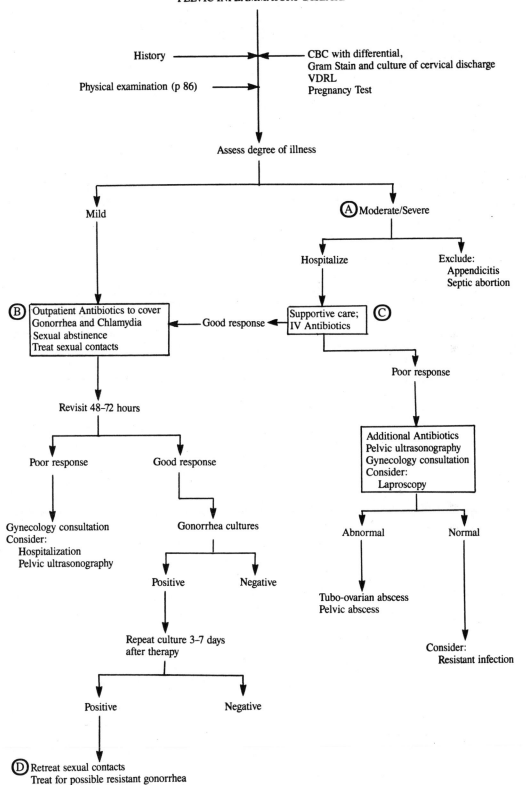

History ——————

CBC with differential,
Gram Stain and culture of cervical discharge
VDRL
Pregnancy Test

Physical examination (p 86) ——→

Assess degree of illness

Mild

Ⓐ Moderate/Severe

Hospitalize

Exclude:
Appendicitis
Septic abortion

Ⓑ Outpatient Antibiotics to cover
Gonorrhea and Chlamydia
Sexual abstinence
Treat sexual contacts

←— Good response —

Supportive care;
IV Antibiotics Ⓒ

Poor response

Revisit 48–72 hours

Additional Antibiotics
Pelvic ultrasonography
Gynecology consultation
Consider:
    Laproscopy

Poor response

Good response

Gynecology consultation
Consider:
    Hospitalization
    Pelvic ultrasonography

Gonorrhea cultures

Abnormal

Normal

Positive

Negative

Tubo-ovarian abscess
Pelvic abscess

Repeat culture 3–7 days
after therapy

Consider:
    Resistant infection

Positive

Negative

Ⓓ Retreat sexual contacts
Treat for possible resistant gonorrhea

89

ABNORMAL URINALYSIS: EVALUATION OF SUSPECTED RENAL DISEASE

A. Determine the onset, duration, and pattern of symptoms. Note precipitating factors including trauma, toxins, medications, foods, dyes, exercise, respiratory infections, streptococcal infections, and gastroenteritis. Identify predisposing conditions such as bleeding disorders (hemophilia), hemoglobinopathies (sickle cell disease), Alport's familial nephritis (with deafness, eye problems, nephritis), and collagen vascular diseases (systemic lupus erythematosus, polyarteritis nodosa, Henoch-Schönlein purpura). Document symptoms which suggest urinary tract infection such as dysuria, frequency, urgency, abdominal pain, and fever. Symptoms of diabetes include polyuria, polydipsia, and weight loss. Note symptoms which suggest hemolytic uremic syndrome (bloody diarrhea) or collagen vascular disease (rash, pallor, abdominal pain, and arthritis). Note symptoms which suggest glomerular disease (dark-colored urine, decreased urine output, or edema). Symptoms which suggest hypertensive encephalopathy include headache, vomiting, confusion, visual disturbances, memory loss, convulsions, and coma. Symptoms which suggest circulatory overload include cough, shortness of breath, dyspnea, and orthopnea.
B. Note vital signs and evidence of circulatory overload such as tachypnea, tachycardia, rales, wheezes, and hepatomegaly. Document signs of renal disease, such as edema and hypertension. Signs of collagen vascular disease or malignancy include lymphadenopathy, hepatosplenomegaly, abdominal mass, rash, and arthritis. Jaundice and hepatomegaly suggest hepatobiliary disease. Suspect a coagulation disorder when petechiae, purpura, or mucous membrane bleeding are present. Note bruises or other signs of trauma.

ABNORMAL URINALYSIS

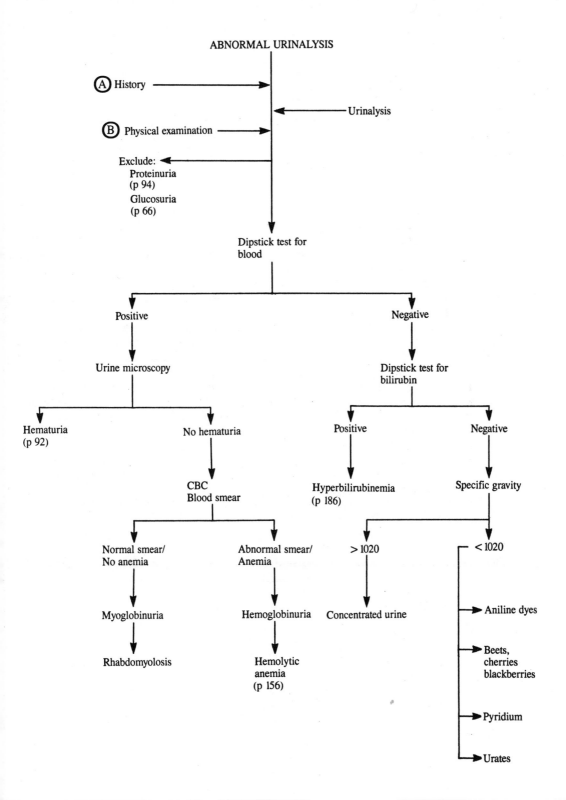

(A) History

Urinalysis

(B) Physical examination

Exclude:
  Proteinuria
  (p 94)
  Glucosuria
  (p 66)

Dipstick test for blood

Positive

Urine microscopy

Hematuria
(p 92)

No hematuria

CBC
Blood smear

Normal smear/
No anemia

Myoglobinuria

Rhabdomyolosis

Abnormal smear/
Anemia

Hemoglobinuria

Hemolytic
anemia
(p 156)

Negative

Dipstick test for bilirubin

Positive

Hyperbilirubinemia
(p 186)

Negative

Specific gravity

> 1020

Concentrated urine

< 1020

Aniline dyes

Beets,
cherries
blackberries

Pyridium

Urates

HEMATURIA

A. Findings that suggest a nonglomerular pattern of hematuria include the presence of bright red blood with or without clots, a varying degree of hematuria during stages of urination, and the absence of red blood cell casts. Typically, edema and hypertension are not present.

B. Findings which suggest a glomerular pattern include a brown or cola colored appearance of the urine, proteinuria, red blood cell casts, and edema or hypertension.

C. Renal function tests include BUN, creatinine, electrolytes, serum albumin, calcium phosphorus, creatinine clearance, 24-hour urine for protein, and a fractional excretion of sodium. Anemia, red cell fragmentation, and thrombocytopenia suggest hemolytic uremic syndrome.

D. When a nonglomerular pattern of hematuria is associated with a normal IVP, consider urethral trauma, penile excoriation, hemorrhagic cystitis, or a foreign body in the urethra or bladder. When microscopic hematuria is associated with a normal IVP and normal renal function, consider idiopathic hematuria, exercise-induced hematuria, and benign recurrent hematuria. When hematuria persists for more than 6 months, refer the patient for a renal biopsy to identify cases of Berger's disease (IgG-IgA nephropathy).

E. Systemic diseases suggested by the history and physical examination include Henoch-Schönlein purpura, systemic lupus erythematosus, familial nephritis, acute interstitial nephritis, sickle cell disease or trait, and Goodpasture's syndrome. Subacute bacterial endocarditis and infected ventricular shunts are also associated with hematuria.

F. The presence of nephrotic syndrome, acute renal failure, or a normal complement is atypical for poststreptococcal acute glomerulonephritis (GN); other entities which should be considered include membranoproliferative nephritis, focal glomerulonephritis, Berger's disease, rapidly progressive acute glomerulonephritis, and renal vein thrombosis. Refer these patients to a pediatric nephrologist for renal biopsy and appropriate therapy.

G. Acute poststreptococcal glomerulonephritis is the most common type of acute glomerulonephritis. It usually presents in children between 3 and 7 years of age with evidence of a recent infection with *S. pyogenes* (impetigo, positive throat culture, positive streptozyme or anti-Dnase B). Physical findings usually include edema and moderate hypertension. Urinalysis reveals red cell casts and the serum complement level is decreased. The presence of nephrotic syndrome, normal complement, acute renal failure, or a positive ANA is atypical and suggests another etiology.

H. A course is atypical when either acute renal failure or severe hypertension develops. It is also unusual for active glomerular disease to persist beyond 2 months. Signs of active disease include decreased renal function, depressed serum complement, and urinalysis with significant hematuria (>20 RBC hPF) or proteinuria ($>2-3+$). Microscopic hematuria which persists longer than 18 months is also unusual.

REFERENCES

Bergstein JM. Hematuria, proteinuria, and urinary tract infections. Pediatr Clin North Am 1982; 29:55.

Jordan SC, Lemire JM. Acute glomerulonephritis: diagnosis and treatment. Pediatr Clin North Am 1982; 29:857.

McCrory WW. Glomerulonephritis. Pediatrics Rev 1983; 5:19.

Northway JD. Hematuria in children. J Pediatr 1971; 78:381.

HEMATURIA

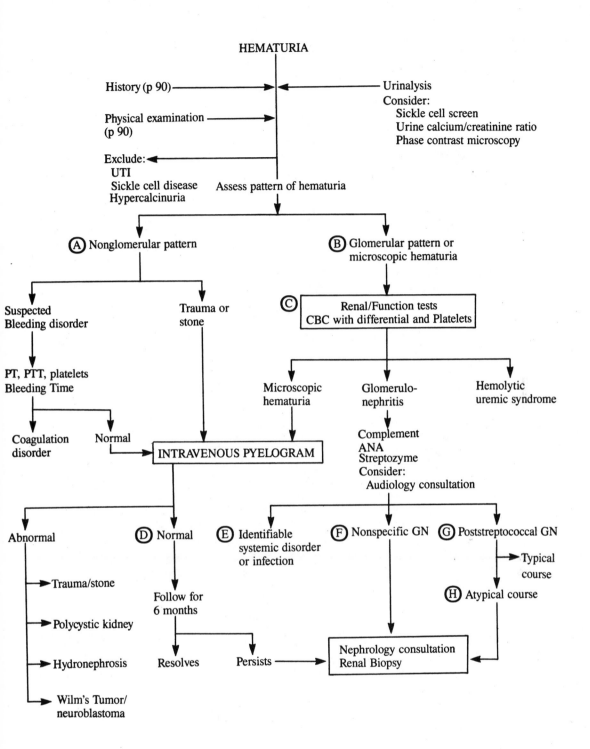

NEPHROTIC SYNDROME

A. Children with a persistent 4+ urinalysis for protein, ≥ 50 mg/kg/day of proteinuria or ≥ 40 mg of proteinuria per hour per square meter of surface area have the nephrotic syndrome. This syndrome is also associated with hypoalbuminemia, hyperlipidemia, and edema. Idiopathic nephrotic syndrome (minimal change nephrotic syndrome) occurs most frequently in children 1–7 years of age. Atypical presentations with acute renal failure, severe hypertension, hematuria, and hypocomplementemia suggest another disease process.

B. Hypoalbuminemia can cause severe edema, ascites, pleural effusions, and hypovolemia with azotemia. Treat hypoalbuminemia with 1–2 gms/kg of 25% salt-poor albumin IV over 60 minutes followed by furosemide 1–2 mg/kg IV. When hypovolemia results in hypotension, do not use furosemide. Complications of the nephrotic syndrome include hypertension, infection (peritonitis, sepsis, cellulitis, urinary tract infections), and coagulation disorders. Use diazoxide 3–5 mg/kg IV bolus to treat severe hypertension. When decreased renal profusion is contributing to hypertension, establish urine output with furosemide, and then consider an albumin infusion. The nephrotic syndrome can be associated with either a hyper- or hypocoagulability. Hypercoagulability is associated with increased levels of procoagulants, thrombocytosis, or increased beta thromboglobulin levels; hypocoagulation results from mild disseminated intravascular coagulation with increased fibrin split products. Correct coagulation abnormalities prior to performing a renal biopsy.

C. Treat children initially with prednisone 2 mg/kg/day (maximum 60 mg), until the urine is protein-free for 5 consecutive days or for a maximum of 8 weeks. Many (73%) cases of idiopathic nephrotic syndrome respond within 2 weeks and most (94%) respond within 1 month. After remission has been achieved, maintain the patient with 2 mg/kg on alternate days for 1–3 months. During the fourth month of therapy, decrease the dose of prednisone to 1 mg/kg, then taper the dose by 5 mg/week. Monitor proteinuria daily with an albumin-sensitive dipstick. Relapse is defined as 3 consecutive days with proteinuria measuring 3+ or more.

D. If the nephrotic syndrome recurs as the prednisone dosage is tapered, steroid-dependent disease is present. These patients, as well as frequent relapsers who experience ≥ 3 relapses per year, require long-term alternate-day prednisone. A maintenance dose of 1.4 mg/kg every other day controls most patients and produces only a minimal steroid toxicity. Alkylating agents, such as cyclophosphamide and chlorambucil, may decrease the relapse rate but are associated with significant side effects, including abnormal gonadal function, alopecia, leukopenia, hemorrhagic cystitis, and predisposition to overwhelming infection with varicella or measles.

REFERENCES

Feld LG, Schoeneman MJ, Kaskel FJ. Evaluation of the child with asymptomatic proteinuria. Pediatr Rev 1984; 5:248.

International study of kidney disease in children: the primary nephrotic syndrome in children. Identification of patients with minimal change nephrotic syndrome from initial response to prednisone. J Pediatr 1981; 98:561.

McEnery PT, Strife CF. Nephrotic syndrome in children. Pediatr Clin North Am 1982; 89:875.

Oliver WJ, Kelsch RC. Nephrotic syndrome due to primary nephropathics. Pediatr Rev 1981; 2:311.

NEPHROTIC SYNDROME

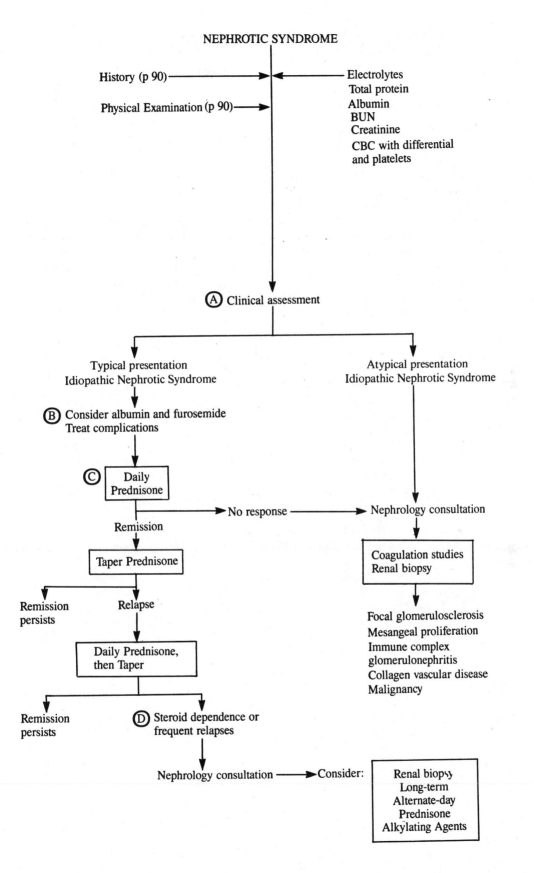

History (p 90) ────→

Physical Examination (p 90) ────→

←──── Electrolytes
Total protein
Albumin
BUN
Creatinine
CBC with differential
and platelets

(A) Clinical assessment

Typical presentation
Idiopathic Nephrotic Syndrome

Atypical presentation
Idiopathic Nephrotic Syndrome

(B) Consider albumin and furosemide
Treat complications

(C) Daily
Prednisone

No response ────→ Nephrology consultation

Remission

Taper Prednisone

Coagulation studies
Renal biopsy

Remission
persists

Relapse

Focal glomerulosclerosis
Mesangeal proliferation
Immune complex
glomerulonephritis
Collagen vascular disease
Malignancy

Daily Prednisone,
then Taper

Remission
persists

(D) Steroid dependence or
frequent relapses

Nephrology consultation ────→ Consider:

Renal biopsy
Long-term
Alternate-day
Prednisone
Alkylating Agents

ACUTE RENAL FAILURE

A. The laboratory helps distinguish prerenal from renal states. Prerenal azotemia results from decreased blood flow to the kidneys with decreased glomerular filtration. Therefore, sodium reabsorption will be high, and a concentrated urine will be produced. The BUN rises rapidly compared to the serum creatinine level, and the fractional excretion of sodium will be decreased. Prerenal states are usually associated with a urine sodium < 20 MEq/L, a urine osmolality > 450 mosm, a plasma BUN/creatinine ratio $< 20:1$, and a fractional excretion of sodium $< 1\%$. Renal disease is usually associated with a urine sodium > 40 mEq/L, urine osmolality < 450 mosm, plasma BUN/creatinine ratio $< 20:1$, and a fractional excretion of sodium $> 3\%$.

B. Suspect a postrenal disorder when acute renal failure is associated with an abdominal or flank mass or when a urinary catheter cannot be passed. Ultrasound and radiologic studies will identify patients with hydronephrosis, ureteropelvic junction obstruction, posterior urethral valves, and other obstructive lesions of the urinary tract. Refer these patients to the urologist and nephrologist for further management.

C. Obtain a chest x-ray to identify congestive heart failure and pulmonary edema. Congestive heart failure may be a primary condition producing prerenal azotemia, or it may be secondary to volume overload and/or severe anemia associated with renal failure.

D. Treat suspected hypovolemia associated with nephrotic syndrome with 1–2 gm/kg of 25% salt-poor albumin over 60 minutes followed by furosemide 1–2 mg/kg IV. Do not use furosemide if hypotension is present. Treat normotensive patients without a nephrotic syndrome but with oligoanuria with furosemide 3–5 mg/kg IV. Consider a trial of isotonic fluids 10 cc/kg/hour in cases resistant to furosemide. When oligoanuria persists despite an adequate trial of furosemide and isotonic fluids, place a central venous pressure line in order to determine the status of the circulatory blood volume.

E. Treat patients with severe hypertension or signs of hypertensive encephalopathy with diazoxide 3–5 mg/kg IV bolus or nitroprusside 3–10 μg/kg/min. Consider Lasix 3–5 mg/kg IV to treat milder forms of hypertension. Acute renal failure can be complicated by hyperkalemia associated with peaked T-waves or arrythmias. Kayexalate enemas can be used to lower potassium. When potassium levels must be reduced quickly, consider using insulin infusions 0.1 units/kg/hour in D1OW and sodium bicarbonate 1–3 mEq/kg IV over 20–30 minutes. Exercise caution in giving sodium bicarbonate to manage hyperkalemia or severe acidosis because of the risk of inducing hypocalcemic tetany. Consider a slow infusion over 2 to 10 minutes of 10% calcium gluconate 0.1–0.5 ml/kg when serious ECG abnormalities are present. When congestive heart failure secondary to anemia complicates renal failure, consider a packed cell exchange transfusion. Treat severe acidosis with sodium bicarbonate 1–3 mEq/kg IV over 20–30 minutes. Give calcium gluconate 100 mg/kg IV every 4–6 hours in order to prevent hypocalcemic tetany.

F. Indications to institute dialysis include severe acidosis with a $NaHCO_3 < 10$ MEq/L, electrolyte abnormalities with Na < 120 MEq/L or a K > 7 MEq/L, severe uremia with a BUN > 100, or circulatory overload causing congestive heart failure or severe hypertension.

REFERENCES

Jordan SC, Lemire JM. Acute glomerulitis: diagnosis and treatment. Pediatr Clin North Am 1982; 29:857.
Schrier RW. Acute renal failure: pathogenesis, diagnosis and management. Hosp Prac 1981; 16:93.

Suspected ACUTE RENAL FAILURE

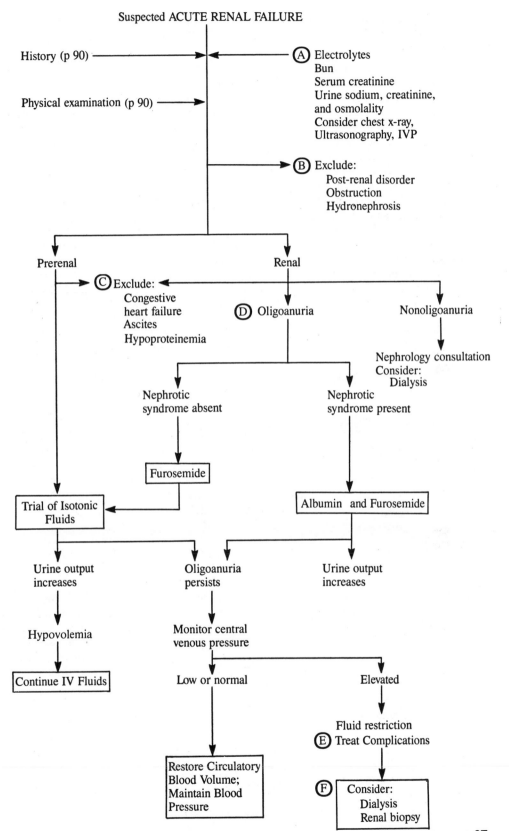

History (p 90) ⟶ Ⓐ Electrolytes
Bun
Serum creatinine
Urine sodium, creatinine,
and osmolality
Consider chest x-ray,
Ultrasonography, IVP

Physical examination (p 90) ⟶

Ⓑ Exclude:
Post-renal disorder
Obstruction
Hydronephrosis

Prerenal

Renal

Ⓒ Exclude:
Congestive
heart failure
Ascites
Hypoproteinemia

Ⓓ Oligoanuria

Nonoligoanuria

Nephrology consultation
Consider:
Dialysis

Nephrotic
syndrome absent

Nephrotic
syndrome present

Furosemide

Trial of Isotonic
Fluids

Albumin and Furosemide

Urine output
increases

Oligoanuria
persists

Urine output
increases

Hypovolemia

Monitor central
venous pressure

Continue IV Fluids

Low or normal

Elevated

Fluid restriction
Ⓔ Treat Complications

Restore Circulatory
Blood Volume;
Maintain Blood
Pressure

Ⓕ Consider:
Dialysis
Renal biopsy

97

URINARY TRACT INFECTION

A. Note dysuria, urgency, frequency, enuresis, abdominal pain, flank pain, or foul-smelling, cloudy urine. Ask about the frequency of recurrent episodes, and document the results of prior urine cultures and radiologic studies. Note associated symptoms such as fever, chills, nausea, vomiting, vaginal or penile discharge, malaise, headaches, visual disturbances. Identify possible predisposing factors including poor perianal hygiene, trauma, pinworms, masturbation, chronic constipation, vaginitis or urethritis, infrequent voiding, tight clothing, exposure to chemicals (bubble bath, soaps), pregnancy and urinary tract abnormalities.

B. Note blood pressure, and do a fundoscopic examination. Determine the presence of vulvovaginitis or urethral discharge. Document suprapubic pain or flank pain.

C. Diagnosis of a urinary tract infection can be based on a suprapubic aspiration which grows any organisms, a catheterized urine specimen with $> 10^4$ organisms (10^3–10^4 organisms is a suspicious infection; $< 10^3$ unlikely infection), or a clean-catch, midstream urine specimen with $> 10^5$ colonies. A clean-catch midstream urine has an 80–97% correlation with a catheterized specimen. Random voids and bagged specimens are useful only if negative, since contamination makes positive cultures uninterpretable; such specimens should not be used to document a urinary tract infection. One positive culture associated with symptoms, or two concurrent positive cultures in an asymptomatic child indicate an infection. The presence of bacteria on unspun, unstained urine specimens examined under oil immersion, or a finding of more than 5 bacteria using a hemocytometer correlates well with positive cultures. The most frequent organisms causing urinary tract infections are *E. coli*, followed by *Klebsiella, Enterobacter, P. mirabilis, Pseudomonas*, and Enterococci.

D. Treat urethritis or cervicitis for *Gonorrhoea* and *Chlamydia* with oral amoxicillin 3 g once plus oral probenecid 1 g once followed by 10 days of tetracycline 500 mg *qid* or an appropriate alternative therapy (pp 84).

E. Reasonable choices for initial oral antibiotic therapy include amoxicillin 50 mg/kg/day, trimethoprim (TMP) 8 mg/kg/day, sulfamethoxazole (SMZ) 40 mg/kg/day, or nitrofurantoin 5–7 mg/kg/day. Treat toxic patients with suspected pyelonephritis with ampicillin 200 mg/kg/day and tobramycin 7.5 mg/kg/day. Antibiotic therapy may require modifications based on the results of the culture and sensitivity tests. The duration of therapy is controversial; recommendations vary from 3 to 14 days. Teach children proper anal hygiene. Children and parents should be instructed to avoid bubble baths, chemical irritants, and tight clothing. Potential predisposing conditions such as constipation and pinworm infections should be treated.

F. Several cost-effective methods of screening for urinary tract infections are available for home use (nitrite dipstick, Microstix, glucose detection strips) or office use (Dipslide or Miniculture). Since all screening tests overdiagnose, positive tests should be confirmed with an appropriately obtained quantitative culture.

G. UTIs may be associated with renal anomalies or reflux nephropathy. UTIs in children under 4 years of age are more likely to be associated with anomalies or reflux nephropathy. Additional risk factors include infections in males, recurrent infections, ear anomalies, and supernumerary nipples. Unfortunately, there is no way of identifying patients with serious underlying disease other than by obtaining an IVP (or renal ultrasonography) and a voiding cystourethrogram (VCUG). One-half of children studied during a UTI episode have mild or moderate reflux; 10–20% of these children have upper urinary tract damage.

H. Antibiotics used for chemoprophylaxis include TMP 2 mg/kg/day/SMZ 10 mg/kg/day or nitrofurantoin 1–2 mg/kg/day.

REFERENCES

Corman LI, Foshee W, Kotchmar G et al. Simplified urinary microscopy to detect significant bacteria. Pediatrics 1982; 70:133.

Hellerstein S, Woods SE, Hodson GJ, et al. Recurrent urinary tract infections in children. Ped Infect Dis 1982; 1:221.

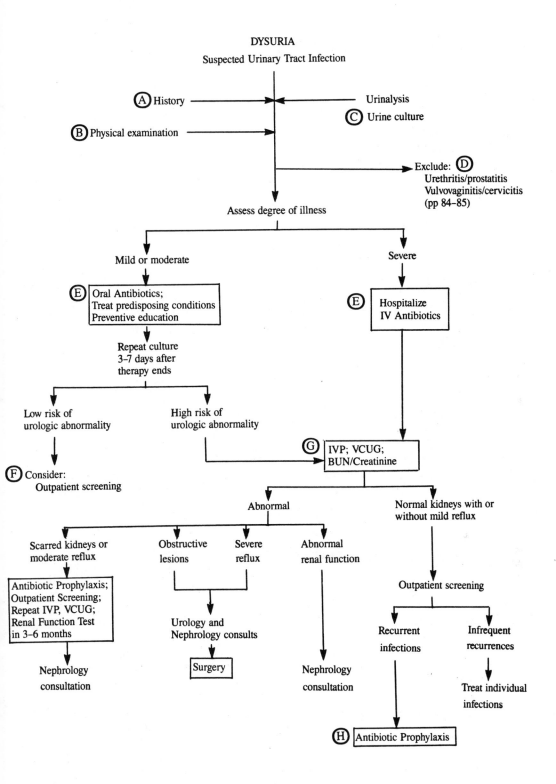

DYSURIA

Suspected Urinary Tract Infection

(A) History — Urinalysis

(C) Urine culture

(B) Physical examination

Exclude: (D)
Urethritis/prostatitis
Vulvovaginitis/cervicitis
(pp 84–85)

Assess degree of illness

Mild or moderate — Severe

(E) Oral Antibiotics;
Treat predisposing conditions
Preventive education

(E) Hospitalize
IV Antibiotics

Repeat culture
3–7 days after
therapy ends

Low risk of
urologic abnormality

High risk of
urologic abnormality

(G) IVP; VCUG;
BUN/Creatinine

(F) Consider:
Outpatient screening

Abnormal — Normal kidneys with or
without mild reflux

Scarred kidneys or
moderate reflux

Obstructive
lesions

Severe
reflux

Abnormal
renal function

Antibiotic Prophylaxis;
Outpatient Screening;
Repeat IVP, VCUG;
Renal Function Test
in 3–6 months

Outpatient screening

Urology and
Nephrology consults

Recurrent
infections

Infrequent
recurrences

Nephrology
consultation

Surgery

Nephrology
consultation

Treat individual
infections

(H) Antibiotic Prophylaxis

Randolph MF, Woods SE, Hodson GJ, et al. Home screening for detection of urinary tract infection in infancy.
    Am J Dis Child 1979; 133:713.
Rapkin RH. Urinary tract infection. Pediatr Rev 1979; 1:133.

SCROTAL SWELLING

A. Note onset, duration, pattern (intermittent or constant), and severity of scrotal swelling. Ask about associated pain radiating to the abdomen (testicular torsion), rectum (orchitis), or inguinal region (epididymitis). Sudden onset of severe pain with nausea, vomiting, and fever suggest testicular torsion. Gradual onset of pain with dysuria, urethral discharge, and fever suggests epididymitis. Note precipitating factors such as trauma, skin infection, or contact dermatitis. Patients with testicular torsion often have a history of mild trauma. Identify predisposing conditions such as Henoch-Schönlein purpura, nephrosis, liver disease, and malignancy, especially leukemia.

B. Inspect and palpate the testis. Examine the standing patient to determine the axis of both testes. An abnormally high-lying horizontal-axis testis that is diffusely tender with discolored, edematous scrotal skin suggests testicular torsion. Elevation of the testis increases pain. Assess blood flow to the testis by Doppler blood pressure monitor. Consider torsion of the testicular appendix when tenderness is limited to the superior lateral aspect of the testis. Occasionally, the blue dot sign of infarction of the appendix may be present. Consider epididymitis when an enlarged tender epididymis is palpated. A varicocele presents as a nontender scrotal mass which feels like a "bag of worms". A soft, fluid-filled mass surrounding the testicle, which transilluminates well, is usually a hydrocele.

C. A hydrocele is fluid within the tunica vaginalis which covers the testis. It may be simple (constant size) or communicating (alterations in size). Simple hydrocele may be present at birth or develop following trauma, torsion, epididymitis, or tumor. Congenital hydroceles usually resolve without complication in 12 to 18 months. Communicating hydroceles that change size are often associated with the development of a hernia. Refer these cases to surgery for correction.

D. Torsion of the testis produces venous engorgement and infarction secondary to loss of arterial blood flow. More than 6 hours of total arterial occlusion will cause irreversible gonadal damage. When testicular torsion is suspected, do not delay surgery in order to perform time-consuming diagnostic studies such as a testicular flow scan. Proceed rapidly even when symptoms have been present more than 6 hours; partial arterial obstruction may allow successful surgery even in cases with prolonged symptoms. The surgeon should perform bilateral orchiopexy in order to correct inadequate fixation of the testes to the intrascrotal subcutaneous tissue. When surgery is performed within 6 hours of torsion, the gonad is always salvaged. Surgery after 7 to 12 hours is successful in 70% of cases, and after 12 hours in 20%. In emergency situations, consider attempting detorsion by rotating the involved testis outward towards the thigh after premedication with IV morphine (0.1 mg/kg). Dramatic relief of pain, return of the testis to its normal position, and return of arterial pulsations as seen on Doppler monitor indicate success.

E. Postpubertal orchitis is associated with several viral infections (mumps, coxsackie and echoviruses) and with gonorrhea. In prepubertal boys, obtain a urology consultation to rule out testicular torsion.

F. Epididymitis, which usually occurs after puberty, is commonly associated with *Chlamydia, E. coli,* or gonorrhea. It often presents with pyuria or hematuria and may be associated with a urinary tract infection. Treat cases with amoxicillin (3 g PO once) plus probenecid (1 g PO once) followed by 10 days of tetracycline or TMP/SMZ. Supportive measures include elevation of the scrotum, sitz baths, and analgesia. Epididymitis may have a 3 to 4 week course. When epididymitis occurs in a prepubertal boy, perform a diagnostic workup for urinary tract abnormalities (IVP, voiding cystourethrogram). When severe pain is present, consult a urologist and consider hospitalization.

G. Idiopathic scrotal edema may be a form of angioneurotic edema. The testes are normal, and the swelling resolves without therapy in 48 hours.

SCROTAL SWELLING/PAIN

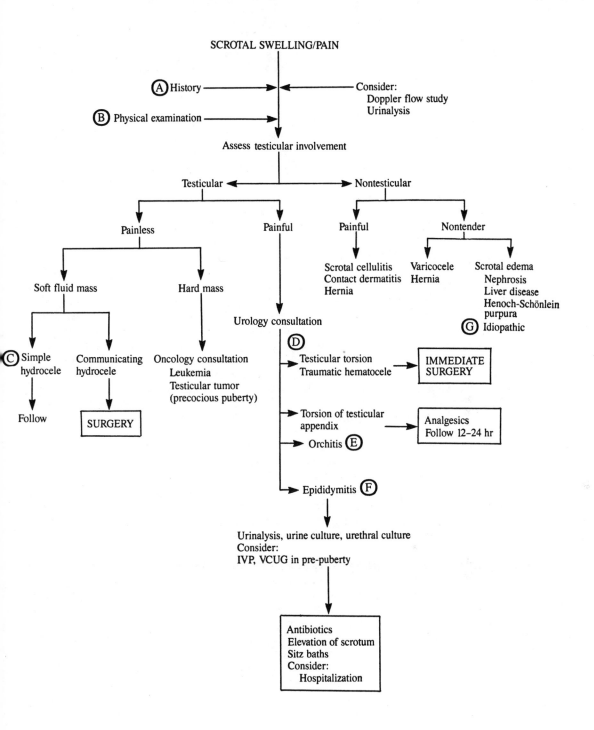

REFERENCES

Snyder HMcC, Caldamone AA, Duckett JW. Scrotal pain/swelling. In: Fleisher G, Ludwig S, eds. Textbook of Pediatric Emergency Medicine. Baltimore: Williams & Wilkins, 1983; 237.

EVALUATION OF SKIN LESIONS

A. Determine the onset, progression, distribution, duration, and recurrence of the lesions. Note the presence of prodromal and associated symptoms including pruritis, fever, cough, coryza, vomiting, diarrhea, jaundice, lymphadenopathy, altered mental status, arthritis, and failure to thrive. Identify precipitating factors or agents including infection, drugs or medications, trauma, sunburn, frostbite, water immersion, foods, soaps, detergents, and new clothes or shoes. Note predisposing conditions such as atopic disease (atopic dermatitis, allergic rhinitis, asthma), malignancy, collagen vascular disease, liver disease, renal disease, and mucocutaneous diseases.

B. Recognize primary lesions including macules, papules, plaques, nodules, wheals, vesicles, and cysts. According to accepted definitions, a macule is a color change in the skin that is flat to the surface and not palpable. A papule is a firm, raised lesion with distinct borders 1 cm or less in diameter. A plaque is a firm, raised, flat-topped lesion with distinct borders and an epidermal change larger than 1 centimeter in diameter. A nodule is a raised lesion with indistinct borders and a deep palpable portion. A large nodule is called a tumor. A wheal is an area of tense edema within the upper dermis producing a flat-topped, slightly raised lesion. A vesicle is a papule filled with clear fluid. A bulla is a lesion larger than 1 centimeter in diameter filled with clear fluid. A cyst is a raised lesion containing a sac filled with liquid or semisolid material. Recognize secondary changes such as pustules, oozing and erosions, crusting, and scaling. With any rash determine its distribution, arrangement, and color. Note the specific location of the rash (generalized, truncal, flexural creases, extremities, hands, and feet). Lesions occurring in a straight line are called linear. Lesions arranged in a circular configuration are annular. Note associated signs of infection or systemic disease such as lymphadenopathy, hepatomegaly, splenomegaly, arthritis, jaundice, and heart murmur.

C. Common laboratory procedures related to dermatologic conditions include KOH preparations to identify fungal infections, exfoliative cytology, and skin biopsy. To perform a KOH prep, scrape scale from the lesion onto a glass slide and add a drop of 10% KOH to dissolve the stratum corneum cells. Heat gently to dissolve the cells more quickly. Cover the slide with a cover slip and examine for branching hyphae. Perform exfoliative cytology by breaking the blister and scraping its base. Place the scrapings on a glass slide. After drying, stain the slide with Wright's or Giemsa stain and examine for the presence of epidermal giant cells (herpes simplex or herpes zoster) or acantholytic cells (pemphigus).

D. Suspect acne when pustules and white papules (closed comedones) are located on the face, upper back, and upper chest in adolescents. Treat acne with benzoyl peroxide gel (5%) or retinoic acid cream (0.05%). In more severe cases consider 2 to 3 months of tetracycline 500 mg daily. Drug-induced acne can be produced by glucocorticosteroids, androgens, ACTH, diphenylhydantoin, or isoniazid. In bacterial or chemical folliculitis, all lesions are in the same stage at the same time. Suspect candidiasis when satellite papulopustule lesions are present around a central, raised erythematous area. Suspect bacteremia with gonococcus or meningococcus when the patient presents with fever, signs of toxicity, and an acral distribution of pustules.

REFERENCES

Weston W. Practical Pediatric Dermatology. Boston: Little, Brown, 1984.

SKIN LESIONS

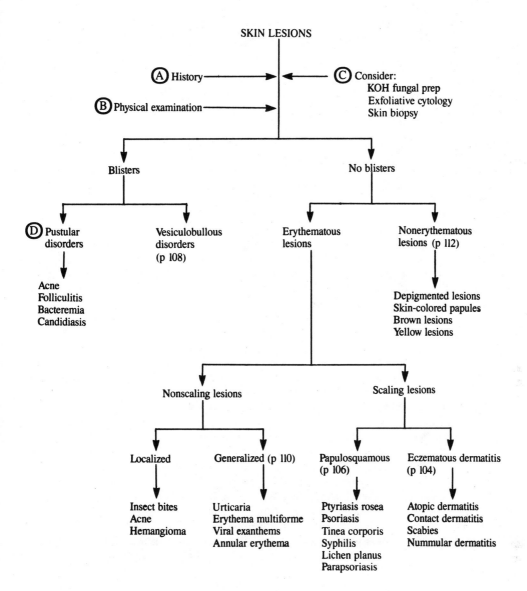

ECZEMATOUS DERMATITIS

A. Dermatitis or inflammation of the epidermis and superficial dermis presents with pruritis and secondary skin changes of marked dryness, oozing, crusting, erosions, vesiculations, and epidermal thickening.

B. Identify substances which cause contact dermatitis by direct irritation or an allergic mechanism. Underlying skin disorders such as severe dryness or atopic dermatitis disrupts the normal epidermal barrier and increases susceptibility to irritants and infection. The most common form of irritant dermatitis is diaper rash which is related to prolonged contact with urine and feces. The presence of satellite lesions or erosions suggests secondary infection with candida. Treat diaper rash by exposing the skin to air, frequent dry diaper changes, 1% hydrocortisone cream, and mycostatin cream.

C. Suspect allergic contact dermatitis when the rash has a localized distribution, especially one involving the hands or feet. Secondary changes of vesiculation, oozing, and excoriation are common. A linear arrangement on the arms or legs suggests contact with plants such as poison ivy or poison oak. Allergic contact dermatitis is related to cell-mediated immunity. Common allergens which act as haptenes include pentadecacatechol found in poison oak and poison ivy, nickel in jewelry and zippers, dichromates in tanned leather, and several chemicals in glues, rubber, dyes, cosmetics, shampoos, and topical medications. When appropriate, consider patch testing to identify a specific allergen. Treat cases with topical steroids for 2 to 3 weeks. Use wet dressings for severe generalized pruritis; water evaporation relieves the pruritis, causes vasoconstriction, and debrides crusting. Instruct the parent to place cotton pajamas in tepid water and wring out the excess water. Have the child wear dry pajamas over the damp ones. Consider oral prednisone 1 mg/kg once daily for 14 to 21 days when allergic contact dermatitis is severe.

D. Suspect atopic dermatitis when its characteristic age-dependent distribution is seen. Involvement of the feet is especially common in school-aged children and adolescents; eyebrows may be involved at any age. Approximately half of the children with atopic dermatitis have an associated history of allergic rhinitis or asthma. Treat acute exacerbations with topical steroids and antihistamines. Recognize and treat secondary infections with S. aureus and S. pyogenes. Consider wet dressings when oozing, excoriations, and crusting are marked. Avoid using fluorinated steroids on the face because of dermal atrophy, telangiectasia, hypopigmentation, and acne. Maintain adequate skin hydration with routine use of 10% urea creams (i.e., aqua care) and lubricant creams (Eucerin), and cetaphil lotions. Use antihistamines when necessary for pruritis. Avoid occlusive clothing, frequent soaping, wool clothes, and cleaning agents and chemicals.

E. Suspect nummular eczema when coin-like lesions 1 to 10 cm in diameter are distributed symmetrically on the extremities or trunk. The lesions can be dry and scaly or wet and oozing. Dry lesions can be confused with tinea corporis and wet lesions with impetigo. Treat both lesions with topical steroids *tid* for 1 to 2 weeks.

F. Greasy scale on the face and scalp of infants and also in the nasolabial folds of the face, posterior auricular areas, scalp or chest in adolescents suggests seborrheic dermatitis. This condition is caused by an overproduction of sebum which traps scale. Treat these cases with topical steroids *tid* for 1 to 2 weeks.

REFERENCES

Esterly NB. Contact dermatitis. Pediatr Rev 1979; 1:85.
Esterly NB. Fungal infections in children. Pediatr Rev 1981; 3:23.
Hurwitz S. Eczematous eruptions in childhood. Pediatr Rev 1981; 3:23.
Munz D, Powell KR, Parr CH. Treatment of candidal diaper dermatitis: a double-blind placebo-controlled comparison of topical nystatin with oral nystatin. J Pediatr 1982; 101:1022.
Weston W. Practical Pediatric Dermatology. Boston: Little, Brown, 1979.

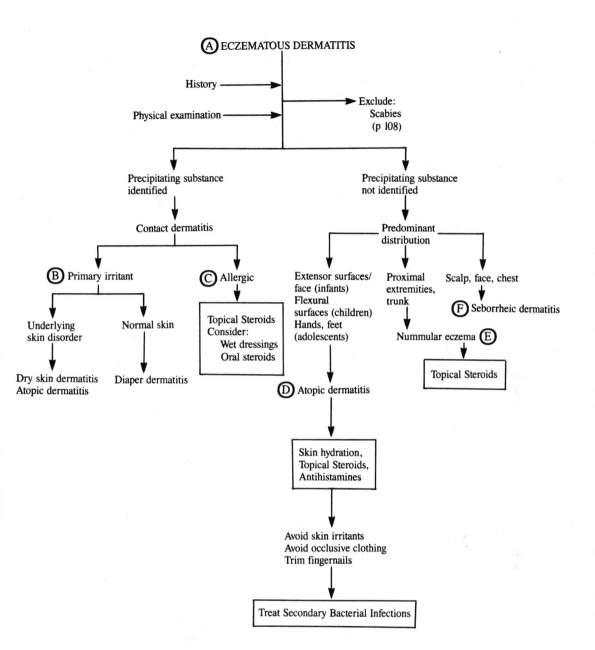

(A) ECZEMATOUS DERMATITIS

History ⟶

Physical examination ⟶

Exclude:
Scabies
(p 108)

Precipitating substance identified

Precipitating substance not identified

Contact dermatitis

Predominant distribution

(B) Primary irritant

(C) Allergic

Extensor surfaces/ face (infants)
Flexural surfaces (children)
Hands, feet (adolescents)

Proximal extremities, trunk

Scalp, face, chest

(F) Seborrheic dermatitis

Underlying skin disorder

Normal skin

Topical Steroids
Consider:
　Wet dressings
　Oral steroids

Nummular eczema **(E)**

Dry skin dermatitis
Atopic dermatitis

Diaper dermatitis

(D) Atopic dermatitis

Topical Steroids

Skin hydration,
Topical Steroids,
Antihistamines

Avoid skin irritants
Avoid occlusive clothing
Trim fingernails

Treat Secondary Bacterial Infections

PAPULOSQUAMOUS LESIONS

A. Papulosquamous disorders are skin lesions consisting of red or purple macules, papules with scale, and often, plaque formation.

B. Suspect pityriasis rosea when red oval lesions appear in the lines of skin stress oriented with their long axis in parallel planes. A large, erythematous, scaly lesion called the herald patch occurs in 80% of the cases. The herald patch is easily confused with tinea corporis when present before the outbreak of other lesions. A viral-like prodrome with fever and malaise may occur with pityriasis rosea, its lesions usually occur on the trunk but in black children may be mostly in the inguinal and axillary areas and extremities. Lesions persist for 4 to 8 weeks, but pruritus usually resolves within 1 week. Treat with sun exposure or ultraviolet light (UVL) therapy to reduce the pruritus and quicken resolution.

C. Parapsoriasis, a rare type of skin disease, occurs in 2 forms: guttate parapsoriasis and acute parapsoriasis. Guttate parapsoriasis resembles pityriasis rosea but can persist for 2 to 3 years. Suspect guttate parapsoriasis when pityriasis rosea fails to clear within 2 to 3 months. The acute form of parapsoriasis, also called Mucha-Habermann disease, presents with red papules that have central petechiae and crusting. The rash, which can be initially confused with varicella, persists for more than 9 months. When the diagnosis is doubtful consider skin biopsy. No definitive therapy for parapsoriasis is currently available.

D. Suspect psoriasis when plaque associated with silver scaling and a red base involves the elbows, knees, or scalp. Other common sites include ears, eyebrows, gluteal creases, genitalia, and nails. Involvement of the scalp with non-greasy thick scale is not associated with hair loss. Nail changes include pitting, yellowing, thickening, and separation of the nail plate from the nail bed. The presence of multiple discrete drop-like papules with scales suggests guttate psoriasis which is seen in approximately one-third of the cases of psoriasis. Skin biopsy in cases of psoriasis is characterized by signs of epidermal proliferation. Treat mild cases with tar gel preparations *bid* for 1 to 3 months and ultraviolet light from natural or artificial sources. Topical fluorinated steroids may provide relief but systemic steroids are contraindicated because of the rebound effect. Recognize and treat secondary staphylococcal infection of the lesions. Avoid using antimetabolites in children.

E. Suspect lichen planus when flat-topped pruritic, purple, polygonal papules are present. Oral, penile and scalp lesions are common. Scalp lesions are associated with hair loss. Nail involvement, although rare, can occur. Treat cases with topical steroids from 4 to 8 weeks. Consider oral prednisone 1 mg/kg daily for 1 to 2 weeks in severe generalized cases. Skin biopsy shows epidermal basal cell injury of unknown cause.

REFERENCES

Cavanaugh RM. Pityriasis rosea in children. Clin Pediatr 1983; 22:201.
Weston W. Practical Pediatric Dermatology. Boston: Little,Brown, 1979.

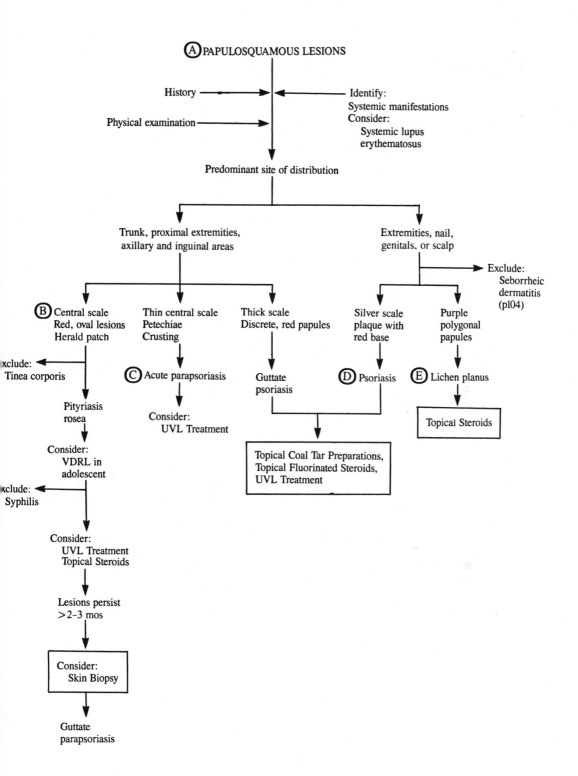

A PAPULOSQUAMOUS LESIONS

History ⟶ ⟵ Identify:
⟶ Systemic manifestations
Physical examination ⟶ Consider:
⟶ Systemic lupus
⟶ erythematosus

Predominant site of distribution

Trunk, proximal extremities,
axillary and inguinal areas

Extremities, nail,
genitals, or scalp

⟶ Exclude:
Seborrheic
dermatitis
(pl04)

B Central scale
Red, oval lesions
Herald patch

Thin central scale
Petechiae
Crusting

Thick scale
Discrete, red papules

Silver scale
plaque with
red base

Purple
polygonal
papules

Exclude: ⟵
Tinea corporis

C Acute parapsoriasis

Guttate
psoriasis

D Psoriasis

E Lichen planus

Pityriasis
rosea

Consider:
UVL Treatment

Consider:
VDRL in
adolescent

Topical Coal Tar Preparations,
Topical Fluorinated Steroids,
UVL Treatment

Topical Steroids

Exclude: ⟵
Syphilis

Consider:
UVL Treatment
Topical Steroids

Lesions persist
>2–3 mos

Consider:
Skin Biopsy

Guttate
parapsoriasis

VESICULOBULLOUS DISORDERS

A. Epidermolysis bullosa has 3 nonscarring and 2 scarring forms. Epidermolysis bullosa simplex (autosomal dominant, nonscarring) junctional epidermolysis bullosa (autosomal recessive, nonscarring) and recessive dystrophic epidermolysis bullosa (autosomal recessive, scarring) present in the newborn period. Forms which present in infancy and childhood include dominant dystrophic epidermolysis bullosa (autosomal dominant, scarring) and recurrent bullous eruption of the hands and feet (Weber-Cocayne disease: autosomal dominant, nonscarring).

B. Urticaria pigmentosa (mastocytosis) is a blistering disease with macular and nodular pigmented lesions occurring in the newborn period and during infancy. Suspect systemic mastocytosis when hepatomegaly, flushing episodes, and peptic ulcer disease are present. When necessary, treat cases with hydroxyzine hydrochloride 2 to 4 mg/kg/day divided in 4 doses. Consider oral cromolyn sodium when severe GI symptoms are present.

C. Epidermolytic hyperkeratosis (congenital bullous ichthyosiform erythroderma) is a blistering disorder associated with erythroderma and thickened, scaling skin lesions. The predominant sites of involvement are the flexural areas, palms, and soles. The mode of inheritance is autosomal dominant.

D. Incontinentia pigmenti usually occurs in girls and presents with blisters arranged in a linear pattern on extremities. The lesions develop a warty appearance and last until approximately one year of age. Swirls of brown pigmentation can also be found on the trunk. Mental retardation, seizures, microcephaly, and ocular and skeletal abnormalities are associated with this disorder.

E. Suspect bacterial impetigo when moist honey-colored crusts on each lesion cover an area of skin greater than 1 cm. Early bullous impetigo looks like an acute burn, contact dermatitis, or a friction blister. Viral infections which present with a vesicular eruption include varicella, herpes zoster, hand-foot-mouth disease (Coxsackie), enteroviral infections, and herpes simplex. Grouped vesicles with a dry crust suggest herpes simplex. Consider obtaining bacterial and/or viral cultures and staining a smear of the blister's contents with Wright's stain to identify epidermal giant cells associated with viral infections.

F. The presence of lesions on the palms and soles suggests scabies. Search the interdigital webs, palms, and soles. Diagnostic S-shaped burrows are obscured in most infants and young children. Scrape several lesions to attempt to identify the scabies mite feces or ova under the microscope. Treat cases with Quell lotion or Eurax cream.

G. When blistering lesions persist for longer than 1 month, obtain a skin biopsy to clarify the diagnosis. Treat chronic bullous disease of childhood and dermatitis herpetiformis with sulfapyridine or dapsone; treat bullous pemphigoid disease with systemic corticosteroids.

REFERENCES

Esterly NB. Infantile acropustulosis and granuloma gluteale infantum. Pediatr Rev 1983; 5:59.
Ginsburg CM. Scalsies. Ped Infect Dis 1984; 3:133.
Ramsdell W, Jarratt M, Fuerst J et al. Bullous disease of childhood. Am J Dis Child 1979; 133:791.
Weston WL. Practical Pediatric Dermatology. 2nd ed. Boston: Little, Brown, 1984.

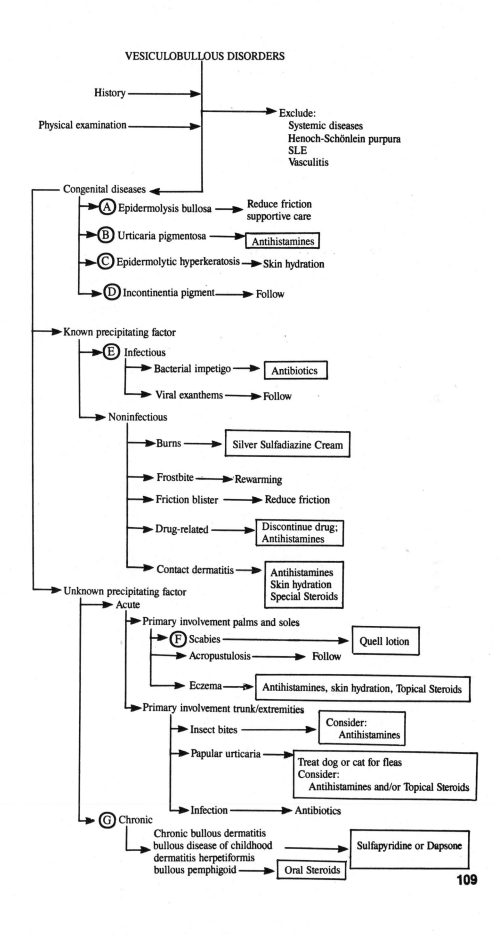

VESICULOBULLOUS DISORDERS

History ⟶

Physical examination ⟶

Exclude:
  Systemic diseases
  Henoch-Schönlein purpura
  SLE
  Vasculitis

Congenital diseases
  Ⓐ Epidermolysis bullosa ⟶ Reduce friction supportive care
  Ⓑ Urticaria pigmentosa ⟶ Antihistamines
  Ⓒ Epidermolytic hyperkeratosis ⟶ Skin hydration
  Ⓓ Incontinentia pigment ⟶ Follow

Known precipitating factor
  Ⓔ Infectious
    ⟶ Bacterial impetigo ⟶ Antibiotics
    ⟶ Viral exanthems ⟶ Follow
  Noninfectious
    ⟶ Burns ⟶ Silver Sulfadiazine Cream
    ⟶ Frostbite ⟶ Rewarming
    ⟶ Friction blister ⟶ Reduce friction
    ⟶ Drug-related ⟶ Discontinue drug; Antihistamines
    ⟶ Contact dermatitis ⟶ Antihistamines Skin hydration Special Steroids

Unknown precipitating factor
  Acute
    Primary involvement palms and soles
      Ⓕ Scabies ⟶ Quell lotion
      Acropustulosis ⟶ Follow
      Eczema ⟶ Antihistamines, skin hydration, Topical Steroids
    Primary involvement trunk/extremities
      ⟶ Insect bites ⟶ Consider: Antihistamines
      ⟶ Papular urticaria ⟶ Treat dog or cat for fleas Consider: Antihistamines and/or Topical Steroids
      ⟶ Infection ⟶ Antibiotics
  Ⓖ Chronic
      Chronic bullous dermatitis
      bullous disease of childhood ⟶ Sulfapyridine or Dapsone
      dermatitis herpetiformis
      bullous pemphigoid ⟶ Oral Steroids

109

ERYTHEMATOUS MACULOPAPULAR LESIONS

A. Insect bite reactions generally occur in crops and are usually few in number. Observe for signs of secondary infection. Urticaria are transient lesions that usually last less than one hour. Lesions of erythema multiforme have a symmetrical distribution, begin as red papules and progress over 7 to 10 days to lesions with a dusky center and a red border. They may form blisters. Prescribe a trial of oral antihistamines such as hydroxyzine hydrochloride 2 to 4 mg/kg/day (*qid*), diphenhydramine hydrochloride 5 mg/kg/day (*qid*) for urticaria or erythema multiforme. Erythema infectiosum (Fifth disease) presents in childhood without systemic symptoms. The rash first appears on the face as a bright red erythema, then evolves into an erythematous maculopapular rash distributed primarily over the extremities. As the rash fades, it develops a lace-like appearance.

B. The presence of high fever of unknown origin over 3 to 4 days followed by development of a rash suggests roseola or echovirus 16. The rash usually appears first on the trunk then spreads to involve the neck, upper extremities, face, and lower extremities. The rash lasts 1 to 2 days. Roseola occurs most frequently in children between 6 months and 3 years of age. Consider enterovirus in cases with an associated aseptic meningitis.

C. Mononucleosis presents with a rash in 10 to 15% of cases. The rash is most commonly an erythematous maculopapular eruption but can appear scarlatiniform, urticarial, or hemorrhagic. Associated findings may include pharyngitis, lymphadenopathy, splenomegaly, hepatitis, pneumonitis, and CNS involvement (meningitis, encephalitis, or Guillain-Barré syndrome). Follow patients for the development of severe complications such as acute airway obstruction (p 44), ruptured spleen, hemolytic anemia, thrombocytopenia, carditis, and orchitis.

D. Suspect scarlet fever when pharyngitis, fever, abdominal pain, and malaise are associated with an erythematous, punctiform (sandpaper) rash. Associated findings include circumoral pallor, flushed cheeks, a strawberry tongue, and Pastia's sign (transverse lines in antecubital fossae). The rash often desquamates. At least 3 types of erythrogenic toxin have been identified. Treat scarlet fever patients under 30 lbs with 10 days of 125 mg Pen VK *qid* or 300,000 units Benzathine Penicillin IM; patients between 30 and 60 lbs with 250 mg Pen VK *qid* or 600,000 Benzathine Penicillin IM; patients between 60 and 90 lbs with 500 mg Pen VK *qid* or 900,000 Benzathine Penicillin IM; and patients over 90 lbs with 500 mg Pen VK *qid* or 1,200,000 Benzathine Penicillin IM.

REFERENCES

Weston WL. Practical Pediatric Dermatology. 2nd ed. Boston: Little, Brown, 1984.
Krugman S, Ward R, Katz SL. Infectious Diseases of Children. St. Louis: CV Mosby, 1977.

ERYTHEMATOUS MACULOPAPULAR LESIONS

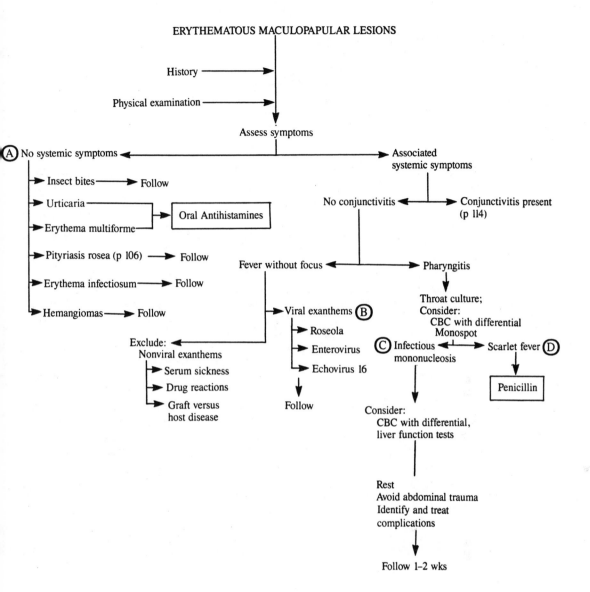

NONBLISTERING NONERYTHEMATOUS SKIN LESIONS

A. Warts usually appear on the extremities, especially hands and feet as solitary papules with an irregular scaly surface. Keratosis pilaris represents a follicular plug of scale within a body hair opening. Lesions usually develop on the extensor surfaces of the extremities and on the cheeks in children between 18 months and 3 years of age. The lesions are rarely erythematous or pustular. Epidermal nevi have a warty appearance and are arranged in a linear pattern. They may be present at birth or become evident at 6 or 12 months of age.

B. Microcomedones of acne appear as solitary discrete dome-shaped papules which are skin colored or slightly whitish in appearance. They first appear between the ages of 8 and 10 years and are located over the forehead and cheeks. Treat with topical keratolytic agents, retinoic acid cream 0.05%, or benzoyl peroxide gel 5%. Flat warts are broad skin colored papules usually grouped together and found on the face and extremities. Flat warts have a smooth surface which is flat or planar rather than dome-shaped as seen in microcomedones. Molluscum contagiosum appear as dome-shaped solitary papules with central umbilication which may be grouped together anywhere on the skin surface. The lesions are produced by a DNA virus, the molluscum virus. Lesions are contagious and may be passed from person to person by skin to skin contact. Molluscum contagiosum are larger than microcomedones and have a central plug of scale.

C. Pityriasis alba usually presents in late childhood as multiple oval scaly flat hypopigmented patches on the face, extensor surface of the arms and upper trunk. The lesions have indistinct borders, do not itch, and are usually distributed symmetrically. Lesions of tinea versicolor are smaller and have distinct borders, and a fine scale. They are distributed most often on the upper chest and back. Diagnose these cases with a KOH examination of a lesion which will show short curved hyphae and numerous spores. Vitiligo is associated with complete depigmentation rather than the hypopigmentation of pityriasis alba or tinea versicolor. A Wood's lamp examination will reveal a dramatic porcelain-white change in vitiligo compared to only subtle changes in color with pityriasis alba or tinea vesicolor.

D. Cafe-au-lait spots are tan in color and are usually located in sun protected areas. They are larger than freckles and are not sun responsive. Suspect neurofibromatosis when 6 cafe-au-lait spots are present or multiple cafe-au-lait spots are found in the axilla or groin area. Junctional nevi are usually dark brown or black in color rather than tan. Mongolian spots are blue or blue-black in color and have indistinct borders.

E. Juvenile xanthogranulomas commonly present at birth as yellow papules or nodules on the head or neck. Juvenile xanthogranuloma may have associated eye lesions which can be misdiagnosed as retinoblastoma. A nevus sebaceous lesion appears as a yellow linear plaque located on the face or scalp. A nevus sebaceous lesion is a hamartoma of the sebaceous glands. At puberty the lesion develops a warty appearance and has a cancerous predisposition.

REFERENCES

Weston WL. Practical Pediatric Dermatology, 2nd ed. Boston: Little, Brown, 1984.

NONBLISTERING, NONERYTHEMATOUS SKIN LESIONS

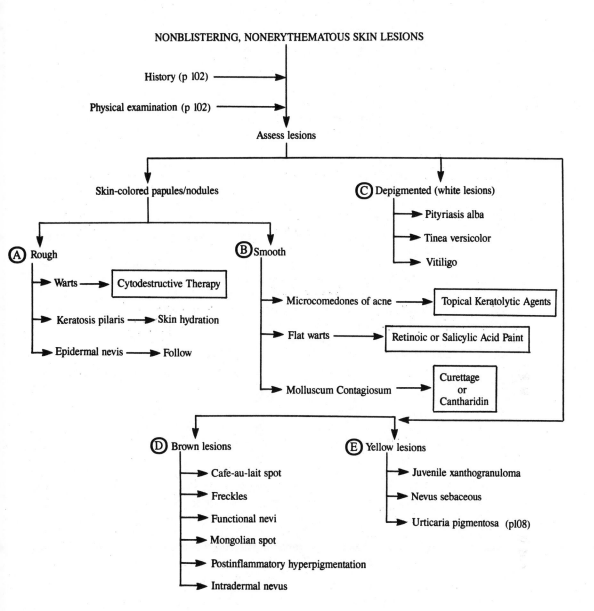

History (p 102)

Physical examination (p 102)

Assess lesions

Skin-colored papules/nodules

Ⓒ Depigmented (white lesions)
→ Pityriasis alba
→ Tinea versicolor
→ Vitiligo

Ⓐ Rough
→ Warts → Cytodestructive Therapy
→ Keratosis pilaris → Skin hydration
→ Epidermal nevis → Follow

Ⓑ Smooth
→ Microcomedones of acne → Topical Keratolytic Agents
→ Flat warts → Retinoic or Salicylic Acid Paint
→ Molluscum Contagiosum → Curettage or Cantharidin

Ⓓ Brown lesions
→ Cafe-au-lait spot
→ Freckles
→ Functional nevi
→ Mongolian spot
→ Postinflammatory hyperpigmentation
→ Intradermal nevus

Ⓔ Yellow lesions
→ Juvenile xanthogranuloma
→ Nevus sebaceous
→ Urticaria pigmentosa (pl08)

RED EYES, RED SKIN

A. Measles is associated with a 3 or 4 day prodrome of cough, coryza, fever, and conjunctivitis. The rash which starts on the head and face moves downward to involve the trunk and extremities. Lesions on the face, neck and upper trunk become confluent. Koplik spots are usually present on the buccal mucosa. The rash resolves in approximately 1 week.

B. Rubella is not usually associated with a prodrome. A red macular rash starts on the face and progresses downward becoming generalized within 24 to 48 hours. Lesions are usually discrete rather than confluent; clearing is noted on the face and trunk by day 3 or 4. Mild conjunctivitis may be present.

C. Suspect Kawasaki's disease (mucocutaneous lymph node syndrome) when an erythematous rash and conjunctival hyperemia are associated with fever for more than 5 days, mouth lesions (fissuring and crusting of the lips, strawberry tongue, or oropharyngeal injection), alterations of the hands and/or feet (erythema and induration followed by desquamation), and lymphadenopathy. Additional findings which may present after 1 to 3 weeks include arthritis or arthralgia, diarrhea, abdominal pain, hepatitis, obstructive jaundice, acute hydrops of the gall bladder, aseptic meningitis, urethritis, and cardiac disease. Cardiac disease occurs in 20% of cases as carditis, congestive heart failure, pericardial effusions, arrythmias, mitral insufficiency, and coronary artery aneurysms. Coronary artery aneurysms can be detected in 14 to 20% of cases and can cause angina and myocardial infarction. Screen all cases with 2-dimensional echocardiograms to identify aneurysms. Therapy with aspirin and steroids is controversial. This multisystem disease may be related to a hypercoagulable state with thrombocytosis.

D. Suspect toxic shock syndrome when erythroderma is associated with fever, altered mental status, diarrhea, hypotension, DIC and renal failure. Tampon use and nasal packing are associated with toxic shock syndrome. Hospitalize these patients, stabilize their circulation, and begin IV antistaphylococcal antibiotic coverage. This syndrome is caused by a phage-related toxin.

E. Stevens-Johnson syndrome (SJS) or toxic epidermal necrolysis (TEN), presents with bullous lesions, a positive Nikolsky sign, and mucous membrane involvement. Unlike SSSS, it is often preceded by erythema multiforme with iris and target lesions and evolves over 3 to 5 days rather than a few hours. SJS is associated with epidermal necrosis and subepidermal blister formation. The most frequent precipitating factors are infections, medications, and drugs. Agents most frequently associated with erythema multiforme and TEN are herpes simplex, *Mycoplasma pneumoniae, S. pyogenes*, EB virus, and tuberculosis. The most commonly associated drugs are sulfonamides, barbiturates, dilantin, salicylate, and penicillin. The use of steroids in SJS is controversial.

F. Suspect staphylococcal scalded skin syndrome (SSSS) when lateral pressure on the edge of the blister enlarges and extends the blister (Nikolsky sign) or bullous impetigo is present. The rash may be localized or generalized such as in Ritter's disease of the newborn. A toxin associated with *S. aureus* of the phage group II causes separation of the granular layer of the stratum corneum of the skin (intraepidermal blister formation). Treat patients with antistaphylococcal antibiotics; hospitalize those with signs of generalized or severe involvement.

REFERENCES

Melish ME, Hicks RV, Ready V. Kawasaki syndrome: an update. Hosp Pract 1982; March:99.
Todd J, Fishout M. Toxic shock syndrome associated with phage group I staphylococci. Lancet 1978; Nov 25: 1116.
Weston W. Practical Pediatric Dermatology. Boston: Little, Brown, 1979.

RED EYES, RED SKIN

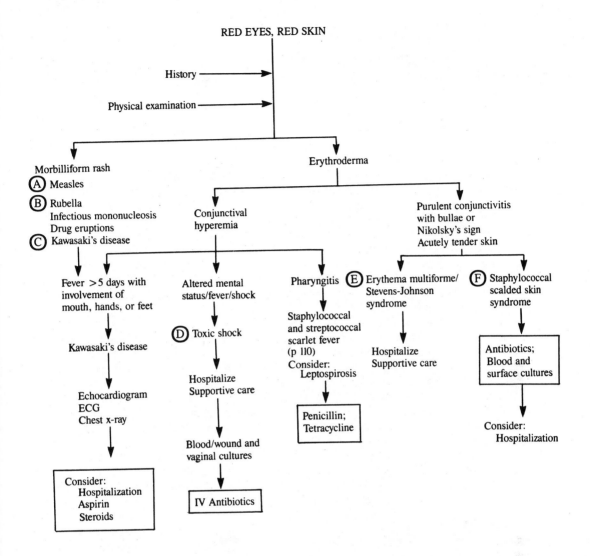

History

Physical examination

Morbilliform rash
(A) Measles
(B) Rubella
    Infectious mononucleosis
    Drug eruptions
(C) Kawasaki's disease

Erythroderma

Conjunctival
hyperemia

Purulent conjunctivitis
with bullae or
Nikolsky's sign
Acutely tender skin

Fever >5 days with
involvement of
mouth, hands, or feet

Kawasaki's disease

Echocardiogram
ECG
Chest x-ray

Consider:
  Hospitalization
  Aspirin
  Steroids

Altered mental
status/fever/shock

(D) Toxic shock

Hospitalize
Supportive care

Blood/wound and
vaginal cultures

IV Antibiotics

Pharyngitis

Staphylococcal
and streptococcal
scarlet fever
(p 110)
Consider:
  Leptospirosis

Penicillin;
Tetracycline

(E) Erythema multiforme/
Stevens-Johnson
syndrome

Hospitalize
Supportive care

(F) Staphylococcal
scalded skin
syndrome

Antibiotics;
Blood and
surface cultures

Consider:
  Hospitalization

115

EVALUATION OF MUSCULOSKELETAL DISORDERS

A. Note the onset, severity and pattern of musculoskeletal pain or arthritis. Identify precipitating factors such as new shoes, local bacterial infections, recent immunizations, viral illness, exercise, and trauma. Ask about exacerbating positions or activities. When pain is associated with acute trauma, determine the patient's activity at the time of the injury (weightbearing vs non-weightbearing). Ask about associated sensations or sounds such as pops, snaps, tearing, or ripping. Rapid onset of hemarthrosis and the inability to bear weight immediately following trauma suggest a grade III sprain, acute dislocation, or intra-articular fracture. Looseness, laxity, or instability of the joint following trauma suggests grade III sprains (complete ligamentous tear). Locking of the knee joint indicates mechanical impingement resulting from an osteochondral loose body or a torn fragment of meniscus. Note any associated symptoms of systemic disease including fever, failure to thrive, chronic diarrhea, and rash. Identify predisposing conditions such as sickle cell disease and other hemoglobinopathies, malignancies, immunodeficency syndromes, or prolonged steroid therapy.

B. Determine the location of all areas of pain and possible joint involvement. Elicit the pain with palpation and movement (active and passive). Note the presence of ecchymosis, bruising, effusion, or hemarthrosis. Document the range of motion (active and passive) of involved joints. Assess the degree of stability of the involved joints. When examining the knee, compress the popliteal space and suprapatellar space to confirm the presence of effusion. Palpate for localized tenderness. Circumferential tenderness indicates a possible intra-articular fracture. Assess the integrity of the medial and lateral collateral ligaments by noting a definite end-point when medial and lateral pressure is applied to the knee in the fully extended and flexed (20°-25°) position. Document the integrity of the anterior cruciate ligament by assessing anterior movement of the tibia (anterior drawer) with the knee flexed 90° and 30°. Document the integrity of the posterior cruciate ligament by observing if the tibia sags backwards with the knee flexed at 90° (posterior drawer sign). When the ankle is involved, assess stability by stabilizing the lower leg and holding the heel firmly in the opposite hand. Pull forward on the heel to determine whether the calcaneus and tallus sublux anteriorly. This determines the intactness of the anterior talofibular ligament. The intactness of the fibulocalcaneal ligament is evaluated by inverting the foot and palpating for tenderness over the ligament. An increased degree of inversion indicates a possible grade III sprain. Widening of the malleoli with the fibula and tibia spread apart suggests a third degree tear of the syndesmosis. Recognize signs of systemic disease including muscle weakness or atrophy, abnormal neurologic reflexes, jaundice and hepatomegaly (hepatitis), mucosal ulcers and rectal fissures (inflammatory bowel disease), lymphadenopathy, vaginal discharge (gonococcal tenosynovitis/arthritis), palpable purpura (Henoch-Schönlein), heart murmurs, bruises, or multiple fractures.

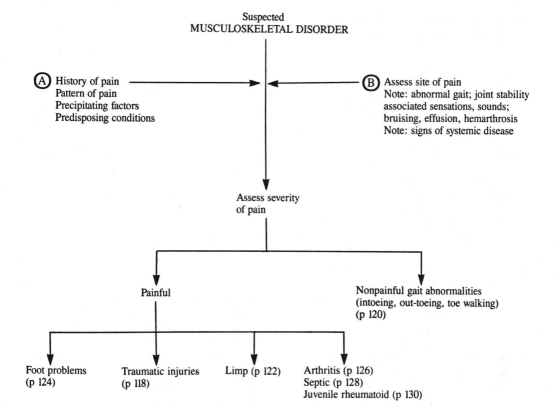

Suspected
MUSCULOSKELETAL DISORDER

Ⓐ History of pain
Pattern of pain
Precipitating factors
Predisposing conditions

Ⓑ Assess site of pain
Note: abnormal gait; joint stability
associated sensations, sounds;
bruising, effusion, hemarthrosis
Note: signs of systemic disease

Assess severity
of pain

Painful

Nonpainful gait abnormalities
(intoeing, out-toeing, toe walking)
(p 120)

Foot problems
(p 124)

Traumatic injuries
(p 118)

Limp (p 122)

Arthritis (p 126)
Septic (p 128)
Juvenile rheumatoid (p 130)

TRAUMATIC INJURIES

A. Treat acute injuries with ice during the first 24–36 hours to provide mild anesthesia, decrease muscle spasm, and reduce effusion or bleeding. Wet part of an Ace bandage and wrap firmly around the injured area. Place an ice bag over the injury and wrap in place with the remainder of the Ace bandage. Elevate the extremity and leave the ice in place for 20 minutes. After 20 minutes remove the ice bag, rewrap the area, and keep the limb elevated. Reapply the ice bag for 20 minutes out of every hour.

B. Consider x-ray examination of the involved joint to identify fractures, bony avulsions, or dislocations. Knee films should include 4 views: AP, lateral, tunnel of the intrachondilar notch, and sunrise of patella. Ankle views should include AP, true lateral, and 45° internal oblique (mortise view). When ligamentous injury is suspected, consider obtaining an AP stress view of the ankle in forced inversion and eversion. Lateral stress views of the ankle are obtained by pulling forward on the calcaneus.

C. Assess the degree of injury. Severe injuries are characterized by a rapid onset of hemarthrosis, inability to bear weight, ligamentous instability, mechanical blockage of the joint, or frozen joint. A moderate injury is characterized by a small and slowly developing effusion or hemarthrosis, crepitation, and moderate pain with specific tenderness. Mild injuries have diffuse pain without a specific area of tenderness and no effusion or hemarthrosis.

D. A compartment syndrome in the musculature of the leg or forearm presents with swelling and severe pain associated with paresthesia which persists after stopping activity. Refer these patients to the orthopedist for fasciotomy.

E. Shin splints resulting from microtears at the origin of the anterior tibialis muscle along the tibia present with diffuse tenderness along the anterior lateral tibia. Suspect a stress fracture when chronic pain progresses to point tenderness over bone. Common areas of involvement include the metatarsals, the distal fibula, the proximal tibia, and the femoral neck. Initial x-rays may be normal, but the bone scan will be diagnostic. Small partial tears of the Achilles tendon result in a tendonitis syndrome.

F. Suspect patellofemoral pain (chondromalacia of the patella) when tenderness is associated with crepitation, a mild effusion, and atrophy of the vastus medialis muscle. Patellar tendinitis (jumper's knee) presents with tenderness over the patellar tendon which is exacerbated by activity. Osgood-Schlatter disease presents with tenderness over the anterior tibial tubercle caused by stress fractures. In osteochondritis dissecans, a fragment of bone beneath the anterior cartilage becomes avascular. The fragment may occasionally become dislodged and cause locking of the knee joint.

G. Implement a rehabilitation program which includes exercises to promote an active range of motion, appropriate muscle strengthening exercises, and stretching exercises. For knee injuries, encourage quadriceps strengthening exercises. Resume ambulation without a knee splint when painless range of motion between extension and 100° of flexion is present (usually 2–3 days).

REFERENCES

Garrick JG. Knee problems in adolescents. Pediatr Rev 1983; 4:235.

Garrick JG. Sports medicine. Pediatr Clin North Am 1977; 24:737.

Harvey J. Ankle injuries in children and adolescents. Pediatr Rev 1981; 2:217.

Sports Medicine: Health Care for Young Medicine, American Academy of Pediatrics, Editor Nathan T. Smith, 1983.

TRAUMATIC INJURY

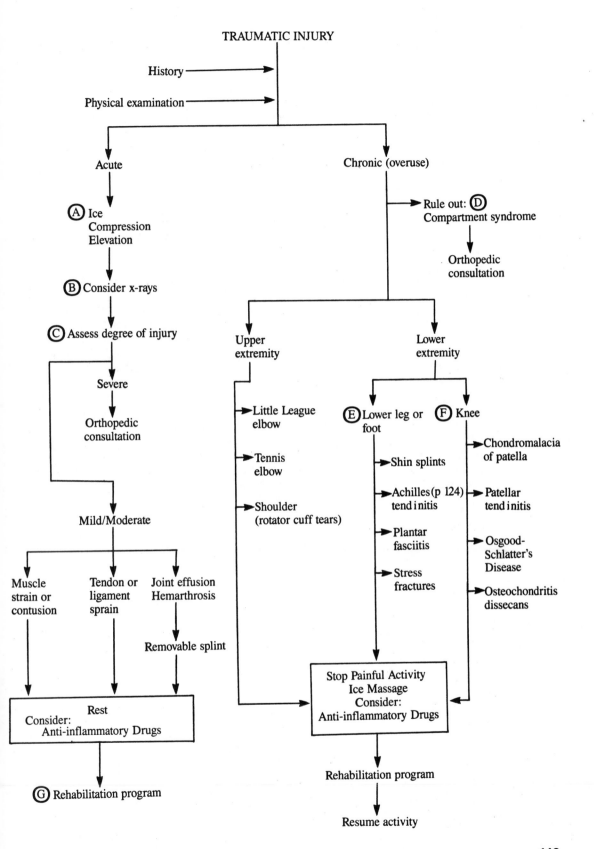

History

Physical examination

Acute

(A) Ice
Compression
Elevation

(B) Consider x-rays

(C) Assess degree of injury

Severe

Orthopedic
consultation

Mild/Moderate

Muscle
strain or
contusion

Tendon or
ligament
sprain

Joint effusion
Hemarthrosis

Removable splint

Rest
Consider:
Anti-inflammatory Drugs

(G) Rehabilitation program

Chronic (overuse)

Rule out: (D)
Compartment syndrome

Orthopedic
consultation

Upper
extremity

Lower
extremity

Little League
elbow

Tennis
elbow

Shoulder
(rotator cuff tears)

(E) Lower leg or
foot

(F) Knee

Shin splints

Achilles (p 124)
tendinitis

Plantar
fasciitis

Stress
fractures

Chondromalacia
of patella

Patellar
tendinitis

Osgood-
Schlatter's
Disease

Osteochondritis
dissecans

Stop Painful Activity
Ice Massage
Consider:
Anti-inflammatory Drugs

Rehabilitation program

Resume activity

ABNORMAL GAIT

A. Observe as the child walks along a straight line. Toe walking or tiptoeing is the sign of a tight heel cord. Assess the angle of gait by estimating the angle of each step within a straight line of progression. Define intoeing as a negative angle and out-toeing as a positive angle. A normal angle of gait has a range of 0°–30°. Note the position of the patella when the child walks. Medial deviation indicates the problem is above the knee.

B. Signs of metatarsus adductus or medial deviation of the forefoot include a convexity of the lateral side of the foot, a wide space between the first and second toes, and a prominence at the base of the fifth metatarsal. A fixed crease at the base of the metatarsals suggests a fixed deformity. Treat a flexible deformity with home exercises. Have the mother stabilize the heel with one hand and repeatedly abduct the forefoot with the other into the correct position. Refer children with fixed or rigid deformities to the orthopedist for serial plaster casting followed by braces or outflared shoes to maintain the correction.

C. Femoral anteversion produces intoeing because of excessive internal rotation of the hip. Assess the degree of rotation of the hip with the child prone, the pelvis flat on the table, and the hips in a neutral position. Allow each leg to drop by gravity into full internal and external rotation. Internal rotation should not exceed 70°; the sum of internal and external rotation should approximate 100°. Femoral anteversion should correct spontaneously. The parents should encourage the child to sit cross-legged. Exercises, braces and orthopedic shoes are not indicated. Consider a derotational osteotomy (major surgery) only in children older than 8 years who suffer a severe impairment.

D. Internal tibial torsion commonly occurs in children under 2 years of age. The amount of internal tibial torsion can be estimated by measuring the angle formed by the axis of the thigh and the foot with the child prone and the knee flexed 90°. The normal range of the angle is between 0° and 30° of external rotation. A severe degree of internal tibial torsion prevents the child from walking normally. Refer these patients to the orthopedist for a Denis Browne splint. Advise parents of children with mild or moderate disease to prevent their child from sleeping or sitting on their legs with in-turned toes.

REFERENCES

Staheli LT. Torsional deformity. Pediatr Clin North Am 1977; 24:799.

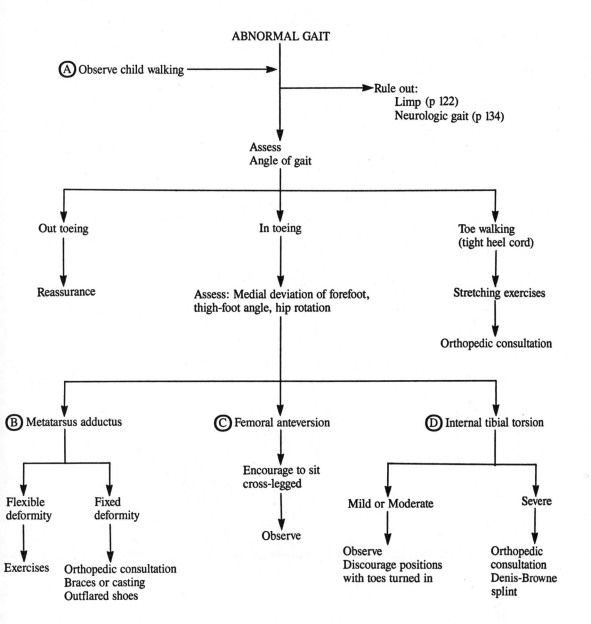

ABNORMAL GAIT

(A) Observe child walking ⟶ Rule out:
Limp (p 122)
Neurologic gait (p 134)

Assess
Angle of gait

Out toeing

In toeing

Toe walking
(tight heel cord)

Reassurance

Assess: Medial deviation of forefoot,
thigh-foot angle, hip rotation

Stretching exercises

Orthopedic consultation

(B) Metatarsus adductus

(C) Femoral anteversion

(D) Internal tibial torsion

Flexible
deformity

Fixed
deformity

Encourage to sit
cross-legged

Mild or Moderate

Severe

Exercises

Orthopedic consultation
Braces or casting
Outflared shoes

Observe

Observe
Discourage positions
with toes turned in

Orthopedic
consultation
Denis-Browne
splint

121

LIMP

A. Suspect congenital hip dislocation when a limp is associated with asymmetry of buttock and thigh creases, decreased external rotation of the hip, and unequal leg lengths. Measure leg length from the anterior superior iliac crest to the medial malleolus.

B. Suspect neurologic disease when muscle weakness or atrophy is present. Note signs of spinal cord or peripheral nerve involvement. Do a rectal examination to determine the presence of a sacral mass.

C. Causes of myalgia which present with limp include exercise, trauma, recent immunization, viral infections (Coxsackie virus, influenza virus), bacterial infections (trichinosis, toxoplasmosis), and collagen vascular diseases (dermatomysitis, lupus erythematosus, polyarteritis nodosa, rheumatoid arthritis, polymyositis).

D. Obtain an x-ray of the involved bones or joints to identify infection, fracture, aseptic necrosis, or mass. When knee pain is present, consider hip disease; pelvic osteomyelitis, discitis, neuroblastoma, or acute leukemia when pain is difficult to localize. Consider a bone scan to diagnose bone or joint infections when initial x-rays are normal since bone destruction and periosteal reaction secondary to infection may not be seen for 10–14 days. Deep soft–tissue swelling at the metaphysis and muscle swelling with loss of intermuscular planes may be seen after 3–5 days. Bone scans may fail to identify early infection or infection in children under 2 years of age.

E. Aseptic necrosis can occur in the vertebral body (Scheuermann's disease), the hip (Legg-Calvé-Perthes disease), the knee (Osgood-Schlatter's disease), or the foot (Freiberg's disease). Cases associated with severe pain should be referred to the orthopedist for immobilization.

F. Malignant tumors include osteogenic sarcoma, Ewing's sarcoma, lymphoma, soft tissue sarcoma, histiocytosis, neuroblastoma, and rabdomyosarcoma. Benign tumors include osteoid osteoma, unicameral cyst, Baker's cyst, fibrous dysplasia, aneurysmal bone cysts, giant–cell tumor, osteochrondroma, hemangioma, and lymphangioma.

G. Osteomyelitis occurs in long bones, the pelvis, or the vertebral bodies. Neonatal osteomyelitis is most frequently associated with streptococci (43%), staphlococci (29%), and gram–negative enterics (19%). After the neonatal period, *S. aureus* is the most common cause of osteomyelitis. Suspect *H. influenzae* infection when osteomyelitis occurs in children under two years of age in association with septic arthritis. Suspect Pseudomonas infection when osteomyelitis of the foot is related to puncture wounds through tennis shoes. Consider salmonella infection in children with sickle cell disease. Subperiosteal aspirates are positive in 70% of cases and blood cultures in 60% of cases. Initial antibiotic therapy is based on Gram stain results, clinical presentation, and patient age. Treat neonatal osteomyelitis with a penicillinase-resistant penicillin and an aminoglycoside. After the neonatal period, use a semisynthetic penicillin. Treat Pseudomonas infections with carbenicillin or ticarcillin in combination with an aminoglycoside. Surgical curettage is necessary when a sequestrum (segment of bone has been separated from its blood supply) has developed.

H. Discitis can cause limp. The etiology of this disorder is unclear since aspirates of the disc space are often negative. When positive *S. aureus* is usually isolated. Tuberculosis, nonstaphylococcal gram–positive organisms, and gram–negative organisms are rare causes. Therapy consists of antibiotics and immobilization. Persistent severe pain indicates the need for needle aspiration of the joint space.

REFERENCES

Berkowitz ID, Wenzel W. Normal technetium bone scans in patients with acute osteomyelitis. Am J Dis Child 1980; 134:828.

Doughty RA. Limp. In: Fleisher G, Ludwig S, eds. Pediatric Emergency Medicine. Baltimore: Williams & Wilkins, 1983:185.

Hensinger RH. Limp: symposium on common orthopedic problems. Pediatr Clin North Am 1977; 24:723.

Peterson HA. Leg aches: symposium on common orthopedic problems. Pediatr Clin North Am 1977; 24:731.

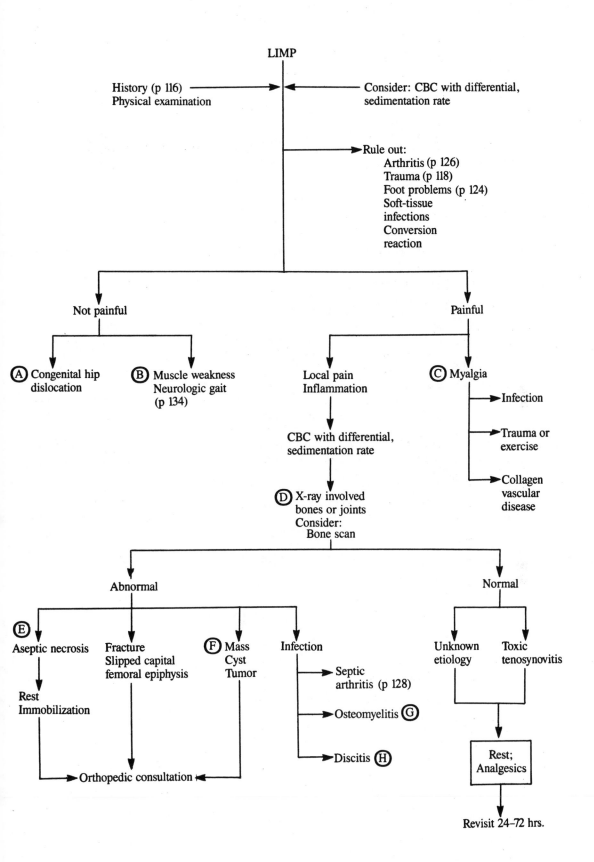

LIMP

History (p 116) → ← Consider: CBC with differential,
Physical examination   sedimentation rate

Rule out:
    Arthritis (p 126)
    Trauma (p 118)
    Foot problems (p 124)
    Soft-tissue
    infections
    Conversion
    reaction

Not painful

Ⓐ Congenital hip
   dislocation

Ⓑ Muscle weakness
   Neurologic gait
   (p 134)

Painful

Local pain
Inflammation

CBC with differential,
sedimentation rate

Ⓓ X-ray involved
   bones or joints
   Consider:
   Bone scan

Ⓒ Myalgia

→ Infection

→ Trauma or
   exercise

→ Collagen
   vascular
   disease

Abnormal

Ⓔ Aseptic necrosis

Rest
Immobilization

Fracture
Slipped capital
femoral epiphysis

Ⓕ Mass
   Cyst
   Tumor

Infection

→ Septic
  arthritis (p 128)

→ Osteomyelitis Ⓖ

→ Discitis Ⓗ

Orthopedic consultation ←

Normal

Unknown
etiology

Toxic
tenosynovitis

Rest;
Analgesics

Revisit 24–72 hrs.

FOOT PAIN

A. Observe the child's effort to avoid pain while walking. Note any sign of soft tissue infection or injury, foreign body, paronychia, or plantar warts. Suspect a problem with shoes if the child can walk normally barefoot. Examine the feet in both the standing and non-weight-bearing positions. Most infants and young children have a plantar fat pad causing a flat foot appearance. In older children, flat feet are most frequently caused by joint hypermobility. In these cases, the longitudinal arch appears in the non-weight-bearing position but disappears on standing. A tight heel cord causing decreased dorsi and plantar flexion at the ankle, results in toe walking. Decreased subtalar motion (inversion and eversion) associated with muscle spasm suggests a tarsal coalition, an accessory navicular bone, or a vertical talus.

B. A mass over the medial aspect of the foot distal to the medial malleolus suggests an accessory navicular bone. This bone may cause spasm of the posterior tibial tendon; when associated with pain, it should be surgically removed. An abnormally high arch or cavus deformity can present with foot pain as weight bearing is located almost entirely on the metatarsal heads and heel. Callouses under the metatarsal heads and claw toes are frequent complications. If metatarsal pads do not provide adequate relief, surgery may be necessary. Consider underlying neurologic disease in cases where the cavus deformity is asymmetric, severe, and progressive. Foot tumors, rare in childhood, include benign osteoid osteoma, Ewing's sarcoma, and synovial sarcoma.

C. A bony ridge between the bones of the mid- or hind foot produces a tarsal coalition. This problem is associated with decreased ankle inversion and eversion and can cause spasm of the peroneal muscles resulting in a rigid, spastic foot. Obtain x-rays, including an oblique non-weight bearing view. Early surgery is indicated prior to the development of secondary degenerative changes.

D. Avascular necrosis of the foot bones is usually asymptomatic. The most common sites of involvement are the navicular or calcaneous bones. Treat a painful heel with a shoe elevation or a heel cup. Aseptic necrosis of the second metatarsal head (Freiberg's disease) can cause severe pain and significant disability.

E. Overuse injuries (p 63) caused by chronic trauma to the foot result in stress fractures or Achilles tendonitis. Stress fractures often have negative x-rays initially, with callus or bone reabsorption only becoming apparent in 10–14 days. Small partial tears of the Achilles tendon result in a tendonitis syndrome.

REFERENCES

Gross RH. Foot pain in children. Pediatr Clin North Am 1977; 24:813.

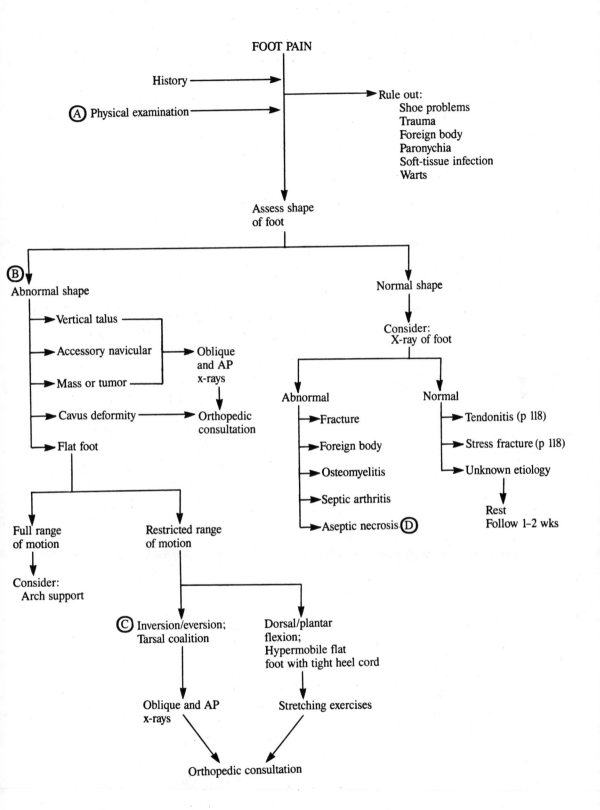

FOOT PAIN

History ─────────→

Ⓐ Physical examination ─────────→

Rule out:
  Shoe problems
  Trauma
  Foreign body
  Paronychia
  Soft-tissue infection
  Warts

Assess shape
of foot

Ⓑ Abnormal shape

→ Vertical talus ──────┐
                       │
→ Accessory navicular ─┼──→ Oblique
                       │   and AP
→ Mass or tumor ───────┘   x-rays

→ Cavus deformity ──────→ Orthopedic
                          consultation
→ Flat foot

Full range   Restricted range
of motion   of motion

Consider:
Arch support

Ⓒ Inversion/eversion;   Dorsal/plantar
   Tarsal coalition   flexion;
                             Hypermobile flat
                             foot with tight heel cord

Oblique and AP   Stretching exercises
x-rays

Orthopedic consultation

Normal shape

Consider:
X-ray of foot

Abnormal   Normal

→ Fracture   → Tendonitis (p 118)

→ Foreign body   → Stress fracture (p 118)

→ Osteomyelitis   → Unknown etiology

→ Septic arthritis

→ Aseptic necrosis Ⓓ   Rest
                            Follow 1–2 wks

ARTHRITIS

A. Determine the onset, precipitating factors (drugs, trauma, bacteria), and duration of arthritis. Suspect juvenile rheumatoid arthritis when the duration exceeds 6 weeks. A sudden onset suggests trauma, infection, or vasculitis.

B. Determine the pattern of joint involvement. Consider JRA when symmetrical polyarticular disease is associated with cervical spine involvement. The involvement of sacroiliac joints or the lumbosacral spine in a male suggests ankylosing spondylitis. Sexually active adolescents who present with polyarthralgias and polytendonitis require a workup to diagnose gonococcal disease. Monoarticular or polyarticular involvement suggests septic, postinfectious, traumatic, or juvenile rheumatoid arthritis. The most common sites for septic arthritis are the knees (40%) and hips (20%) followed by the shoulders, elbows, ankles, and wrists.

C. The CBC with differential helps to identify patients with a malignancy, sickle cell disease, or infection. While an elevated sedimentation rate usually suggests an inflammatory process, one-third of patients with JRA can present with a normal sedimentation rate. Findings on joint x-rays include effusions, lytic lesions, bone destruction, fracture, periostitis, leukemic lines, avascular necrosis, and osteoporosis.

D. Signs which suggest systemic disease include jaundice (hepatitis); diarrhea, bloody stools, abdominal pain, perianal disease, and weight loss (bacterial enteritis, inflammatory bowel disease); palpable purpura, abdominal pain, bloody stools, hematuria (Henoch-Schonlein purpura), conjunctivitis, cracked lips, prolonged fever, lymphadenopathy and rash (Kawasaki's disease); hepatosplenomegaly, chronic fevers, weight loss, lymphadenopathy (malignancy); scaly rash and nailbed pitting (psoriasis); vaginal discharge, PID (gonorrhea); multiple bruises (coagulation disorders and nonaccidental trauma); and joint hypermobility (Ehlers-Danlos syndrome).

E. An ANA titer > 1:80 suggests SLE. The diagnosis requires the presence of at least 4 of the following 14 findings; butterfly rash, discoid lesions, alopecia, Raynaud's phenomena, photosensitivity, oral or nasal pharyngeal ulceration, arthritis, LE cells, false positive VDRL, proteinuria, urine cellular casts, pleuritis or pericarditis, seizures or psychosis, hemolytic anemia, leukopenia or thrombocytopenia. Work up suspected SLE with complement, anti DNA antibodies, and urinalysis.

F. Analyze the effusion from joint aspiration for cell count, differential, glucose, mucin clot formation, Gram stain, and CIE. Septic arthritis usually has more than 50,000 WBCs with a predominance of neutrophils (>90%), a glucose <20 mg/100, and a poor mucin clot. Aseptic inflammatory effusions (rheumatoid, postinfectious, and vasculitis) often have 10,000 to 50,000 WBCs with 50–80% neutrophils, glucose 20–50 mg/100, and a fair-to-poor mucin clot. Traumatic effusions have <2000 WBCs with 10–30% neutrophils, glucose >50 mg/100, and a good mucin clot. Xanthocromia and crenated red cells suggest old trauma.

G. The diagnosis of rheumatic fever requires 2 major Jones criteria or 1 major and 2 minor criteria with evidence of an antecedent streptococcal infection (positive culture, ASO titer, or scarlet fever). The major Jones criteria include carditis, migratory polyarthritis, chorea, erythema marginatum, and subcutaneous nodules. The minor criteria are fever, arthralgia, prior rheumatic fever, elevated ESR or CRP and a prolonged PR interval.

REFERENCES

Brewer EJ. Differential diagnoses of arthritis in children. Pediatr Rev 1979; 1:154.
Keat A. Reiter's syndrome and reactive arthritis in perspective. N Engl J Med 1983; 309:1606.
Schaller JG. Arthritis and infections of bones and joints in children. Pediatr Clin North Am 1977; 24:775.
Wedgwood R, Schaller JG. The pediatric arthritides. Hosp Prac 1977; June:83.
Ziai M. Patient management problems: arthritis with a rash. Pediatr Rev 1979; 1:173.

ARTHRITIS

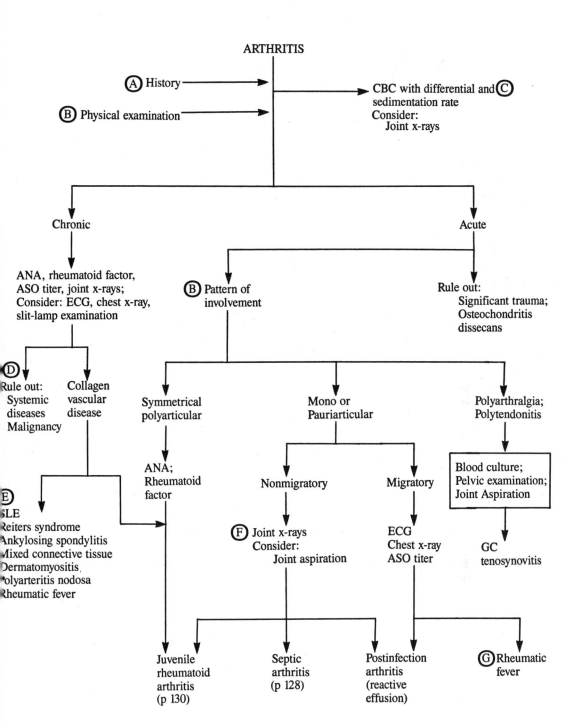

(A) History

(B) Physical examination

(C) CBC with differential and
sedimentation rate
Consider:
    Joint x-rays

Chronic

ANA, rheumatoid factor,
ASO titer, joint x-rays;
Consider: ECG, chest x-ray,
slit-lamp examination

(D) Rule out:
Systemic
diseases
Malignancy

Collagen
vascular
disease

(E) SLE
Reiters syndrome
Ankylosing spondylitis
Mixed connective tissue
Dermatomyositis
Polyarteritis nodosa
Rheumatic fever

Acute

(B) Pattern of
involvement

Rule out:
Significant trauma;
Osteochondritis
dissecans

Symmetrical
polyarticular

Mono or
Pauriarticular

Polyarthralgia;
Polytendonitis

ANA;
Rheumatoid
factor

Nonmigratory

Migratory

Blood culture;
Pelvic examination;
Joint Aspiration

(F) Joint x-rays
Consider:
    Joint aspiration

ECG
Chest x-ray
ASO titer

GC
tenosynovitis

Juvenile
rheumatoid
arthritis
(p 130)

Septic
arthritis
(p 128)

Postinfection
arthritis
(reactive
effusion)

(G) Rheumatic
fever

127

SEPTIC ARTHRITIS

A. Joint fluid with a white blood cell count >50,000 with a predominance of neutrophils, a low glucose level, and a friable clot, suggests a pyogenic process. Gram stain and culture are positive in 60% of cases with septic arthritis. A CIE for *S. pneumoniae* or *H. influenzae* type B can be positive despite negative cultures. Blood cultures are positive in 40% of cases of septic arthritis. Consider lumbar puncture in children under 2 years of age, because associated *H. influenzae* bacteremia predisposes the child to meningitis.

B. Surgical drainage is the initial treatment of choice for septic arthritis of the shoulder or hip, in order to prevent disruption of the blood supply to the intra-articular epiphysis. Surgical drainage is also recommended for infections associated with *S. aureus* because of the potential destructive effect of this organism on intra-articular cartilage.

C. The choice of initial IV antibiotic therapy is based on the Gram stain and the age of the patient. Neonatal septic arthritis is usually caused by staphylococci, streptococci, or coliform species. A semisynthetic penicillin, oxacillin or nafcillin (150–200 mg/kg/day) and an aminoglycoside, gentamicin (5–7.5 mg/kg/day) or cefotaxime (150 mg/kg/day) provide the broad coverage needed in this age group. In children under age 5 years, *H. influenzae* type B is the most common organism associated with septic arthritis. Other organisms in decreasing frequency are *S. aureus*, *S. pyogenes*, and *S. pneumoniae*. In this age group, use a semisynthetic penicillin plus chloramphenicol (100 mg/kg/day) or cefotaxime. In older children and adolescents, the most common organisms are *S. aureus*, *S. pyogenes*, and *N. gonorrhoeae*; a semisynthetic penicillin provides appropriate therapy. Children with sickle cell disease with septic arthritis should be treated with chloramphenicol in order to cover salmonella infection. Subsequent IV therapy should be based on culture results.

D. Signs of adequate clinical response include: decreased swelling and pain, decreased sedimentation rate, and loss of fever. Oral therapy may then be started and the dosage designed to produce a peak serum bactericidal titer >1:8. Treat *N. gonorrhoeae* infections for 7–10 days, *H. influenzae* infections 14–21 days, and other bacterial infections for at least 30 days.

REFERENCES

Aronoff SC, Scoles PV. Treatment of childhood skeletal infections. Pediatr Clin North Am 1983; 30:271.
DeLiberti JH, Tarlow S. Bone and joint complications of *Hemophilus influenzae* meningitis. Clin Ped 1983; 22:7.
Telzlaff TR, McCracken GR Jr, Nelson JD. Oral antibiotic therapy for skeletal infections of children. J Pediatr 1978; 92:485.

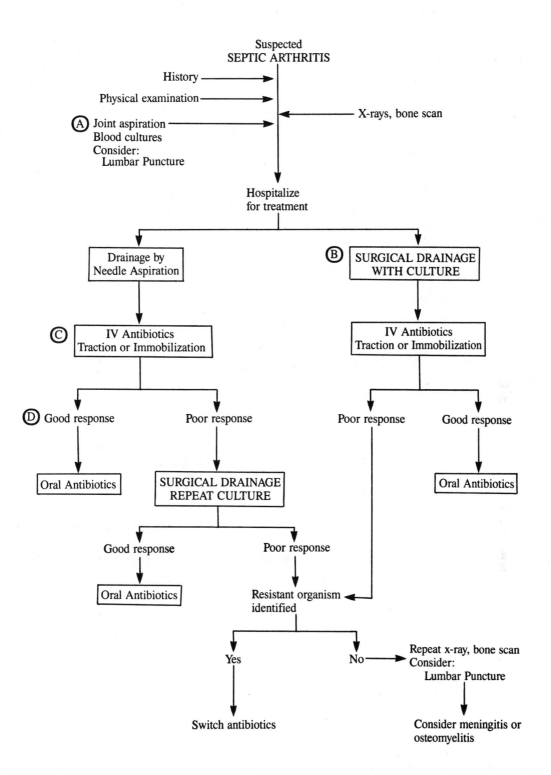

Suspected
SEPTIC ARTHRITIS

History ⟶

Physical examination ⟶

Ⓐ Joint aspiration ⟶   ⟵ X-rays, bone scan
Blood cultures
Consider:
  Lumbar Puncture

Hospitalize
for treatment

Drainage by
Needle Aspiration

Ⓑ SURGICAL DRAINAGE
WITH CULTURE

Ⓒ IV Antibiotics
Traction or Immobilization

IV Antibiotics
Traction or Immobilization

Ⓓ Good response   Poor response

Poor response   Good response

Oral Antibiotics

SURGICAL DRAINAGE
REPEAT CULTURE

Oral Antibiotics

Good response   Poor response

Oral Antibiotics

Resistant organism ⟵
identified

Yes   No ⟶ Repeat x-ray, bone scan
Consider:
  Lumbar Puncture

Switch antibiotics   Consider meningitis or
osteomyelitis

JUVENILE RHEUMATOID ARTHRITIS

A. History, physical examination, and laboratory screening are intended to categorize children into one of three forms of juvenile rheumatoid arthritis (JRA): systemic, pauciarticular, or polyarticular. *Systemic* JRA is characterized by spiking fever, hepatosplenomegaly, lymphadenopathy, pericarditis, and cervical spine involvement. The pauciarticular form presents with a history of asymmetrical arthritis for >72 hours and is often associated with a positive ANA and/or HLA B27 antigen. Iridocyclitis is most frequently associated with this type of JRA. The polyarticular form is subdivided into rheumatoid factor seronegative and seropositive disease. Seronegative disease has a more favorable prognosis and is characterized by symmetrical polyarthritis, low grade fever, mild anemia, moderate hepatosplenomegaly, and a positive ANA in 25% of cases. Seropositive disease has a poor prognosis and is characterized by destructive symmetrical polyarthritis, rheumatoid nodules, and a positive ANA in 75% of cases. In mild cases of JRA, the child is afebrile and experiences mild pain with minimal limitation of activity. Moderate involvement is characterized by recurrent fevers and pain, with moderate limitation of activity. In severe JRA, the child has incapacitating fever, anemia, iridocyclitis, pericarditis, or incapacitating pain.

B. Salicylate therapy should be instituted and therapeutic blood levels of 20–30 mg/100 ml documented. Liver function tests should be followed during therapy. A good response is achieved when fever is controlled and pain, joint swelling, and range of motion improve. Definite improvement should occur in 2–6 weeks.

C. Use alternative anti-inflammatory agents when the desired therapeutic response is not achieved. In addition to tolectin, consider ferroprofen (Nalfen), ibuprofen (Motrin), naproxen (Naprosyn), or sulindac (Clinerol). Failure of these agents to relieve symptoms is an indication for gold therapy and possibly steroids.

D. If symptoms of severe disease persist or develop with salicylate therapy (pericarditis, severe anemia, high fever, iridocyclitis), consider starting prednisone 1–2 mg/kg/day after obtaining bone marrow to rule out occult malignancy. Use systemic steroids with great caution because of their adverse affects on bone mineralization.

REFERENCES

Schaller JG. Juvenile rheumatoid arthritis. Pediatr Rev 1980; 2:163.

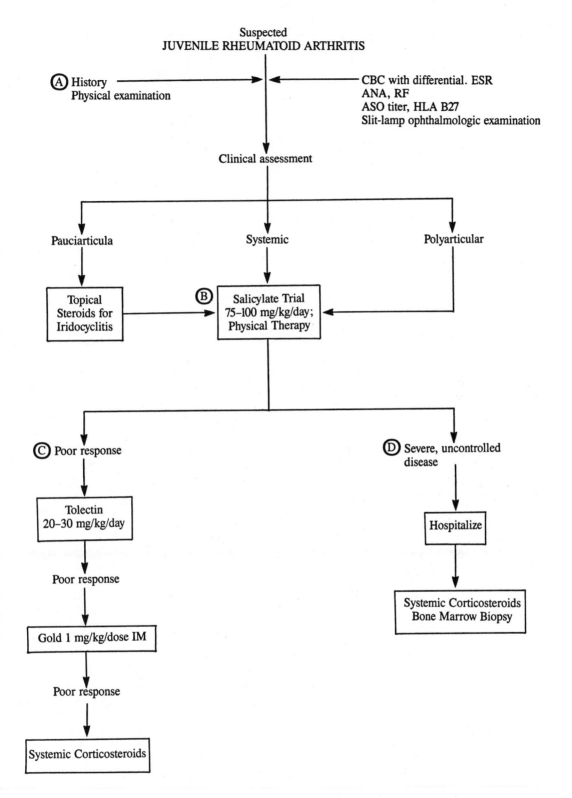

Suspected
JUVENILE RHEUMATOID ARTHRITIS

(A) History
Physical examination

CBC with differential. ESR
ANA, RF
ASO titer, HLA B27
Slit-lamp ophthalmologic examination

Clinical assessment

Pauciarticula — Systemic — Polyarticular

Topical
Steroids for
Iridocyclitis

(B) Salicylate Trial
75–100 mg/kg/day;
Physical Therapy

(C) Poor response

Tolectin
20–30 mg/kg/day

Poor response

Gold 1 mg/kg/dose IM

Poor response

Systemic Corticosteroids

(D) Severe, uncontrolled
disease

Hospitalize

Systemic Corticosteroids
Bone Marrow Biopsy

EVALUATION OF A SUSPECTED NEUROLOGIC DISORDER

A. Determine the onset, duration, frequency, course, and severity of neurologic symptoms. Symptoms that suggest increased intracranial pressure include nausea and protracted vomiting, severe headache, and altered mental status. Focal neurologic signs and visual disturbances suggest a cerebral mass lesion. Personality changes (recent memory loss, decreased attention span, regressive behavior, emotional lability, and decline in school performance) suggest a mass lesion or degenerative process. Document the attainment of appropriate developmental milestones. Determine the history of any perinatal or subsequent cerebral insults (anoxia, hypoglycemia, intracranial hemorrhage, head trauma), central nervous system infections, and CNS anomalies (hydrocephalus, AV malformations, tumors, cysts, Arnold-Chiari syndrome, myelomeningocele). Note systemic diseases such as collagen vascular disease, malignancy, renal disease, bleeding disorders, immune deficiency syndromes, and cardiac disease (right to left shunt and bacterial endocarditis). Document adequate vaccination against polio and diphtheria. Identify relevant precipitating factors such as medication or drug ingestion, bacterial infection, viral infection, tick exposure, child abuse or nonaccidental trauma, and significant family or school problems. Determine the family history for CNS disorders (migraine headaches, seizure disorders), myopathies, hypertension, bleeding disorders, and inborn errors of metabolism.
B. Assess mental status, cranial nerves, the motor and sensory systems, cerebellar function, and deep tendon reflexes. Check for signs of meningeal irritation (stiff neck, Kernig's sign, and Brudzinski's sign) and the presence of pathological reflexes. Document the blood pressure and vital signs. Evaluate patients with an altered mental status with an assessment of brain dysfunction (level of consciousness, pattern of breathing, pupillary size and reflexes, oculomotor function, and motor responses; determine the Glasgow coma score (p 148). Assess weakness during infancy by suspending the infant in the horizontal position. Observe the older child while walking, and test muscle strength by having the child walk on both toes and heels noticing a positive Gower's sign (inability to rise directly from the floor without climbing up on oneself). Palpate the muscles to assess tone, increased firmness, hypertrophy, or atrophy. Evaluate the resistance in each extremity noting differences in upper and lower extremity tone. Note the type of posturing (frog leg), the amount of spontaneous antigravity movement, and the presence of fasciculations, ptosis, contractures, and hip dislocation. Distinguish weakness from paralysis (absent movements and deep tendon reflexes), and document the distribution of the affected muscles (symmetrical vs asymmetrical and proximal vs distal).
C. Assess cerebellar function (motor coordination) by observing the child walk and turn quickly, stand with the feet together, sit without support, perform finger to nose and heel to knee tests, and rapid alternating movements of the hands and feet. Note the presence or absence of nystagmus. Assess the sensory system. Loss of sensation and the distribution of a nerve (stocking glove) suggest a peripheral neuropathy. Assess the deep tendon reflexes. The knee reflexes are innervated at the L3-L4 level and the ankle reflexes at the S1 level. The absence of an anal wink reflex suggests spinal cord or conus involvement. Observe the skin for signs of a neurocutaneous disorder, and note the presence of a defect on the spine such as a hairy patch or hemangioma that may overlie a deeper abnormality. Perform a complete ophthalmologic evaluation. Note the size and reactivity of the pupils and integrity of the extraocular eye movements. Visualize the fundi to identify papilledema, retinal hemorrhages, exudates, or abnormal pigmentation.

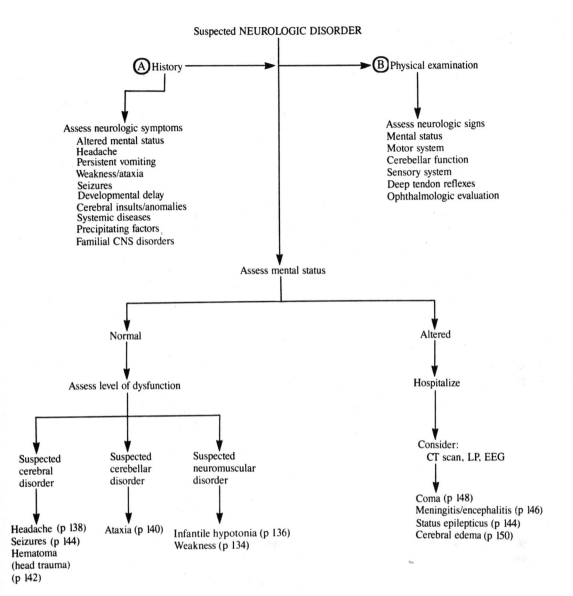

Suspected NEUROLOGIC DISORDER

(A) History → → (B) Physical examination

Assess neurologic symptoms
  Altered mental status
  Headache
  Persistent vomiting
  Weakness/ataxia
  Seizures
  Developmental delay
  Cerebral insults/anomalies
  Systemic diseases
  Precipitating factors
  Familial CNS disorders

Assess neurologic signs
  Mental status
  Motor system
  Cerebellar function
  Sensory system
  Deep tendon reflexes
  Ophthalmologic evaluation

Assess mental status

Normal

Assess level of dysfunction

Altered

Hospitalize

Suspected cerebral disorder

Suspected cerebellar disorder

Suspected neuromuscular disorder

Consider:
  CT scan, LP, EEG

Headache (p 138)
Seizures (p 144)
Hematoma (head trauma) (p 142)

Ataxia (p 140)

Infantile hypotonia (p 136)
Weakness (p 134)

Coma (p 148)
Meningitis/encephalitis (p 146)
Status epilepticus (p 144)
Cerebral edema (p 150)

CHILDHOOD WEAKNESS

A. Causes of myoglobinuria with weakness include physical overexertion, infection, genetic disorders, and idiopathic rhabdomyolysis. Suspect acute intermittent porphyria when abdominal pain and altered mental function are associated with porphyrins in the urine. Periodic paralysis, an autosomal dominant familial disorder, can be associated with hypokalemia.

B. Paralysis is identified by the absence of active movement and deep tendon reflexes. The acute sudden onset of paralysis suggests a CNS hemorrhage or spinal cord trauma. A spinal mass, tumor, or infarction may be associated with symmetrical involvement, loss of the anal reflex, rectal or urinary incontinence and recurrent urinary tract infections. Asymmetrical involvement is most likely due to lesions at, or distal to, the nerve root. Loss of sensation in the distribution of a nerve or a stocking-glove distribution suggests a peripheral neuropathy. Consider the possibility of a conversion reaction when paralysis or weakness occurs in a nonanatomical pattern and the patient is capable of withdrawal movements to appropriate stimuli.

C. Neurotoxins that prevent the release of acetylcholine at the nerve endings are produced by ticks, diphtheria, and *C. botulinum*. Removal of the offending tick brings a rapid relief of symptoms. Botulism presents with blurred vision, loss of accommodation, diplopia, and constipation in association with weakness or paralysis of the extremities. Consider *C. diphtheriae* in the inadequately immunized child with a prior history of severe exudative pharyngitis and myocarditis. Myasthenia gravis results from failure of neuromuscular transmission caused by antibodies against acetylcholine receptors. The administration of Tensilon produces improvement in patients with myasthenia.

D. A motor unit consists of an anterior horn cell, its axon, and the muscle fibers it innervates. In myopathic disorders, individual muscle fibers are destroyed and electromyography reveals small motor unit potentials. In neuropathic disorders involving the anterior horn cells or peripheral nerves, the motor units are increased in size and electrical potentials are large. Nerve conduction studies assess the function of motor and sensory nerves. A relatively normal conduction velocity associated with decreased amplitude suggests axonal pathology related to metabolic disorders. Markedly decreased nerve conduction velocity suggests demyelination caused by Guillain-Barré syndrome, inflammatory neuropathies, or leukodystrophies. The muscle biopsy in addition to separating myopathic and neuropathic disorders may be helpful in characterizing the type of myopathy.

E. Myopathic disorders include muscular dystrophy, myotonic dystrophy, central core disease, nemaline rod, myotubular myopathy, fiber type disproportion, and others. Suspect Duchenne's (X-linked) muscular dystrophy in a boy when a Gower sign (inability to rise directly from the floor without climbing up on oneself), difficulty in toe walking, pseudohypertrophy, and a markedly elevated CPK(>2000) are present. Onset is usually between 2 and 5 years of age with a course characterized by progressive weakness, contractures, scoliosis, and eventual cardiac and pulmonary failure.

F. Guillain-Barré syndrome often presents with symmetrical progressive motor weakness and areflexia. Cranial nerve involvement and signs of autonomic dysfunction may be present. CSF examination reveals elevated protein levels in association with absent or slight pleocytosis (<10 WBCs/mm³). Symptoms generally progress for the first 4 weeks, then plateau for 2 to 4 weeks prior to recovery. Transverse myelitis is a parainfectious process resulting in inflammation and infarction of the spinal cord. Suspect this entity when acute flaccid paralysis of lower extremities, sensory loss to pain and temperature, and rectal and bladder incontinence are present. No specific therapy is available. Suspect poliomyelitis in the patient with asymmetric involvement, CSF pleocytosis, and signs of meningeal irritation. Anterior horn cell disease can present in an intermediate form between 6 months and 2 years and in a juvenile form after 2 years of age. Suspect a leukodystrophy when signs of both upper and lower motor neuron disease are present.

CHILDHOOD WEAKNESS

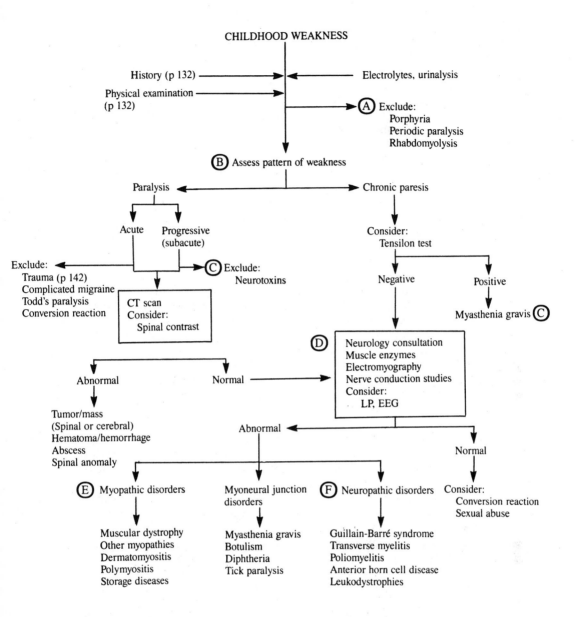

REFERENCES

Freeman JM. Diagnosis and evaluation of acute paraplegia. Pediatr Rev 1983; 4:327.

Kaplan J, Rabinowich L, Burger A. Modern electrodiagnostic studies in infants and children. Pediatr Ann 1984; 13:150.

Nellhaus G, Stumpf DA, Moe PG. Neurologic and muscular disorders. In: Kempe CH, Silver HK, O'Brien D, eds. Current Pediatric Diagnosis and Treatment. 8th ed. Los Altos, California: Lange Medical Publications, 1984.

INFANTILE HYPOTONIA

A. Paralysis (absent or markedly diminished deep tendon reflexes and antigravity movements) suggests lower motor neuron disorders involving the anterior horn cell, peripheral nerve, neuromuscular junction, or muscle. Nonparalytic weakness suggests an upper motor neuron disorder involving the extrapyramidal-pyramidal cortex, basal ganglia, cerebellum, brain stem, or spinal cord.

B. Identifiable congenital syndromes associated with hypotonia include trisomy 21, congenital hypothyroidism, Ehlers-Danlos syndrome, Prader-Willi syndrome, Laurence-Moon-Biedl syndrome, and congenital brain anomalies (hydrocephalus, Dandy-Walker cyst, Arnold-Chiari syndrome).

C. A motor unit consists of the anterior horn cell, its axon and the muscle fibers it innervates. In myopathic disorders, individual muscle fibers are lost and electromyography (EMG) demonstrates small motor unit potentials. In neuropathic disorders involving the anterior horn cell or peripheral nerves, the motor units have increased size and motor unit potentials. Nerve conduction studies assess the function of peripheral motor and sensory nerves. A relatively normal conduction velocity associated with decreased amplitude suggests axonal pathology related to metabolic disorders. A markedly decreased nerve conduction velocity associated with asynchronous evoked potentials suggests demyelinization caused by Guillain-Barré syndrome, inflammatory polyneuropathies, and leukodystrophies. The muscle biopsy, in addition to separating myopathic from neuropathic disorders, may be helpful in characterizing the specific type of myopathy.

D. Myopathic disorders include myotonic dystrophy, muscular dystrophy, central core disease, nemaline rod, myotubular myopathy, fiber type disproportion, and other myopathies. Myotonic dystrophy is the most common infantile genetic myopathy. It presents in early infancy with poor feeding and respiratory distress secondary to diaphragmatic and intercostal weakness. Since electrical myotonia is not present at birth and muscle biopsy findings are nonspecific, the diagnosis of myotonic dystrophy depends on the identification of electrical myotonia in the mother. Surviving infants can eventually stand and walk independently but have a high incidence of mental retardation and speech difficulties.

E. Myasthenia gravis results from failure of neuromuscular transmission caused by antibodies against acetylcholine receptors. Infantile myasthenia can be transient or congenital. Transient disease occurs in infants born to mothers with myasthenia. Consider a test dose of neostigmine when myasthenia is suspected. Botulism toxin impairs acetylcholine release from nerve endings. EMG findings are suggestive but a definitive diagnosis requires isolation of the organism in the stool. Honey has been implicated as the source of the botulism spores. Avoid drugs that worsen neuromuscular blockade, such as aminoglycoside antibiotics. Consider the use of human-derived antitoxin.

F. The most common infantile neuropathic disorder is infantile spinal muscular atrophy or Werdnig-Hoffman disease. Suspect this disorder when the infant presents with tongue fasiculations and absent deep tendon reflexes. The infantile form has a very poor prognosis; progressive weakness leads to respiratory compromise at an early age. When anterior horn cell loss has occurred *in utero*, the infant may have arthrogryposis multiplex congenita. Consider the possibility of a leukodystrophy when both upper and lower motor neuron manifestations are present. Lumbar puncture and EEG are useful in identifying these disorders.

G. Failure to demonstrate abnormalities in muscle biopsy, nerve conduction studies or electromyography suggests the diagnosis of essential hypotonia which may be related to "immaturity" of the motor end-plates. At least half of these infants recover fully.

REFERENCES

Brown LW. Infant botulism. Pediatr Ann 1984; 13:135.
Hansen PA. Myotonic dystrophy in infancy and childhood. Pediatr Ann 1984; 13:123.

INFANTILE HYPOTONIA

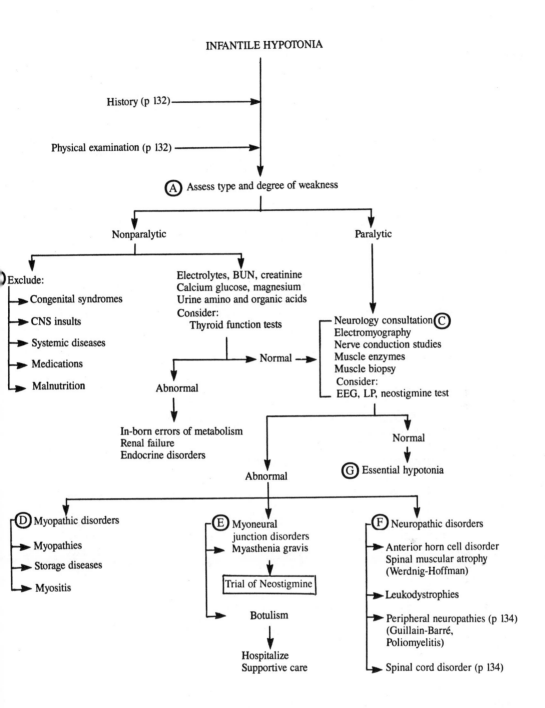

History (p 132) ——→

Physical examination (p 132) ——→

(A) Assess type and degree of weakness

Nonparalytic / Paralytic

Exclude:
- Congenital syndromes
- CNS insults
- Systemic diseases
- Medications
- Malnutrition

Electrolytes, BUN, creatinine
Calcium glucose, magnesium
Urine amino and organic acids
Consider:
  Thyroid function tests

→ Normal →

Abnormal

In-born errors of metabolism
Renal failure
Endocrine disorders

(C) Neurology consultation
Electromyography
Nerve conduction studies
Muscle enzymes
Muscle biopsy
 Consider:
 EEG, LP, neostigmine test

Normal

Abnormal

(G) Essential hypotonia

(D) Myopathic disorders
- Myopathies
- Storage diseases
- Myositis

(E) Myoneural
junction disorders
Myasthenia gravis

Trial of Neostigmine

Botulism

Hospitalize
Supportive care

(F) Neuropathic disorders
- Anterior horn cell disorder
  Spinal muscular atrophy
  (Werdnig-Hoffman)
- Leukodystrophies
- Peripheral neuropathies (p 134)
  (Guillain-Barré,
  Poliomyelitis)
- Spinal cord disorder (p 134)

Kaplan J, Rabinowich L, Berger A: Modern electrodiagnostic studies in infants and children. Pediatr Ann 1984; 13:150.

Peterson H. Diagnosis of hypertonia in children: types, differential diagnosis and management. Pediatr Ann 1976; May: 31.

Rumack BH. Poisoning. In: Kempe CH, Silver HK, O'Brien DO, eds. Current Pediatric Diagnosis and Treatment. 8th ed. Los Altos, California: Lange Medical Publications, 1984.

HEADACHE

A. Mildly ill patients have normal neurologic and ophthalmologic examinations and minimal impairment of normal activity. Moderately ill patients have a headache associated with abnormal focal neurologic findings (aphasia, hemiparesis, paresthesia, hemisensory loss, visual disturbances, ataxia, seizures), personality changes (recent memory loss, decreased attention span, emotional liability, regressive behavior, poor school performance), papilledema, growth failure or diabetes insipidus. Severely ill patients have a severe headache associated with an altered mental status (confusion, delirium, coma) and other signs of increased intracranial pressure (vomiting, bradycardia, impending herniation). Their course suggests a CNS infection, intracranial hemorrhage, or vascular accident.

B. Typical migraine presents as a throbbing unilateral headache associated with an aura and/or nausea and vomiting. A positive family history for migraine is present in most cases. In children, a migraine headache is often generalized and associated with nausea, vomiting, malaise, and dizziness. The classic aura of blurred vision, scotomata, flashing lights, hemianopsia is unusual. Suspect a complicated migraine syndrome when the headache is associated with transient hemiplegia or hemianopsia, eye pain, third-nerve palsy (ophthalmoplegic migraine), visual disturbances, vertigo, ataxia, syncope (basilar artery migraine), combativeness, hyperactivity, delirium (acute confusional state), or distortions of body image, spatial relations, and time sense (Alice in Wonderland syndrome). Treat mild episodes of migraine with aspirin and a sedative such as chloral hydrate or fiorinal. In an older child who experiences an aura, use cafergot PB ½ to 1 tablet at the onset of the aura followed by ½ to 1 tablet every 3 hours for a maximum of 2 to 4 tablets. When vomiting is present, consider using cafergot suppositories or a sublingual preparation (Ergomar). Institute migraine prophylaxis for frequent debilitating headaches with propranolol 5 to 20 mg *tid*, cyproheptadine (Periactin) 0.2 to 0.4 mg/kg/day *bid* or *tid*, or phenytoin (Dilantin) 5 to 7 mg/kg/day *bid*. Other alternatives include imipramine, Elavil, and phenobarbital.

C. Tension headaches, common in children, are caused by the sustained contraction of muscles of the neck and scalp. The headache may persist for weeks. Normal activity is not usually impaired. Treat these patients with aspirin or acetaminophen, and recommend adequate sleep and rest.

D. Suspect brain tumors when headache is associated with neurologic deficits, personality change, or signs of increased intracranial pressure (papilledema). Childhood brain tumors have different peak ages of occurrence. In infancy, the most common tumors are medulloblastoma, ependymoma, astrocytoma, and choroid plexus tumors. In preadolescence, the common tumors are cerebellar astrocytoma, medulloblastoma, ependymoma and craniopharyngioma. In adolescence, the common tumors are cerebellar astrocytoma, craniopharyngioma, and medulloblastoma. More than 50% of childhood tumors are infratentorial, of which 40% have their origin in the cerebellum. Treatment modalities include surgery, chemotherapy, and radiation therapy.

REFERENCES

Nellhaus G, Stumpf DA, Moe PG. Neurologic and muscular disorders. In: Kempe CH, Silver HK, O'Brien DO, eds. Current Pediatric Diagnosis and Treatment. 8th ed. Los Altos, California: Lange Medical Publications, 1984:628.

Scheff D, Vannucci R. Headaches in children. Pediatr Ann 1975; 4:51.

Shinnar S, D'Souza B. Migraine in children and adolescents. Pediatr Rev 1982; 3:257.

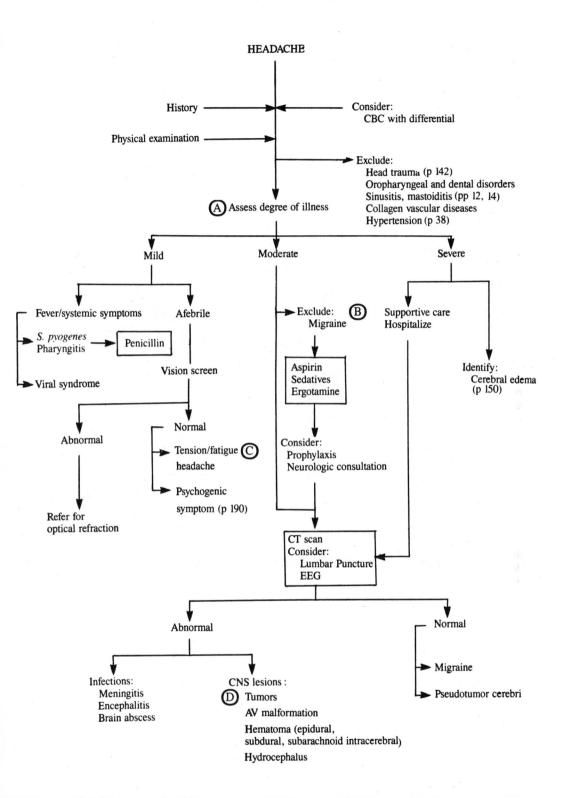

HEADACHE

History ────→├←──── Consider:
                     CBC with differential

Physical examination ────→

                     Exclude:
                       Head trauma (p 142)
                       Oropharyngeal and dental disorders
                       Sinusitis, mastoiditis (pp 12, 14)
                       Collagen vascular diseases
                       Hypertension (p 38)

(A) Assess degree of illness

Mild   Moderate   Severe

Fever/systemic symptoms   Afebrile   Exclude: (B)   Supportive care
                                            Migraine   Hospitalize
S. pyogenes ──→ Penicillin
Pharyngitis   Identify:
                        Vision screen   Aspirin   Cerebral edema
Viral syndrome   Sedatives   (p 150)
                                           Ergotamine

                        Normal
Abnormal   Consider:
              Tension/fatigue (C)   Prophylaxis
              headache   Neurologic consultation

              Psychogenic
Refer for   symptom (p 190)
optical refraction

                        CT scan
                        Consider:
                          Lumbar Puncture
                          EEG

Abnormal   Normal

Infections: CNS lesions: Migraine
  Meningitis   (D) Tumors
  Encephalitis   AV malformation   Pseudotumor cerebri
  Brain abscess
                      Hematoma (epidural,
                      subdural, subarachnoid intracerebral)

                      Hydrocephalus

139

ATAXIA

A. Note the onset, course, frequency, and severity of ataxia. Note the presence of associated symptoms such as vertigo, fever, earache, vomiting, and irritability, meningeal signs, headache, weakness, and altered mental status. Identify precipitating factors such as drug or toxin ingestions (phenytoin, phenobarbital, alcohol, carbamazepine, lead).

B. Assess motor coordination and cerebellar function. Consider a neural crest tumor (neuroblastoma) when opsoclonus myoclonus (dancing eyes, dancing feet) are present. Nystagmus suggests a labyrinthitis or involvement of a deep cerebellar structure.

C. Severely ill patients have marked ataxia associated with an altered mental status or signs of increased intracranial pressure, respiratory distress, or circulatory instability. Moderately ill patients have ataxia which may be associated with neurologic signs such as weakness, abnormal sensation, cranial nerve abnormalities. Mildly ill patients have ataxia associated with vertigo without neurologic signs.

D. Vertigo, an altered feeling of whirling or rotation, is associated with alterations in vestibular function which may be peripheral (secondary to dysfunction of the vestibular apparatus) or central (abnormalities of the vestibular nuclei or their brain stem/cerebellar connections). Examination of the tympanic membrane will identify cases of peripheral vertigo caused by acute otitis media or cholesteatoma. Benign *paroxysmal* vertigo presents with sudden episodes of ataxia (several seconds to minutes) usually in children between 1 and 3 years of age. Viral labyrinthitis in older children and adolescents is often associated with a viral infection and usually resolves within 2 weeks. Benign *positional* vertigo is triggered by rapid changes of head position. Drug-related vertigo (toxic labrynthitis) has been associated with aminoglycosides, ethycrinic acid, salicylates, and quinine. Head trauma may also result in vestibular damage that produces both immediate vertigo and post-traumatic vertigo which can last for days or weeks. Central vertigo may be a sign of brain tumors, acoustic neuromas, encephalitis, or multiple sclerosis. Consider treating peripheral vertigo in older children with meclizine (12.5 to 25 mg *bid*) and younger children with diphenhydramine (5 mg/kg/day).

E. Work up patients with polymyoclonus opsoclonus with x-rays (chest, abdominal, and skeletal), an IVP, urinary catecholamine metabolites, cystathionine, and organic acids. Consider performing an inferior vena cavagram to localize the neural crest neoplasms.

F. Suspect acute cerebellar ataxia when children between 2 and 6 years of age develop ataxia following a prodromal illness without any associated neurologic signs or alteration in mental status. The only abnormality in the workup may be a slight lymphocytosis or increased protein in the CSF. In most cases, the course is benign; 80 to 90% of patients recover full function within 6 to 8 weeks.

G. Causes of a chronic progressive ataxia include spinal cerebellar degenerative diseases such as Friedreich's ataxia (dysarthria, pes cavus, cardiomyopathy, scoliosis, and diabetes mellitus), dominant hereditary ataxia, ataxia telangectasia (associated increased α-fetoprotein and immune defects), Wilson's disease, Refsum's disease (ichthyosis, cardiomyopathy, retinitis pigmentosa) and abetalipoproteinemia (diarrhea, acanthocytosis, and retinitis pigmentosa). Chronic nonprogressive ataxia may be caused by a cerebral insult (hypoxia, bleed) or kernicteris.

REFERENCES

Berman PH, Packer FJ. Ataxia. In: Fleisher G, Ludwig S, eds. Textbook of Pediatric Emergency Medicine. Baltimore: Williams and Wilkins, 1983.

Nellhaus G, Stumpf DA, Moe P. Neurologic and muscular disorders. In: Kempe CH, Silver HK, O'Brien DO, eds. Current Pediatric Diagnosis and Treatment. 8th ed. Los Altos, California: Lange Medical Publications, 1984.

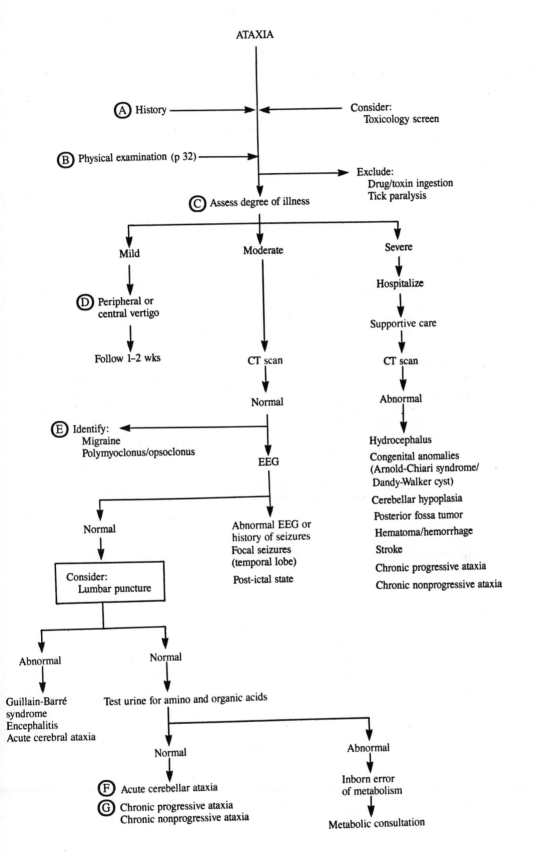

ATAXIA

(A) History

Consider:
    Toxicology screen

(B) Physical examination (p 32)

Exclude:
    Drug/toxin ingestion
    Tick paralysis

(C) Assess degree of illness

Mild

Moderate

Severe

Hospitalize

(D) Peripheral or
    central vertigo

Supportive care

Follow 1–2 wks

CT scan

CT scan

Normal

Abnormal

(E) Identify:
    Migraine
    Polymyoclonus/opsoclonus

Hydrocephalus

Congenital anomalies
    (Arnold-Chiari syndrome/
    Dandy-Walker cyst)

EEG

Cerebellar hypoplasia

Posterior fossa tumor

Normal

Abnormal EEG or
history of seizures
Focal seizures
(temporal lobe)

Post-ictal state

Hematoma/hemorrhage

Stroke

Chronic progressive ataxia

Chronic nonprogressive ataxia

Consider:
    Lumbar puncture

Abnormal

Normal

Guillain-Barré
syndrome
Encephalitis
Acute cerebral ataxia

Test urine for amino and organic acids

Normal

Abnormal

(F) Acute cerebellar ataxia

(G) Chronic progressive ataxia
    Chronic nonprogressive ataxia

Inborn error
of metabolism

Metabolic consultation

141

HEAD TRAUMA

A. Determine the time, circumstances, and severity of the trauma. Note presence and duration of loss of consciousness, altered mental status, retrograde amnesia, seizure activity, vomiting, ataxia, or headache. Identify predisposing conditions, especially bleeding disorders and underlying CNS pathology (hydrocephalus, AV malformations).

B. Assess the patient for multiple trauma. The presence of orbital ecchymosis (raccoon sign), mastoid erythema and swelling (battle sign), or hemotympaneum suggest a basilar skull fracture. Carefully palpate the skull for evidence of a depressed skull fracture. Note presence of possible CSF discharge from the nose or ears. Examine the optic fundi to identify papilledema, hemorrhages, and venous pulsations. Perform a thorough neurologic evaluation to identify neurologic signs (paralysis, paresis, ataxia, pathologic reflexes, meningeal signs). In patients with altered level of consciousness, determine the level of brain dysfunction and the Glasgow coma score. Findings which suggest a subdural hematoma include increased head size, bulging fontanel, retinal hemorrhages, extraocular palsy, hemiparesis, and anemia. Suspect an acute epidural hematoma when rapid deterioration in level of consciousness follows a 12- to 48-hour lucid period.

C. Severely ill patients have respiratory distress, circulatory instability, altered mental status (unresponsiveness, coma), marked irritability, or signs of increased intracranial pressure (severe headache, protracted vomiting, altered mental status). Moderately ill patients have experienced more than 10 minutes of post-traumatic unconsciousness, have post-traumatic seizures, focal neurologic deficits, retrograde amnesia for more than 30 minutes, evidence of a depressed skull fracture, basilar skull fracture, CSF leak, signs of severe headache, and irritability. Mildly ill patients are asymptomatic or have had less than 5 to 10 minutes loss of consciousness with rapid clearing of the mental status. They may have 1 to 3 episodes of vomiting and continue to have a mild headache for 24 to 48 hours.

D. Indications for skull x-rays include open head injuries, possible depressed compound or basilar fractures, possible foreign body, cases of suspected child abuse, and cases in which moderate to severe injury has occurred and a CT scan cannot be performed.

E. Home follow-up includes instructing the parents to waken their child during the night, check the pupils for size and response to light, and note any alteration in mental status, difficulty in speaking, blurring of vision, unsteadiness in walking, difficulty in using the arms, fever, persistent vomiting, or seizures. Recommend a clear liquid diet until the child has gone 6 hours without vomiting.

F. Post-traumatic seizures may be immediate, early, or late. Impact seizures that occur immediately with head trauma are benign and not associated with subsequent epilepsy. Early post-traumatic seizures occur during the first week after head trauma; 35% occur within the first hour after trauma, 40% within 24 hours, and 25% within one week. Treat early post-traumatic seizures with anticonvulsants for 6 months. Late post-traumatic seizures which occur after 1 week have a high rate of recurrence and require treatment for 3 to 4 seizure-free years.

G. CSF leaks usually heal spontaneously within 2 weeks of trauma. Prophylactic antibiotics are not efficacious in preventing secondary infection. When signs of meningeal irritation or fever develop, perform a spinal tap to diagnose meningitis. Consider surgical repair when a CSF leak has failed to resolve within 2 weeks. Skull fractures may be complicated by a leptomeningeal cyst when CSF accumulates under the scalp because of a tear in the dura and arachnoid membranes. Refer these patients to a neurosurgeon. Severe head trauma may be associated with a post-concussion syndrome characterized by behavior disturbances (aggressiveness), poor impulse control, emotional lability, phobias, headaches, vertigo, dizziness, and deteriorating school performance.

HEAD TRAUMA

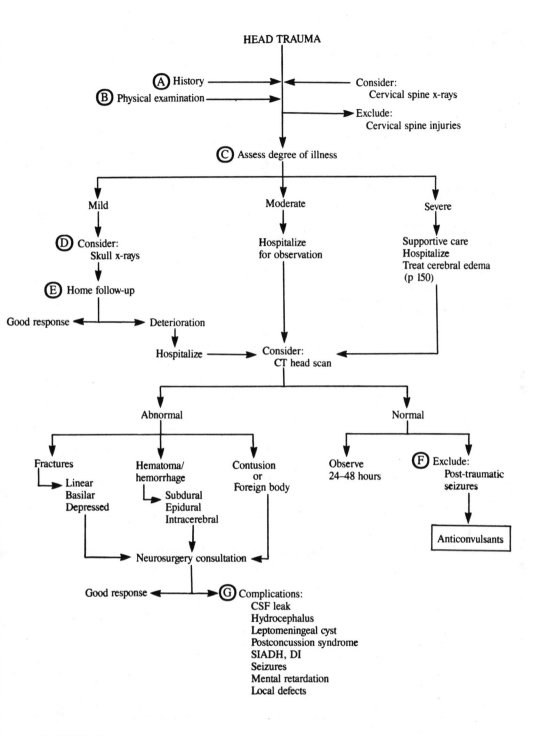

(A) History

(B) Physical examination

Consider:
Cervical spine x-rays

Exclude:
Cervical spine injuries

(C) Assess degree of illness

Mild

Moderate

Severe

(D) Consider:
Skull x-rays

Hospitalize
for observation

Supportive care
Hospitalize
Treat cerebral edema
(p 150)

(E) Home follow-up

Good response   Deterioration

Hospitalize

Consider:
CT head scan

Abnormal

Normal

Fractures

Linear
Basilar
Depressed

Hematoma/
hemorrhage

Subdural
Epidural
Intracerebral

Contusion
or
Foreign body

Observe
24–48 hours

(F) Exclude:
Post-traumatic
seizures

Anticonvulsants

Neurosurgery consultation

Good response

(G) Complications:
CSF leak
Hydrocephalus
Leptomeningeal cyst
Postconcussion syndrome
SIADH, DI
Seizures
Mental retardation
Local defects

REFERENCES

Nellhaus G, Stumpf DA, Moe PG. Neurologic and muscular disorders. In: Kempe CH, Silver HK, O'Brien D, eds. Current Pediatric Diagnosis and Treatment. 8th ed. Los Altos, California: Lange Medical Publications, 1984.

SEIZURES

A. Seizures are classified as general (grand mal, petit mal, and minor motor) or partial (focal motor, sensory, and psychomotor). Generalized grand mal seizures have tonic clonic movements, eye deviation, and unresponsiveness followed by a postictal period with or without stool and/or urine incontinence. Petit mal or absence seizures produce brief (< 30 seconds) staring spells without a postictal period and are associated with an EEG finding of 3/sec spike and wave forms. Minor motor seizures include myoclonic, atonic, and akinetic seizures and infantile spasms. Partial seizures may be simple (no alteration in consciousness) or complex (with alteration in consciousness). Psychomotor seizures may be preceded by an aura and have complex automatisms such as sucking and lip smacking.

B. Determine the onset, duration, frequency, and description (aura, movements, incontinence, postictal period) of the seizure. Note associated symptoms such as fever, vomiting, bloody diarrhea (shigellosis), visual disturbances, and altered mental status. Identify precipitating factors and predisposing conditions.

C. Assess the degree of illness. Severely ill patients are in coma or status (generalized seizure activity lasting >20 minutes or recurrent seizure activity over 20 minutes during which time the patient remains unconscious). Moderately ill patients have atypical febrile seizures (duration >15 minutes, focal features, altered mental status, and repeated seizures during a single febrile illness) or a first afebrile seizure without a known seizure disorder. Mildly ill patients have a simple febrile seizure, immediate post-traumatic seizure, or a breakthrough seizure in a patient with a known seizure disorder without an alteration in the baseline neurologic status.

D. Provide supportive care to patients in status to maintain cerebral tissue oxygenation. Establish an adequate airway, maintain ventilation, and treat shock. Initiate anticonvulsant therapy with diazepam (Valium) 0.3 to 0.5 mg/kg IV over 2 minutes (maximum dose in an infant 4 mg, in an older child 10 mg). If necessary, repeat this dose at 10-minute intervals 3 times. If seizures are controlled, begin phenytoin (Dilantin) to prevent seizure recurrence. If the seizure activity is not interrupted by diazepam, begin an IV infusion of phenytoin (10 to 25 mg/kg) and monitor for cardiac rhythm disturbances. If seizures persist, administer an IV infusion of phenobarbital (15 to 25 mg/kg). Consider paraldehyde or valproic acid for continuing status and general anesthesia when medical therapy fails.

E. Simple febrile seizures have no atypical features or signs of infection or metabolic abnormalities. Since the incidence of unrecognized meningitis or electrolyte abnormalities is less than 1%, an extensive workup is unnecessary. Indications for the treatment of simple febrile seizures with phenobarbital include a positive family history of epilepsy, abnormal neurologic or developmental status, or age of onset under 6 months. Treat cases with atypical febrile seizures (duration >15 minutes, focal features). Complications of phenobarbital therapy include behavioral changes (hyperactivity), sleep disturbances, and altered cognitive functioning. Valproic acid maintenance is an alternative to phenobarbital therapy.

F. Drugs used in maintenance therapy for grand mal seizures include phenobarbital: 4–6 mg/kg/day, therapeutic range 10–25 mg/L); carbamazepine (Tegretal): 10–30 mg/kg/day, therapeutic range 5–14 mg/L; phenytoin (Dilantin): 4–10 mg/kg/day, therapeutic range 10–20 mg/L; and valproic acid (Depakene): 20–60 mg/kg/day, therapeutic range 60–115 mg/L. Treat petit mal seizures with ethosuximide (Zarontin): 20 to 40 mg/kg/day, therapeutic range 40–100 mg/L; valproic acid (Depakene) or clonazepam (Clonopin): 0.1–0.2 mg/kg/day, therapeutic range 10–70 ng/ml.

REFERENCES

Barbosa E, Freeman JM. Status epilepticus. Pediatr Rev 1982; 4:185.
Freeman JM, Vining EPG. Focal epileptic seizures. Pediatr Rev 1979; 1:141.
Holmes GL. Therapy of petit mal (absence seizures). Pediatr Rev 1982; 4:150.

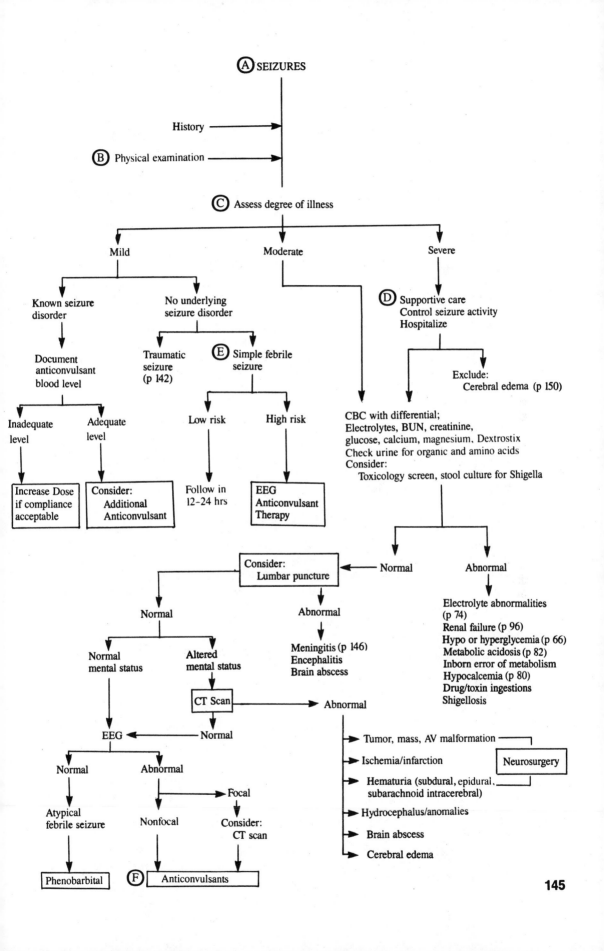

Ⓐ SEIZURES

History ⟶

Ⓑ Physical examination ⟶

Ⓒ Assess degree of illness

Mild — Moderate — Severe

Mild:

Known seizure disorder ⟶ Document anticonvulsant blood level

Inadequate level ⟶ Increase Dose if compliance acceptable

Adequate level ⟶ Consider: Additional Anticonvulsant

No underlying seizure disorder

Traumatic seizure (p 142)

Ⓔ Simple febrile seizure

Low risk ⟶ Follow in 12-24 hrs

High risk ⟶ EEG Anticonvulsant Therapy

Severe:

Ⓓ Supportive care
Control seizure activity
Hospitalize

Exclude:
Cerebral edema (p 150)

CBC with differential;
Electrolytes, BUN, creatinine,
glucose, calcium, magnesium, Dextrostix
Check urine for organic and amino acids
Consider:
Toxicology screen, stool culture for Shigella

Normal — Abnormal

Abnormal:

Electrolyte abnormalities (p 74)
Renal failure (p 96)
Hypo or hyperglycemia (p 66)
Metabolic acidosis (p 82)
Inborn error of metabolism
Hypocalcemia (p 80)
Drug/toxin ingestions
Shigellosis

Normal:

Consider: Lumbar puncture

Normal — Abnormal

Abnormal ⟶ Meningitis (p 146)
Encephalitis
Brain abscess

Normal:

Normal mental status — Altered mental status

Altered mental status ⟶ CT Scan ⟶ Abnormal

CT Scan ⟶ Normal

EEG

Normal — Abnormal

Normal ⟶ Atypical febrile seizure ⟶ Phenobarbital

Abnormal ⟶ Nonfocal / Focal

Focal ⟶ Consider: CT scan

Nonfocal ⟶ Ⓕ Anticonvulsants

Consider: CT scan ⟶ Ⓕ Anticonvulsants

Abnormal (CT):

Tumor, mass, AV malformation ⟶ Neurosurgery
Ischemia/infarction
Hematuria (subdural, epidural, subarachnoid intracerebral) ⟶ Neurosurgery
Hydrocephalus/anomalies
Brain abscess
Cerebral edema

MENINGITIS

A. The most useful test performed on cerebrospinal fluid is the CSF Gram stain. It is positive in 85–90% of cases of bacterial meningitis diagnosed by culture. The Gram stain will still be positive in the great majority of cases of bacterial meningitis despite antibiotic therapy prior to diagnosis.

B. If the Gram stain and CIE are negative, it may be difficult to distinguish viral from bacterial infection until culture results become available. The risk of bacterial meningitis is <1% regardless of prior antibiotic therapy when the CSF cell count is <200 cells with <50% PMN and the CSF glucose is >40 mg percent. After the neonatal period, consider a CSF sample with >8–10 cells abnormal. High CSF cell counts with a low CSF glucose are not diagnostic of bacterial disease without confirmation by culture since enteroviral meningitis may have a CSF count >500 in 45% of cases and a glucose <40 mg percent in 18% of cases.

C. Consider withholding antibiotic therapy and performing a repeat lumbar puncture, if the patient is stable and the initial LP was traumatic, an increased percentage of bands is present on the CSF differential, or if the patient received prior antibiotic therapy.

D. Start IV antibiotic therapy with ampicillin 200–400 mg/kg/day in 4 divided doses and either cefotaxime 200 mg/kg/day in 4 divided doses or chloramphenicol 75–100 mg/kg/day in 4 divided doses in order to cover ampicillin-resistant *H. influenzae*. If gram-positive cocci are seen on Gram stain, use ampicillin and chloramphenicol. If chloramphenicol is given, monitor blood levels to maintain a therapeutic level of 10–20 mg/ml and follow CBCs to identify bone marrow suppression. Antibiotic therapy should be based on culture results; continue IV therapy for 10–14 days. In uncomplicated cases, a repeat LP at the completion of therapy is not necessary.

E. Approximately two-thirds of the cases of diagnosed meningitis are viral and one-third bacterial. The enteroviruses (coxsackie virus, echovirus, mumps, and poliomyelitis) and herpes simplex are the most common viral agents. In early infancy, the bacterial organisms which cause meningitis are group *B streptococcus, S. pneumoniae, H. influenzae, Salmonella, N. meningitidis,* and *E. coli.* Later *H. influenzae, S. pneumoniae* and *N. meningitidis* are the predominant organisms.

F. Assess hearing and neurologic states at discharge. Follow-up studies of infants and children who have had bacterial meningitis indicate that 50% appear normal, 9% have behavioral problems, and 28% have significant handicaps (hearing loss, language disorder, vision loss, seizures, MR, motor disorder). The prognosis is worse in patients presenting with complications. Follow-up studies of children who have had enteroviral meningitis showed 58% normal, 26% with possible impairments such as behavioral problems, speech disorder, or mild retardation, and 15% with definite significant problems. Children who had meningitis before 1 year of age were at greater risk for sequelae than were older children.

G. Signs of severe complications include shock, purpura, respiratory distress, persistent seizures, focal neurologic signs, and coma. If these are present, consider septic shock, adrenal failure, cardiogenic shock, purulent pericarditis, pulmonary edema, severe pneumonia, severe anemia, disseminated intravascular coagulation. Suspect a CNS complication if seizures, signs of increased intracranial pressure, or an altered level of consciousness persist after 3 days of therapy. Complications include subdural effusion or empyema, cerebral abscess, acute hydrocephalus, cerebritis, cerebral infarct, cerebral edema, inappropriate secretion of antidiuretic hormone or diabetes insipidus.

REFERENCES

Bodino J, Lylyk P, Del Valle M. Computed tomography in purulent meningitis. Am J Dis Child 1982; 136:495.

Davis SD, Hill HR, Feigl P. Partial antibiotic therapy in Haemophilus influenzae meningitis. Am J Dis Child 1975; 129:802.

Dillon HC. Studies of moxalactam for gram-negative and Haemophilus influenzae meningitis: an appraisal. J Pediatr 1981; 99:907.

Sell SH. Long-term sequelae of bacterial meningitis in children. Ped Infect Dis 1983; 2:90.

Singer JI, Maur PR, Riley JP, et al. Management of central nervous system infections during an epidemic of enteroviral aseptic meningitis. J Pediatr 1980; 96:559.

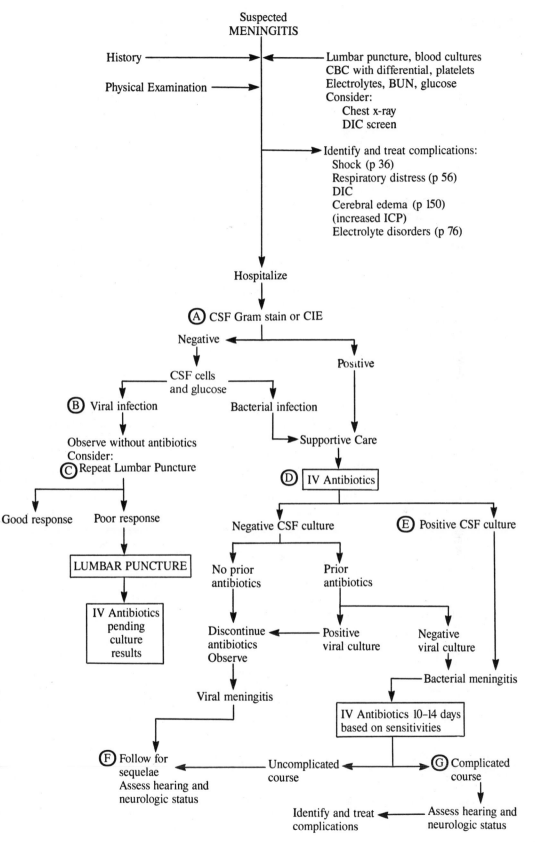

Suspected
MENINGITIS

History ⟶

Physical Examination ⟶

Lumbar puncture, blood cultures
CBC with differential, platelets
Electrolytes, BUN, glucose
Consider:
　　Chest x-ray
　　DIC screen

Identify and treat complications:
　Shock (p 36)
　Respiratory distress (p 56)
　DIC
　Cerebral edema (p 150)
　(increased ICP)
　Electrolyte disorders (p 76)

Hospitalize

Ⓐ CSF Gram stain or CIE

Negative　　　　　　　　Positive

CSF cells
and glucose

Ⓑ Viral infection　　　Bacterial infection

Observe without antibiotics
Consider:
Ⓒ Repeat Lumbar Puncture

Supportive Care

Good response　Poor response

Ⓓ IV Antibiotics

LUMBAR PUNCTURE

Negative CSF culture　　　Ⓔ Positive CSF culture

IV Antibiotics
pending
culture
results

No prior
antibiotics　　　Prior
antibiotics

Discontinue
antibiotics
Observe　　⟵　Positive
viral culture　　　Negative
viral culture

Viral meningitis

Bacterial meningitis

IV Antibiotics 10–14 days
based on sensitivities

Ⓕ Follow for
sequelae
Assess hearing and
neurologic status　　⟵　Uncomplicated
course　　⟶　Ⓖ Complicated
course

Identify and treat　⟵　Assess hearing and
complications　　　　neurologic status

COMA

A. Coma results from brain dysfunction, that is, inadequate interaction between the cerebral hemispheres and the reticular activating systems of the diencephalon, midbrain, and pons.

B. In the physical examination note vital signs. Assess the level of brain dysfunction by evaluating the level of consciousness, pattern of breathing, pupillary size and reflexes, oculomotor function, and motor responses. Involvement limited to the cerebral hemispheres and basal ganglia presents with confusion, or delirium associated with a normal breathing pattern, normal- or small-sized reactive pupils, roving eye movements, and spontaneous movements of the extremities. Diencephalic dysfunction presents with stupor and unresponsiveness, periodic or Cheyne-Stokes breathing, small reactive pupils, positive oculocephalic (doll's eye movements) and oculovestibular reflexes, and decorticate posturing. Signs of midbrain and upper pons dysfunction include hyperventilation, moderate pupillary dilatation (3–5 mm), dysconjugate gaze with loss of oculocephalic and oculovestibular reflexes, and decerebate posturing. Dysfunction of the lower pons and medullary level presents with a shallow and irregular breathing pattern, fixed and dilated pupils, absent eye movements, and flaccid paralysis. Rapid rostral-caudad deterioration suggests herniation through the tentorial notch (central herniation syndrome). Unilateral pupillary dilatation associated with signs of midbrain dysfunction is caused by compression of the third nerve with displacement of the temporal lobe through the tentorial notch (uncal herniation syndrome).

C. Suspect a toxic metabolic disease when the neurologic assessment demonstrates inconsistencies in the level of dysfunction among breathing pattern, pupillary reflexes, eye movements, and motor responses. Hypoglycemia and herpes simplex encephalitis may present with focal neurologic signs that suggest structural mass lesions.

D. Suspect a supratentorial mass lesion when focal neurologic signs are present or the clinical course suggests central or uncal herniation. Causes include intracranial hematomas (subdural, epidural, intracerebral), brain tumors, contusions, or infarctions. Subtentorial mass lesions present with brain stem signs such as cranial nerve palsies and altered oculovestibular reflexes. Causes include a posterior fossa hematoma or tumor, basilar aneurysm, or brain stem or pontine hemorrhage.

E. Toxins that produce a metabolic acidosis include salicylate (treat with alkaline diuresis), carbon monoxide (treat with oxygen), cyanide (treat with sodium nitrate followed by sodium thiosulfate), heavy metals (treat with chelating agents), methyl alcohol (treat with ethanol), ethylene glycol (treat with ethanol), and paraldehyde. When respiratory acidosis is present in association with pinpoint or small pupils, suspect narcotics (except meperidine) or organophosphates (cholinesterase inhibitors). Treat suspected narcotic overdoses with naloxone 5–10 μg/kg/dose IV (adult dose 0.4 mg) repeated every 30 minutes as needed. Document cases of organophosphate intoxication with a red cell cholinesterase level. Treat with atropine (0.01–0.05 mg/kg IV), and consider the use of a cholinesterase reactivator, pralidoxime (Protopam). Suspect CNS sedatives such as alcohol, barbiturates, chlordiazepoxide, diazepam, meprobamate, or methaqualone with small- or normal-sized pupils. Meperidine ingestions present with normal or large pupils, glutethimide (Doriden) with fixed pupils. Suspect an anticholinergic ingestion when a normal acid-base status is associated with fixed and dilated pupils and dry mouth. Compounds with anticholinergic effects include atropine, scopolamine, Jimson weed, and many of the cyclic antidepressants (Elavil, Tofranil). Treat these patients cautiously with physostigmine (0.5 to 2 mg IV). Avoid the use of physostigmine in patients with asthma, urinary obstruction, or vascular compromise. When the pupils are dilated but not fixed, suspect amphetamines, cocaine, methylphenidate, or phenothiazines. Consider dialysis when the patient fails to respond to other conservative measures.

REFERENCES

Plum F, Posner JB. The Diagnosis of Stupor and Coma. Philadelphia: FA Davis, 1972.

Rumack BH. Poisoning. In: Kempe CH, Silver HK, O'Brien DO, eds. Current Pediatric Diagnosis and Treatment. 8th ed. Los Altos, California: Lange Medical Publications, 1984.

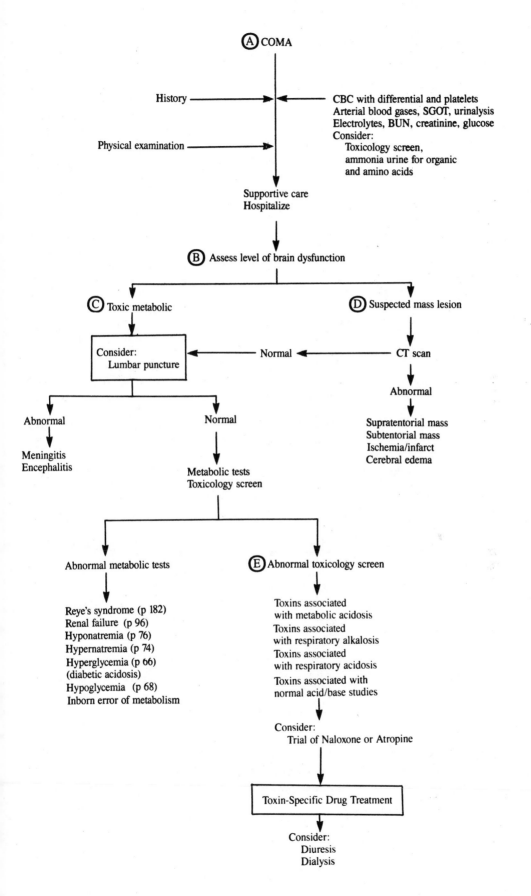

$\textcircled{A}$ COMA

History ⟶

Physical examination ⟶

CBC with differential and platelets
Arterial blood gases, SGOT, urinalysis
Electrolytes, BUN, creatinine, glucose
Consider:
    Toxicology screen,
    ammonia urine for organic
    and amino acids

Supportive care
Hospitalize

$\textcircled{B}$ Assess level of brain dysfunction

$\textcircled{C}$ Toxic metabolic

$\textcircled{D}$ Suspected mass lesion

Consider:
    Lumbar puncture ⟵ Normal ⟵ CT scan

Abnormal

Supratentorial mass
Subtentorial mass
Ischemia/infarct
Cerebral edema

Abnormal

Meningitis
Encephalitis

Normal

Metabolic tests
Toxicology screen

Abnormal metabolic tests

$\textcircled{E}$ Abnormal toxicology screen

Reye's syndrome (p 182)
Renal failure (p 96)
Hyponatremia (p 76)
Hypernatremia (p 74)
Hyperglycemia (p 66)
(diabetic acidosis)
Hypoglycemia (p 68)
Inborn error of metabolism

Toxins associated
with metabolic acidosis
Toxins associated
with respiratory alkalosis
Toxins associated
with respiratory acidosis
Toxins associated with
normal acid/base studies

Consider:
    Trial of Naloxone or Atropine

Toxin-Specific Drug Treatment

Consider:
    Diuresis
    Dialysis

CEREBRAL EDEMA

A. Cerebral edema or brain swelling is categorized into three forms: cytotoxic, vasogenic, and interstitial. Cytotoxic edema is produced by conditions that disrupt intracellular metabolism and allow sodium and water to accumulate intracellularly. Causes include Reye's syndrome, viral encephalitis, hypoxic or ischemic insults, lead intoxication, SIADH, and hexachloraphene toxicity. Vasogenic or extracellular edema occurs with capillary leakage through a disrupted blood brain barrier. Causes include tumors, hematomas, trauma, abscess, cerebritis, and infarction. In interstitial edema, acute hydrocephalus forces CSF to pass through the ependymal lining of the ventricles.

B. Note symptoms of cerebral edema and increased intracranial pressure such as nausea, vomiting, headache, irritability, confusion, and altered mental status.

C. Visualize the fundi for venous pulsations, papilledema, hemorrhage, and exudates, and assess the level of brain dysfunction (p 148). Note the presence of focal neurologic signs, seizure activity, or abnormal reflexes. Severe bradycardia suggests increased intracranial pressure.

D. The Glasgow coma score is a useful guide in management and prognosis. Sum the score of each of the 3 categories to give a total score. *Eye opening*: 4 spontaneous, 3 to speech, 2 to pain, and 1 none. *Verbal response*: 5 oriented, 4 confused, 3 inappropriate, 2 incomprehensible, 1 none. *Motor response*: 6 obeys commands, 5 localizes pain, 4 withdraws, 3 flexion to pain, 2 extension to pain, 1 none. Patients with scores of 3 or 4 have a poor prognosis and, if they survive, often suffer severe sequelae.

E. Consider elective intubation to prevent aspiration and sudden respiratory arrest. Intubation should be performed by an experienced anesthesiologist using paralyzing agents in order to prevent marked increases in intracranial pressure. Hyperventilate to a lower PCO_2 to a range of 25 to 30 torr to produce mild cerebrovasoconstriction and reduce cerebral blood flow and edema formation. Avoid maintaining PCO_2 <20 torr to prevent severe vasoconstriction and inadequate cerebral blood flow. Manage acute high pressure waves with manual hyperventilation.

F. Monitor intracranial pressure with a pressure-sensitive device that can be placed in the epidural, subdural, or subarachnoid spaces or the lateral ventricle. The normal intracranial pressure is <10 to 15 torr. Normally, cerebral blood flow is unaffected by minor alterations in systemic arterial pressures between 50 and 150 torr. When cerebral dysfunction disrupts autoregulation, the cerebral perfusion pressure is determined by the difference between mean systemic arterial pressure and intracranial pressure.

G. Treat an elevation of intracranial pressure >20 with IV mannitol 0.5 to 1 g/kg. Follow vital signs and urine output, serum osmolality, and electrolytes closely. Avoid serum osmolalities >300. Consider using Lasix. The efficacy of steroids has been demonstrated for vasogenic edema but not for cytotoxic edema. Consider using morphine and Pavulon to reduce increased intracranial pressure secondary to agitation and muscle spasm. Osmotic agents remove fluid only from uninjured brain tissue. Avoid using osmotic agents in the first 24 hours after trauma or in the presence of renal failure.

H. Consider barbiturate therapy with doses of sodium thiopental, pentobarbital, or phenobarbital sufficient to suppress EEG activity when intracranial pressure cannot otherwise be adequately controlled. Hypothhermia to 32°C will also reduce cerebral metabolism and cerebral blood flow.

REFERENCES

Bruce DA. Management of cerebral edema. Pediatr Rev 1983; 4:217.

Griffith JF, Brassfield JC. Increased intracranial pressure. Pediatr Rev 1981; 2:269.

Mickell JJ, Reigel DH, Cook DR, et al. Intracranial pressure monitoring in normalization therapy in children. Pediatrics 1977; 59:606.

Miller JD. Barbiturates in raised intracranial pressure. Ann Neurol 1979; 6:189.

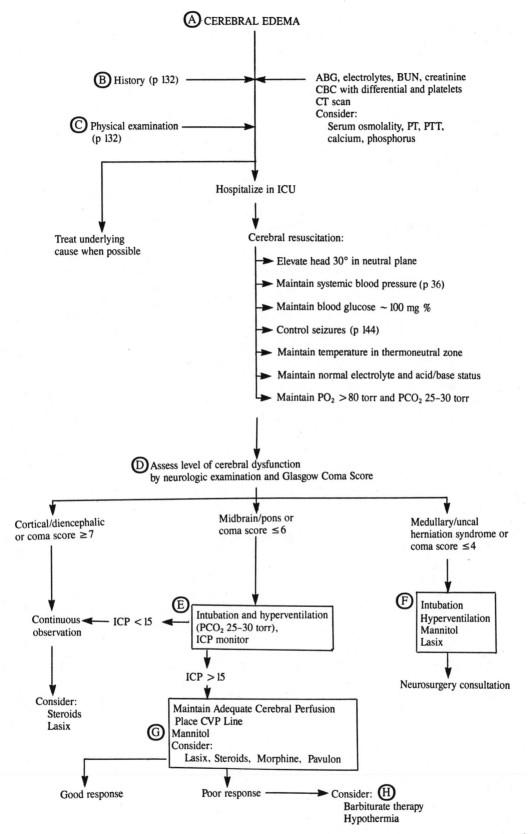

Ⓐ CEREBRAL EDEMA

Ⓑ History (p 132)

ABG, electrolytes, BUN, creatinine
CBC with differential and platelets
CT scan
Consider:
    Serum osmolality, PT, PTT,
    calcium, phosphorus

Ⓒ Physical examination
(p 132)

Hospitalize in ICU

Treat underlying
cause when possible

Cerebral resuscitation:

→ Elevate head 30° in neutral plane

→ Maintain systemic blood pressure (p 36)

→ Maintain blood glucose ~ 100 mg %

→ Control seizures (p 144)

→ Maintain temperature in thermoneutral zone

→ Maintain normal electrolyte and acid/base status

→ Maintain PO_2 >80 torr and PCO_2 25–30 torr

Ⓓ Assess level of cerebral dysfunction
by neurologic examination and Glasgow Coma Score

Cortical/diencephalic
or coma score ≥7

Midbrain/pons or
coma score ≤6

Medullary/uncal
herniation syndrome or
coma score ≤4

Continuous ← ICP < 15
observation

Ⓔ Intubation and hyperventilation
(PCO_2 25–30 torr),
ICP monitor

Ⓕ Intubation
Hyperventilation
Mannitol
Lasix

Consider:
Steroids
Lasix

ICP > 15

Neurosurgery consultation

Ⓖ Maintain Adequate Cerebral Perfusion
 Place CVP Line
Mannitol
Consider:
    Lasix, Steroids, Morphine, Pavulon

Good response

Poor response ⟶ Consider: Ⓗ
Barbiturate therapy
Hypothermia

MICROCYTIC ANEMIA
Peter A. Lane, M.D.

A. Note the presence or absence of jaundice (thalassemia), chronic illness, recurrent infections, or fever (anemia of chronic disease), irritability or pica (iron deficiency or lead poisoning), vomiting or seizures (lead poisoning), and blood loss (iron deficiency). A diet deficient in iron commonly causes iron deficiency anemia in children aged 6 to 36 months, particularly if large volumes of cow's milk are consumed. Note any family history of anemia or jaundice. Consider the possibility of a hemoglobinopathy in black, Mediterranean and Arab children (α thalassemia, β thalassemia, sickle cell-β thalassemia) and in Southeast Asian children (α thalassemia, β thalassemia, hemoglobin E disease).

B. Note the presence of jaundice or splenomegaly (thalassemia), hypertension, altered mental status, or signs of increased intracranial pressure (lead poisoning) or delayed growth and development (chronic disease). Assess the circulatory status, and note signs of high-output congestive heart failure.

C. Normal values for hemoglobin, hematocrit, and MCV vary with age: in the newborn, hematocrit $>45\%$ and MCV >94; at 6 months, hematocrit $>33\%$ and MCV >72; at 2 years, hematocrit $>34\%$ and MCV >72; at 5 years, hematocrit $>35\%$ and MCV >75. Thereafter, normal values for hematocrit and MCV gradually increase until they reach adult normals after puberty.

D. Institute a trial of oral iron (6 mg/kg/day of elemental iron *tid*). Do not give with milk or formula. A response to oral iron is the single best test of iron deficiency.

E. In the face of moderately severe microcytic anemia, a presumptive diagnosis of iron deficiency should be made *only* with a history of an iron-poor diet (age 6–36 months) or explained blood loss (age >36 months) *and* a history and physical examination which do not suggest another cause of microcytosis.

F. Obtain a hematology consultation. Consider hospitalization and cautious transfusion if the hemoglobin is <6 mg/dl or if there are signs of cardiac decompensation.

G. In iron deficiency, oral iron therapy causes a reticulocytosis within 5 to 7 days. Documentation of this reticulocyte response is a relatively inexpensive way to confirm the diagnosis and assess the adequacy of therapy.

H. Severe microcytosis (MCV <60) and hypochromia suggest significant iron deficiency or β thalassemia; numerous target cells suggest thalassemia (including sickle cell-β thalassemia) or hemoglobin E disease. Basophilic stipling is often present with lead poisoning but is not specific for this diagnosis. The erythrocyte protoporphyrin is mildly elevated in iron deficiency and markedly elevated with lead poisoning. The serum ferritin is typically low in iron deficiency (low serum iron) but high in the anemia of chronic disease (low serum iron). The absence of anemia or microcytosis in both parents excludes the diagnosis of β thalassemia or sickle cell-β thalassemia, but not α thalassemia, in their child. A quantitative hemoglobin electrophoresis shows an elevated A_2 and/or F hemoglobin in β thalassemia, a hemoglobin S level greater than the hemoglobin A_1 level in sickle cell-β thalassemia, and hemoglobin E in hemoglobin E disease. The hemoglobin electrophoresis is usually normal in α thalassemia, except in the newborn where Bart's hemoglobin is detected.

I. Iron therapy should be continued until body stores are replenished. The possibility of blood loss should be thoroughly investigated when iron deficiency occurs in children over 3 years of age.

REFERENCES

Dallman PR, Siimes MA. Percentile curves for hemoglobin and red cell volume in infancy and childhood. J Pediatr 1979; 94:26.

Dallman PR, Reeves JD, Driggers DA, Lo EYT. Diagnosis of iron deficiency: the limitations of laboratory tests in predicting response to iron treatment in 1-year-old infants. J Pediatr 1981; 99:376.

MICROCYTIC ANEMIA

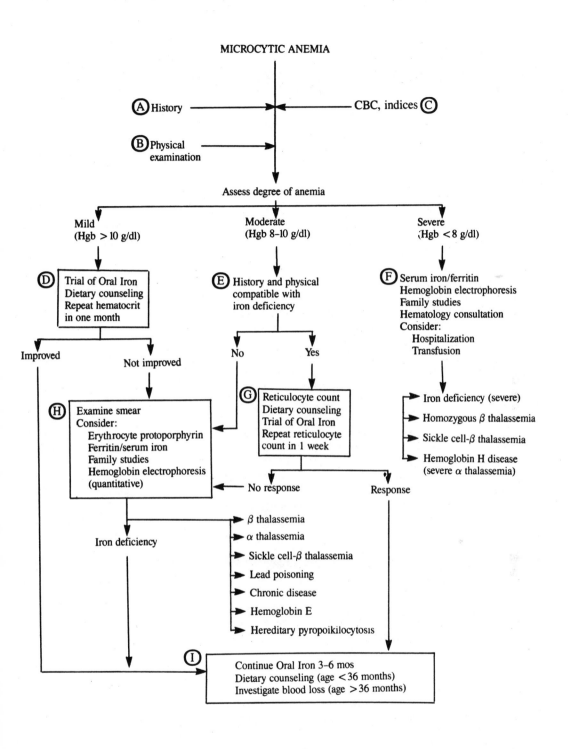

Ohene-Frempong K, Schwartz E. Clinical features of thalassemia. Pediatr Clin North Am 1980; 27:403.

Oski FA, Stockman JA. Anemia due to inadequate iron sources or poor iron utilization. Pediatr Clin North Am 1980; 27:237.

Reeves JD, Driggers DA, Lo EYT, Dallman PR. Screening for iron deficiency anemia in one-year-old infants: Hemoglobin alone or hemoglobin and mean corpuscular volume as predictors of response to iron treatment. J Pediatr 1981; 98:894.

NORMOCYTIC OR MACROCYTIC ANEMIA

Peter A. Lane, M.D.

A. Note symptoms such as jaundice (hemolysis or liver disease), persistent or recurrent fever (chronic infection, juvenile rheumatoid arthritis, malignancy), epistaxis or easy bruising (leukemia, aplastic anemia, hemolytic uremic syndrome), limp or limb pain (JRA, leukemia, neuroblastoma, sickle cell disease), chronic diarrhea (malabsorption), or acute diarrhea (HUS). Note any medications. An unusual dietary history may suggest B_{12} or folate deficiency. Obtain a family history for anemia, jaundice, splenomegaly, or unexplained gallstones (hereditary hemolytic disorders).

B. Document short stature (severe chronic anemia, renal disease, hypothyroidism, Blackfan-Diamond anemia, Fanconi's anemia) or the presence of microcephaly or congenital anomalies (Fanconi's anemia, Blackfan-Diamond anemia). Note signs of systemic diseases such as petechiae or bruising (leukemia, aplastic anemia, HUS), jaundice (hemolysis or liver disease), generalized lymphadenopathy (JRA, leukemia), or splenomegaly (leukemia, sickle syndromes, hereditary spherocytosis, liver disease, hypersplenism).

C. Note the MCV and use age-adjusted normal values for determining the presence or absence of microcytosis (p 152) or macrocytosis. Macrocytosis suggests a megaloblastic anemia, a bone marrow failure state (Fanconi's, Blackfan-Diamond, preleukemia), liver disease, hypothyroidism, or a significant reticulocytosis caused by hemolysis or hemorrhage.

D. The reticulocyte count helps differentiate anemias caused by increased peripheral red cell destruction from those caused by underproduction. A low or "normal" reticulocyte count in the face of significant anemia is inappropriate and suggests bone marrow failure. However, a low reticulocyte count does *not* exclude the possibility of hemolysis; hemolytic anemias frequently present in "aplastic" or "hypoplastic" crisis.

E. Review the peripheral smear. The presence of sickle forms, red cell fragmentation (disseminated intravascular coagulation, hemolytic uremic syndrome), or spherocytes (hereditary spherocytosis, autoimmune hemolytic anemia) suggests hemolysis.

F. Consider the possibility of malignancy or aplastic anemia when a low neutrophil and/or platelet count coexists with the anemia or underproduction. A normal or elevated neutrophil and platelet count suggests a pure red cell aplasia.

G. Consult a hematologist prior to performing a bone marrow to avoid omitting important special studies (e.g., biopsy, chromosomes, lymphoid markers).

H. Pure red cell aplasia of unknown etiology usually requires a bone marrow examination. However, if the anemia is mild (Hgb >9–10 g/dl) and occurs in a well-appearing child (normal physical examination), the bone marrow may be delayed and the child followed closely with weekly examinations and CBCs.

REFERENCES

Alter P. Childhood red cell aplasia. Am J Pediatr Hematol/Oncol 1980; 2:121.

Chu JY, Monteleone JA, Peden VH, et al. Anemia in children and adolescents with hypothyroidism. Clin Pediatr 1981; 20:696.

Dallman PR, Siimes MA. Percentile curves for hemoglobin and red cell volume in infancy and childhood. J Pediatr 1979; 94:26.

Lipton JM, Nathan DG. Aplastic and hypoplastic anemia. Pediatr Clin North Am 1980; 27:217.

NORMOCYTIC OR MACROCYTIC ANEMIA

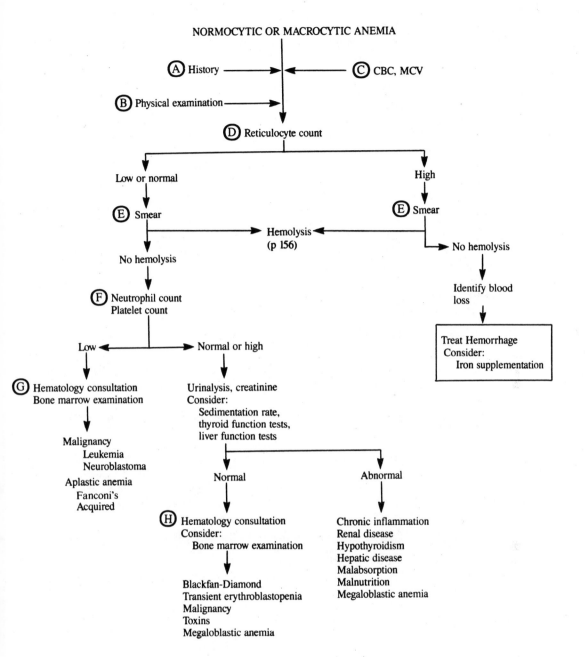

(A) History

(B) Physical examination

(C) CBC, MCV

(D) Reticulocyte count

Low or normal

High

(E) Smear

(E) Smear

Hemolysis
(p 156)

No hemolysis

No hemolysis

Identify blood
loss

(F) Neutrophil count
Platelet count

Treat Hemorrhage
Consider:
Iron supplementation

Low

Normal or high

(G) Hematology consultation
Bone marrow examination

Urinalysis, creatinine
Consider:
Sedimentation rate,
thyroid function tests,
liver function tests

Malignancy
Leukemia
Neuroblastoma

Aplastic anemia
Fanconi's
Acquired

Normal

Abnormal

(H) Hematology consultation
Consider:
Bone marrow examination

Chronic inflammation
Renal disease
Hypothyroidism
Hepatic disease
Malabsorption
Malnutrition
Megaloblastic anemia

Blackfan-Diamond
Transient erythroblastopenia
Malignancy
Toxins
Megaloblastic anemia

155

HEMOLYTIC ANEMIA
Peter A. Lane, M.D.

A. Note symptoms that suggest severe hemolysis such as headache, dizziness, syncope, fever, chills, or abdominal or back pain. Inquire about neonatal jaundice or recurrent jaundice. Note possible precipitating factors such as viral illness or the use of medications. A history of recurrent infections, arthritis, rash, mouth ulcers, or thyroid disease suggests the possibility of autoimmune hemolysis. Black, Mediterranean, or Arab ancestry suggests the possibility of a sickle cell syndrome or G6PD deficiency (in a male). Obtain a family history for anemia, jaundice, splenectomy or unexplained gallstones.

B. Assess the circulatory status. If the hemoglobin is >8.0 mg/dl, significant tachypnea or tachycardia suggests a rapidly falling hemoglobin or shock secondary to sepsis with disseminated intravascular coagulation (DIC) or a splenic sequestration. Note fever (intravascular hemolysis, acute infection, or collagen-vascular disease) or growth retardation (longstanding anemia or diseases associated with autoimmune hemolysis). Note the presence of splenomegaly. Mild splenomegaly is unusual in homozygous sickle cell disease, but common in sickle cell-hemoglobin C disease, sickle-cell-β thalassemia, and hereditary spherocytosis. Moderate to massive splenomegaly suggests a splenic sequestration. Note petechiae or bruising (DIC, HUS) and arthritis or rash (collagen-vascular disease).

C. Perform a CBC and a reticulocyte count. A normal hemoglobin does not exclude the possibility of hemolysis since an increased production of red cells may completely compensate for their increased destruction. Microcytosis (p 152) suggests a thalassemia syndrome, hemoglobin E disease, hereditary pyropoikilocytosis, or coexistent iron deficiency. A low or normal reticulocyte count suggests a hypoplastic crisis.

D. Perform both direct and indirect Coombs tests. Coombs negative autoimmune hemolytic anemias occur but are rare in children.

E. Determine the thermal amplitude (warm or cold) and antigen specificity (e.g., Rh, I) of the antibody, as well as whether IgG, C_3, or both are present on the red cells. Attempt to find compatible units of packed RBCs, but avoid transfusions if possible. Most cases of autoimmune hemolytic anemia in children are idiopathic or related to infection and transient. The presence of neutropenia, thrombocytopenia, a prolonged PTT, or a positive ANA suggests the presence of other autoantibodies and an underlying systemic disease.

F. Spherocytes and elliptocytes occur in many clinical settings. Obtain blood smears on family members; hereditary spherocytosis and elliptocytosis are usually autosomal dominant.

G. In the absence of microcytosis or liver disease, target cells suggest a hemoglobinopathy. A sickle cell prep or solubility test confirms the presence of sickle hemoglobin. Children with sickle cell trait have a positive sickle cell prep but do not have significant hemolysis or an abnormal blood smear. Obtain a *quantitative* hemoglobin electrophoresis to accurately diagnose a sickle cell syndrome.

H. The finding of red cell fragmentation suggests a microangiopathic hemolytic process. Consider DIC or HUS in the acutely ill child. DIC is most commonly associated with overwhelming infection.

REFERENCES

Buchanan GR, Boxer LA, Nathan DG. The acute and transient nature of idiopathic immune hemolytic anemia in childhood. J Pediatr 1976; 88:780.

Lux SE, Wolfe LC. Inherited disorders of the red cell membrane skeleton. Pediatr Clin North Am 1980; 27:463.

Petz LD, Garratty G. Acquired Immune Hemolytic Anemias. New York: Churchhill Livingston, 1980:349.

Sullivan DW, Glader BE. Erythrocyte enzyme disorders in children. Pediatr Clin North Am 1980; 27:449.

Vichinsky EP, Lubin BH. Sickle cell anemia and related hemoglobinopathies. Pediatr Clin North Am 1980; 27:429.

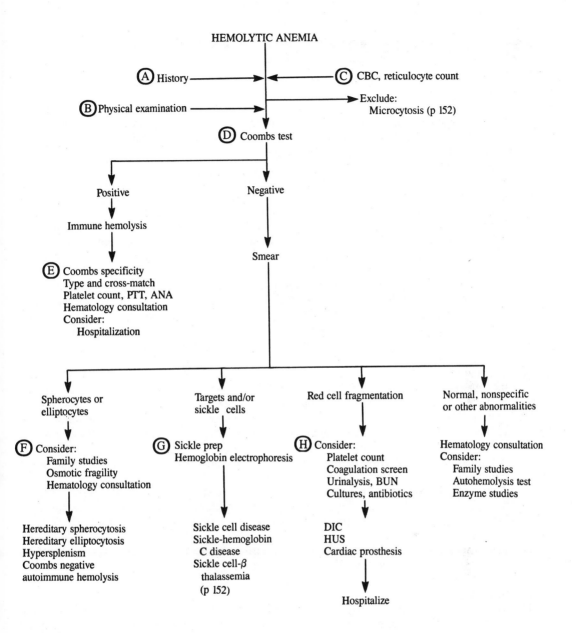

HEMOLYTIC ANEMIA

(A) History

(C) CBC, reticulocyte count

(B) Physical examination

Exclude:
Microcytosis (p 152)

(D) Coombs test

Positive

Immune hemolysis

(E) Coombs specificity
Type and cross-match
Platelet count, PTT, ANA
Hematology consultation
Consider:
    Hospitalization

Negative

Smear

Spherocytes or
elliptocytes

(F) Consider:
    Family studies
    Osmotic fragility
    Hematology consultation

Hereditary spherocytosis
Hereditary elliptocytosis
Hypersplenism
Coombs negative
autoimmune hemolysis

Targets and/or
sickle cells

(G) Sickle prep
Hemoglobin electrophoresis

Sickle cell disease
Sickle-hemoglobin
C disease
Sickle cell-β
    thalassemia
(p 152)

Red cell fragmentation

(H) Consider:
    Platelet count
    Coagulation screen
    Urinalysis, BUN
    Cultures, antibiotics

DIC
HUS
Cardiac prosthesis

Hospitalize

Normal, nonspecific
or other abnormalities

Hematology consultation
Consider:
    Family studies
    Autohemolysis test
    Enzyme studies

BLEEDING DISORDERS
Peter A. Lane, M.D.

A. Note the type and extent of bruising or bleeding as well as the frequency and duration of these symptoms. Epistaxis is a common occurrence in children, but prolonged recurrent nose bleeds (> 10 minutes) suggest the possibility of thrombocytopenia or a platelet function defect. Oral mucous membrane bleeding in infancy suggests hemophilia. Note jaundice (liver disease), poor weight gain (uremia, malabsorption with secondary vitamin K deficiency), recurrent joint pain or swelling (hemophilia, collagen vascular disease), or recent abdominal or joint pain (Henoch-Schönlein purpura-HSP). Breast-fed infants may be at risk for vitamin K deficiency, particularly after a bout of diarrhea. Inquire about excessive bleeding following any operations, especially circumcision, tonsillectomy, or tooth extraction. Note all drug use; ask specifically about aspirin. Consider the possibility of physical abuse (p 202). Review the family history for any clues to congenital bleeding disorders.

B. Perform a complete physical examination. Note petechiae (thrombocytopenia or platelet dysfunction), jaundice (liver disease), lymphadenopathy or hepatosplenomegaly (leukemia, malignancy), rash or joint swelling (collagen vascular disease, HSP, hemophilia).

C. Bleeding is a frequent complication of known systemic disease such as sepsis, liver disease, and uremia. Other diagnoses such as HSP and physical abuse are frequently apparent without laboratory studies.

D. Children with known congenital coagulopathies require the expeditious administration of replacement therapy for significant episodes of bleeding: cryoprecipitate or factor VIII concentrates for factor VIII deficiency (classic hemophilia), cryoprecipatate or desmopressin acetate (stimulates release of factor VIII from storage sites) for von-Willebrand's disease, and platelet transfusions for platelet function defects. Less common hereditary defects are treated with factor IX concentrates or fresh frozen plasma.

E. A normal bleeding screen does not exclude a coagulopathy; significant unexplained bleeding requires a hematology consultation and further evaluation.

F. A prolonged bleeding time in association with a normal platelet count suggests platelet dysfunction. Consult with a hematologist to ensure that appropriate laboratory studies for von-Willebrand's disease are performed. Reconsider the possibility of uremia or a drug effect on platelet function.

G. Prolongation of both prothrombin time and partial thromboplastin time suggests a diffuse coagulopathy such as that caused by vitamin K deficiency, liver disease, DIC, afibrinogenemia, dysfibrinogenemia, or hypofibrinogenemia. Consider giving vitamin K; treat serious bleeding with fresh frozen plasma.

H. Consult a hematologist for assistance in evaluating a prolonged PTT. Repeating the PTT after 1:1 mixing with normal plasma may help differentiate a factor deficiency from an inhibitor of coagulation.

I. An isolated prolongation of the prothrombin time is rare and suggests factor VII deficiency, mild vitamin K deficiency, or liver disease.

REFERENCES

Bachmann F. Diagnostic approach to mild bleeding disorders. Sem Hematol 1980; 17:292.
Buchanan GR. Hemophilia. Pediatr Clin North Am 1980; 27:309.
Montgomery RR, Hathaway WE. Acute bleeding emergencies. Pediatr Clin North Am 1980; 27:327.

BRUISED OR BLEEDING CHILD

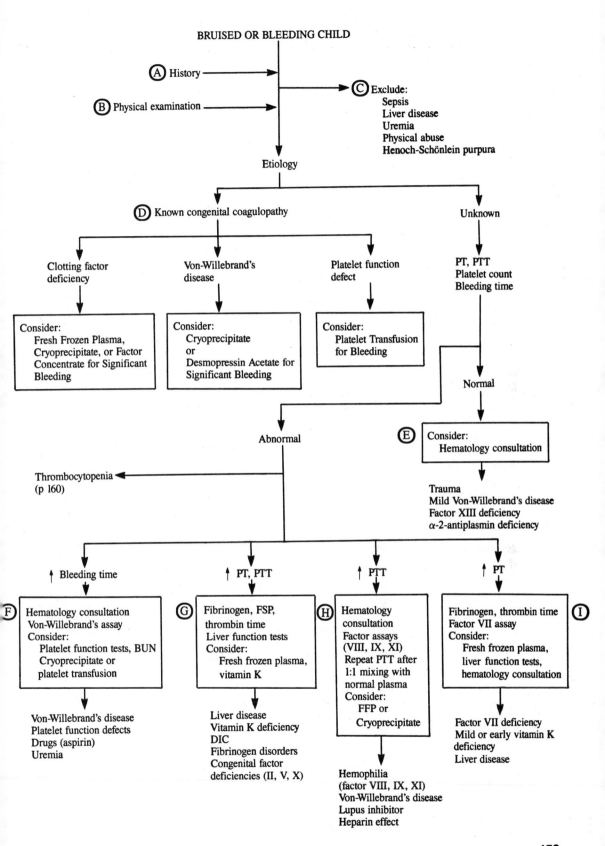

Ⓐ History ⟶

Ⓑ Physical examination ⟶

Ⓒ Exclude:
Sepsis
Liver disease
Uremia
Physical abuse
Henoch-Schönlein purpura

Etiology

Ⓓ Known congenital coagulopathy

Unknown

Clotting factor deficiency

Von-Willebrand's disease

Platelet function defect

PT, PTT
Platelet count
Bleeding time

Consider:
Fresh Frozen Plasma, Cryoprecipitate, or Factor Concentrate for Significant Bleeding

Consider:
Cryoprecipitate or Desmopressin Acetate for Significant Bleeding

Consider:
Platelet Transfusion for Bleeding

Normal

Abnormal

Ⓔ Consider:
Hematology consultation

Thrombocytopenia (p 160)

Trauma
Mild Von-Willebrand's disease
Factor XIII deficiency
α-2-antiplasmin deficiency

↑ Bleeding time

↑ PT, PTT

↑ PTT

↑ PT

Ⓕ Hematology consultation
Von-Willebrand's assay
Consider:
Platelet function tests, BUN
Cryoprecipitate or platelet transfusion

Ⓖ Fibrinogen, FSP, thrombin time
Liver function tests
Consider:
Fresh frozen plasma, vitamin K

Ⓗ Hematology consultation
Factor assays (VIII, IX, XI)
Repeat PTT after 1:1 mixing with normal plasma
Consider:
FFP or Cryoprecipitate

Ⓘ Fibrinogen, thrombin time
Factor VII assay
Consider:
Fresh frozen plasma, liver function tests, hematology consultation

Von-Willebrand's disease
Platelet function defects
Drugs (aspirin)
Uremia

Liver disease
Vitamin K deficiency
DIC
Fibrinogen disorders
Congenital factor deficiencies (II, V, X)

Hemophilia (factor VIII, IX, XI)
Von-Willebrand's disease
Lupus inhibitor
Heparin effect

Factor VII deficiency
Mild or early vitamin K deficiency
Liver disease

THROMBOCYTOPENIA

Peter A. Lane, M.D.

A. Note the type and duration of bruising, bleeding, or petechiae. Note recent illnesses such as diarrhea, hemolytic uremic syndrome (HUS), or sore throat (infectious mononucleosis, acute post streptococcal glomerulonephritis). Document associated symptoms such as fever (infection, leukemia, collagen vascular disease), limp, or limb pain (leukemia, collagen vascular disease). Note any medications. Obtain a family history of bleeding disorders.

B. Note fever and the degree of illness. Acutely ill and toxic-appearing children with thrombocytopenia require expeditious evaluation (DIC, sepsis, HUS, severe internal hemorrhage). Note the extent and type of manifestations of bleeding. Short stature, microcephaly, skeletal anomalies, hyperpigmentation, hypogenitalism, (Fanconi's anemia), absent radii with normal thumbs, and chronic eczema and recurrent infections in a boy (Wiskott-Aldrich syndrome) are all clues to congenital thrombocytopenia. Splenomegaly or generalized lymphadenopathy suggests leukemia, malignancy, infection (infectious mononucleosis), a storage disease, or hypersplenism. Typically, children with idiopathic thrombocytopenic purpura (ITP) do *not* have splenomegaly. Arthritis, mouth ulcers, or a characteristic rash may suggest a collagen vascular disease.

C. Order a CBC with differential and platelet count. The finding of anemia or neutropenia (absolute neutrophil count < 1500/mm³) in association with thrombocytopenia helps direct the subsequent workup. While neutropenia may occur with infection, its association with significant thrombocytopenia suggests bone marrow failure. Anemia suggests bone marrow failure, intravascular hemolysis, autoimmune disease, or blood loss secondary to thrombocytopenic bleeding.

D. Review the peripheral blood smear. Red cell fragmentation suggests intravascular hemolysis. Spherocytes (autoimmune hemolysis) or macrocytes (bone marrow failure, Fanconi's anemia), or brisk reticulocytosis are also helpful clues. Note platelet size and morphology. Boys with Wiskott-Aldrich syndrome have tiny platelets; large platelets suggest rapid platelet turnover, as seen in ITP, or a familial thrombocytopenia such as Bernard-Soulier syndrome or May-Hegglin anomaly.

E. Consult a hematologist prior to performing a bone marrow in order to avoid omitting important special studies (biopsy, chromosomes, lymphoid markers). The absence of lymphadenopathy, organomegaly, and leukemic blasts on the blood smear does not exclude the possibility of leukemia.

F. While ITP is the most common cause of acute thrombocytopenia in an otherwise well child, other diagnostic possibilities must always be entertained. A positive ANA or Coombs test indicates the presence of other autoantibodies and suggests the possibility of an underlying collagen vascular disease. The decision to perform a bone marrow examination may be individualized. Children with platelet counts > 50,000 and an otherwise normal CBC and physical examination may be observed with serial CBCs and platelet counts. Children with severe thrombocytopenia or other blood count abnormalities should be evaluated with a bone marrow examination. No child should ever receive steroid therapy for presumed ITP without first undergoing bone marrow examination to exclude acute leukemia.

G. Because splenomegaly and lymphadenopathy are unusual in children with ITP, these findings in a child with significant thrombocytopenia dictate an early bone marrow examination unless a clear alternative explanation exists (i.e., longstanding splenomegaly with portal hypertension suggesting hypersplenism).

REFERENCES

Corrigan JJ. Disseminated intravascular coagulopathy. Pediatr Rev 1979; 1:37.

Lightsey AL. Thrombocytopenia in children. Pediatr Clin North Am 1980; 27:293.

McWilliams NB, Mauer HM. Acute idiopathic thrombocytopenic purpura in children. Am J Hematol 1979; 7:87.

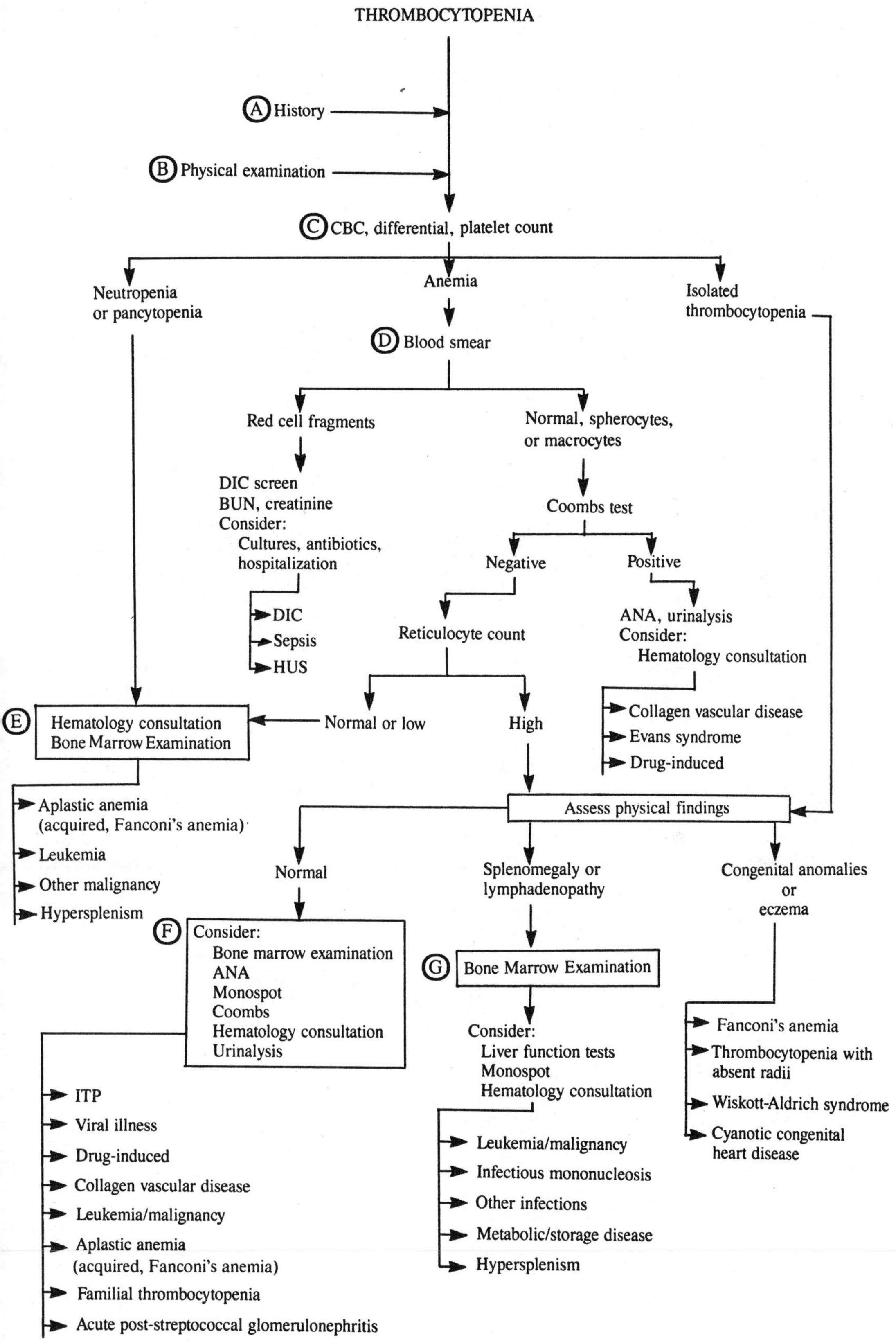

THROMBOCYTOPENIA

(A) History

(B) Physical examination

(C) CBC, differential, platelet count

Neutropenia or pancytopenia

Anemia

(D) Blood smear

Isolated thrombocytopenia

Red cell fragments

Normal, spherocytes, or macrocytes

DIC screen
BUN, creatinine
Consider:
Cultures, antibiotics, hospitalization

→ DIC
→ Sepsis
→ HUS

Coombs test

Negative

Positive

Reticulocyte count

ANA, urinalysis
Consider:
Hematology consultation

→ Collagen vascular disease
→ Evans syndrome
→ Drug-induced

(E) Hematology consultation
Bone Marrow Examination

Normal or low

High

→ Aplastic anemia
(acquired, Fanconi's anemia)
→ Leukemia
→ Other malignancy
→ Hypersplenism

Assess physical findings

Normal

Splenomegaly or lymphadenopathy

Congenital anomalies or eczema

(F) Consider:
Bone marrow examination
ANA
Monospot
Coombs
Hematology consultation
Urinalysis

(G) Bone Marrow Examination

Consider:
Liver function tests
Monospot
Hematology consultation

→ Fanconi's anemia
→ Thrombocytopenia with absent radii
→ Wiskott-Aldrich syndrome
→ Cyanotic congenital heart disease

→ ITP
→ Viral illness
→ Drug-induced
→ Collagen vascular disease
→ Leukemia/malignancy
→ Aplastic anemia
(acquired, Fanconi's anemia)
→ Familial thrombocytopenia
→ Acute post-streptococcal glomerulonephritis

→ Leukemia/malignancy
→ Infectious mononucleosis
→ Other infections
→ Metabolic/storage disease
→ Hypersplenism

161

GENERALIZED LYMPHADENOPATHY

Peter A. Lane, M.D.

A. Note systemic symptoms such as persistent or recurrent fever (infection, malignancy, collagen vascular disease), sore throat (infectious mononucleosis), cough (tuberculosis or fungal infection), epistaxis or easy bruising (leukemia), limp or limb pain (juvenile rheumatoid arthritis, leukemia, neuroblastoma). Note duration and severity of any systemic symptoms and assess whether they are improving or progressing. Obtain a complete history of travel or animal exposures. Note all recent immunizations and medications (serum sickness, drug reaction, phenytoin-induced lymphadenopathy). Document routine immunizations; inquire about possible exposure to tuberculosis.

B. Note the degree and extent of lymphadenopathy. Discrete, mobile, nontender lymph nodes are palpable in most healthy children (young infants excepted). The presence of small inguinal or high cervical nodes ($\leq$1 cm) or occipital, submandibular, or axillary nodes ($\leq$3 mm) is normal. Generalized lymphadenopathy is defined as abnormal lymph node enlargement of more than two noncontiguous lymph node regions with or without hepatosplenomegaly. Note thyromegaly (hyperthyroidism), massive hepatosplenomegaly (malignancy, storage disease), arthritis (collagen vascular disease, leukemia), or a characteristic rash or conjunctivitis (viral exanthem, JRA, systemic lupus, mucocutaneous lymph node syndrome, leptospirosis, or histiocytosis).

C. False negative monospot tests frequently occur early in the course of infectious mononucleosis and are the rule in very young children with EB virus infection.

D. Atypical lymphocytes are frequently associated with many viral illnesses. A differential count with 10–20% atypical lymphocytes suggests infectious mononucleosis, CMV, toxoplasmosis, viral hepatitis, or drug hypersensitivity. Screen titers for EB virus or toxoplasmosis, a urine culture for CMV, or liver function tests may be helpful in selected cases.

E. Children with prolonged fever, unexplained weight loss, persistent cough, known exposure to TB, or significant systemic toxicity are considered moderately to severely ill. Mildly ill children can be followed clinically.

F. Perform a chest x-ray and place a PPD. Further evaluation depends upon the CXR results, age of the child, and diagnostic clues obtained during the history and physical examination. Consider obtaining a bone marrow test, lymph node biopsy, urine VMA, and histoplasmosis titers.

G. Severe anemia, neutropenia, or thrombocytopenia accompanying generalized lymphadenopathy suggests a malignancy, severe infection, or storage disease. Obtain an oncology consultation prior to performing a bone marrow examination in order to avoid omitting important special studies (biopsy, chromosomes, lymphoid markers, fungal cultures).

REFERENCES

Yanagihara R, Todd JK. Acute febrile mucocutaneous lymph node syndrome. Am J Dis Child 1980; 134:603.
Zuelzer WW, Kaplan J. The child with lymphadenopathy. Sem Hematol 1975; 12:323.

GENERALIZED LYMPHADENOPATHY

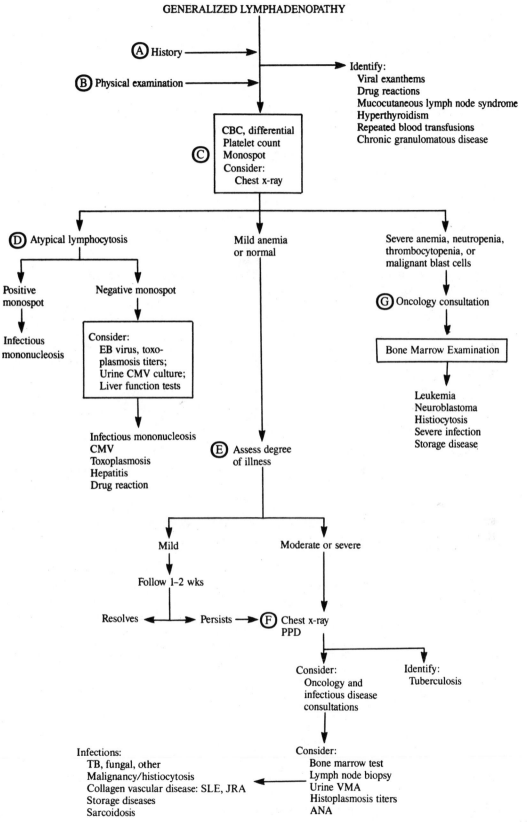

Ⓐ History

Ⓑ Physical examination

Identify:
Viral exanthems
Drug reactions
Mucocutaneous lymph node syndrome
Hyperthyroidism
Repeated blood transfusions
Chronic granulomatous disease

Ⓒ CBC, differential
Platelet count
Monospot
Consider:
Chest x-ray

Ⓓ Atypical lymphocytosis

Mild anemia
or normal

Severe anemia, neutropenia,
thrombocytopenia, or
malignant blast cells

Positive
monospot

Negative monospot

Ⓖ Oncology consultation

Infectious
mononucleosis

Consider:
EB virus, toxo-
plasmosis titers;
Urine CMV culture;
Liver function tests

Bone Marrow Examination

Leukemia
Neuroblastoma
Histiocytosis
Severe infection
Storage disease

Infectious mononucleosis
CMV
Toxoplasmosis
Hepatitis
Drug reaction

Ⓔ Assess degree
of illness

Mild

Moderate or severe

Follow 1–2 wks

Resolves ◄──── Persists ───► Ⓕ Chest x-ray
PPD

Consider:
Oncology and
infectious disease
consultations

Identify:
Tuberculosis

Infections:
TB, fungal, other
Malignancy/histiocytosis
Collagen vascular disease: SLE, JRA
Storage diseases
Sarcoidosis

Consider:
Bone marrow test
Lymph node biopsy
Urine VMA
Histoplasmosis titers
ANA

ACUTE ILLNESS ASSOCIATED WITH SICKLE CELL DISEASE
Peter A. Lane, M.D.

A. Review prior problems associated with sickle cell disease as well as the details of the acute illness. Inquire specifically about fever, pain, cough, shortness of breath, and neurologic symptoms. If pain is present, ask whether the pain is similar or dissimilar to previous "sickle pains". Determine from the patient or from medical records the precise diagnosis of prior disease (homozygous sickle cell disease, sickle-hemoglobin C disease, sickle-β thalassemia) as well as the patient's baseline values for hemoglobin, hematocrit, WBC, and reticulocyte count.

B. Perform a complete physical examination; search carefully for foci of infection. Note fever (infection or infarction), tachypnea (pneumonia, pulmonary infarction), or tachycardia or hypotension (splenic sequestration, severe infection). Significant splenomegaly suggests a diagnosis of sickle-hemoglobin C disease, sickle-β thalassemia or splenic sequestration. Note any neurologic abnormalities (stroke, meningitis), right upper quadrant tenderness (biliary colic, hepatitis, vaso-occlusive crisis), knee or hip pain (aseptic necrosis of the femoral head), or priapism.

C. Assess the risk of infection. Because functional hyposplenia develops at an early age, children with sickle cell disease commonly develop bacterial sepsis and/or meningitis. Patients with a temperature > 102°F or with unexplained lethargy are at high risk for overwhelming sepsis. Immediately draw blood cultures and begin IV antibiotics (pneumococcus, *H. influenzae* are the most common organisms). Perform a lumbar puncture for patients with meningismus or young children with excessive lethargy or toxicity.

D. Consider the possibility of an illness unrelated to sickle cell disease (e.g., appendicitis presenting with abdominal pain). Acute splenic enlargement with a hematocrit below baseline or signs of intravascular volume depletion suggests a splenic sequestration crisis. A lower-than-baseline hematocrit in association with a low reticulocyte count (<5%) suggests an aplastic crisis.

E. Splenic sequestration is a life-threatening emergency requiring IV fluids and red cell transfusions to maintain intravascular volume. Support a hypotensive patient with large volumes of isotonic crystalloid while awaiting whole blood or packed red blood cells (PRBC's) from the blood bank.

F. Aplastic crises occur commonly in association with viral illness and represent a transient inability of erythropoiesis to keep pace with chronic hemolysis. The rapidly falling hemoglobin may result in congestive heart failure; red cell transfusions should be used to support the patient until adequate red cell production resumes.

G. Vaso-occlusive crises with severe pain secondary to ischemia may occur in any part of the body. Treatment includes hydration with one and one-half to twice maintenance fluids (sickle cell patients have hyposthenuria) and adequate analgesia (codeine for mild pain, morphine or hydromorphine for severe pain). Do *not* use meperidine because of its potential to induce seizures. Indications for hospitalization include an inability to maintain hydration orally and the failure of oral analgesics to control pain. Consider the possibility of acute osteomyelitis (*S. aureus*, *Salmonella*) in patients thought to have bone infarctions. Pulmonary infarction is often difficult to distinguish from bacterial pneumonia (*S. pneumoniae*, *H. influenzae*, mycoplasma). A cerebrovascular accident is indication for exchange transfusion and subsequent chronic transfusions. Boys with priapism may also benefit from exchange transfusion.

H. Sickle cell patients who require general anesthesia for major surgical procedures should be first transfused to lower the sickle hemoglobin level to 30% to avoid perioperative sickling complications.

REFERENCES

Giller RH. Sickle cell disease. In: Barkin R, Rosen P, eds. Pediatric Emergencies. St Louis: CV Mosby, 1984.

ACUTE ILLNESS ASSOCIATED WITH SICKLE CELL DISEASE

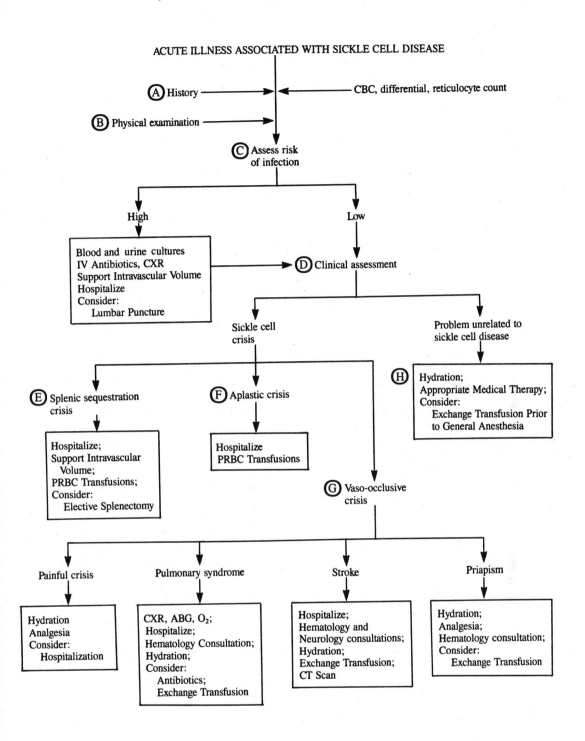

McIntosh S, Rooks Y, Ritchey AK, et al. Fever in young children with sickle cell disease. J Pediatr 1980; 96:199.

Vinchinsky EP, Lubin BH. Sickle cell anemia and related hemoglobinopathies. Pediatr Clin North Am 1980; 27:429.

ACUTE ABDOMINAL PAIN

A. Determine the onset, frequency, severity, pattern, and location of the pain. Note associated symptoms of urinary tract involvement (dysuria, frequency) and the presence of fever, vomiting, diarrhea, rectal bleeding, jaundice, weight loss, or arthritis. Identify precipitating factors or predisposing conditions including constipation, trauma, medications, menses, spider bite, sickle cell disease, pregnancy, prior abdominal surgery, or inflammatory bowel disease.

B. Assess the circulatory and hydration status. Note signs of peritoneal irritation such as ileopsoas rigidity (psoas sign) and pain with external thigh rotation (obturator test). Locate the site of pain and document the presence of point tenderness, rigidity of abdominal muscles, and rebound. Do a rectal examination to identify an impaction, mass, or right lower quadrant tenderness. Note signs of pneumonia and other extraintestinal manifestations of disease.

C. Assess the degree of illness. Severely ill patients appear toxic with signs of shock or peritonitis and are unable to walk. Peritoneal signs include rigidity of the abdominal muscles, rebound tenderness, and decreased bowel sounds. Moderately ill patients have difficulty walking, an intermittent pain pattern characteristic of intussusception, or signs of peritoneal irritation. Peritoneal irritation results in pain with jarring movements, referred pain to the neck or shoulder, a positive psoas sign, or an abnormal obturator test.

D. Infections which can present with abdominal pain include bacterial enteritis, parasitic disease, urinary tract infections, hepatitis, pneumonia, pharyngitis associated with *S. pyogenes* or Ebstein Barr virus, or pelvic inflammatory disease. When extraintestinal manifestations are present, consider inflammatory bowel disease, Henoch-Schönlein purpura, hemolytic uremic syndrome, pseudomembranous colitis, renal disease, malignancy, collagen vascular disease, and sickle cell disease.

E. With epigastric pain, consider peptic ulcer disease, hiatal hernia, gastroesophageal reflux, esophagitis, and pancreatitis. Right upper quadrant pain suggests hepatitis, liver abscess or tumor, Fitz-Hugh Curtis syndrome, cholecystitis, or cholangitis. When mild abdominal pain is diffuse, periumbilical, or left-sided, consider constipation, mesenteric adenitis, food poisoning, pharyngitis, muscle strain, gastroenteritis, and psychogenic pain.

F. Abnormal radiographic findings include fecaliths (appendicitis), pneumatosis intestinalis (NEC), free air (perforation), obstructive patterns (mechanical and functional), air in an abscess, abdominal mass, and abdominal calcifications. Renal stones, pneumonia, or osteomyelitis may also be identified.

G. Appendicitis typically presents with a leucocytosis, elevated sedimentation rate, vomiting, signs of peritoneal irritation, and point tenderness over McBurney's point. Acute appendicitis may cause a low-volume diarrhea. An abscess near the right ureter can cause pyuria.

H. Consider an intussuception when intermittent crampy abdominal pain is associated with vomiting, abdominal distention, or bloody stools. Note the presence of an epigastric sausage-shaped mass. Intussuception may cause an alteration in mental status which suggests CNS disease. Intussuception most commonly occurs in children 4–24 months of age. Attempt a hydrostatic reduction with a barium enema prior to surgery.

REFERENCES

Apley J. The Child with Abdominal Pains. Philadelphia: FA Davis, 1959.

Green M. Abdominal Pain in Pediatric Diagnosis. Philadelphia: WB Saunders, 1980:325–337.

Jones PF. Acute abdominal pain in childhood, with special reference to cases not due to acute appendicitis. Br med J 1969; 1:284–286.

Smith EI. Appendicitis and peritonitis. In: Kelly VC, ed. Practice of Pediatrics. Philadelphia: Harper and Row, 1984:5:1.

ACUTE ABDOMINAL PAIN

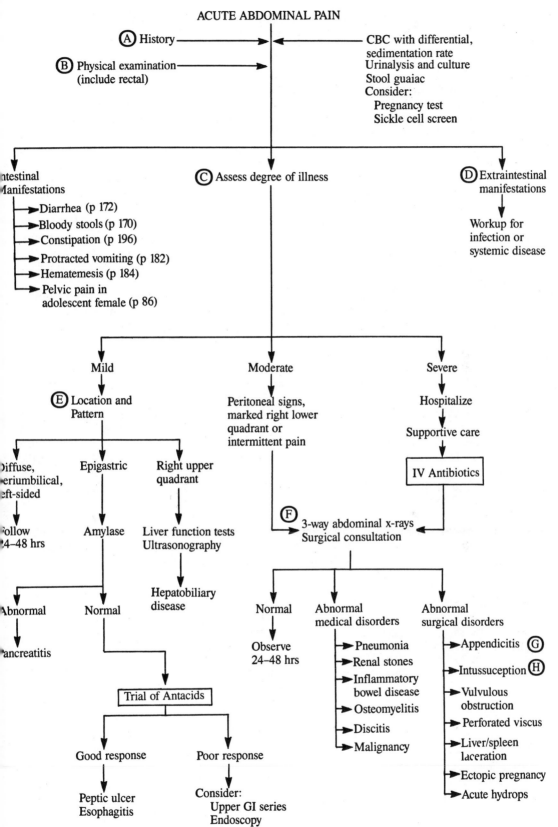

Ⓐ History

Ⓑ Physical examination (include rectal)

CBC with differential, sedimentation rate
Urinalysis and culture
Stool guaiac
Consider:
   Pregnancy test
   Sickle cell screen

Intestinal Manifestations

→ Diarrhea (p 172)
→ Bloody stools (p 170)
→ Constipation (p 196)
→ Protracted vomiting (p 182)
→ Hematemesis (p 184)
→ Pelvic pain in adolescent female (p 86)

Ⓒ Assess degree of illness

Ⓓ Extraintestinal manifestations

Workup for infection or systemic disease

Mild

Ⓔ Location and Pattern

Moderate

Peritoneal signs, marked right lower quadrant or intermittent pain

Severe

Hospitalize

Supportive care

IV Antibiotics

Diffuse, periumbilical, left-sided

Epigastric

Right upper quadrant

Follow 24–48 hrs

Amylase

Liver function tests
Ultrasonography

Ⓕ 3-way abdominal x-rays
Surgical consultation

Abnormal

Pancreatitis

Normal

Hepatobiliary disease

Normal

Observe 24–48 hrs

Abnormal medical disorders

→ Pneumonia
→ Renal stones
→ Inflammatory bowel disease
→ Osteomyelitis
→ Discitis
→ Malignancy

Abnormal surgical disorders

→ Appendicitis Ⓖ
→ Intussuception Ⓗ
→ Vulvulous obstruction
→ Perforated viscus
→ Liver/spleen laceration
→ Ectopic pregnancy
→ Acute hydrops

Trial of Antacids

Good response

Peptic ulcer
Esophagitis

Poor response

Consider:
Upper GI series
Endoscopy

167

CHRONIC ABDOMINAL PAIN

A. Criteria for chronic or recurrent abdominal pain in childhood are vague. Apley defines recurrent abdominal pain as 3 discrete episodes which occur over a minimum 3-month period and which interfere with regular activities. Determine the onset, frequency, severity, pattern, and location of the pain. Note associated gastrointestinal manifestations as well as extraintestinal manifestations such as fever, weight loss, arthritis, hematuria, frequency, and dysuria. Note the presence of nonspecific autonomic symptoms such as headache, limb pains, nausea, pallor, perspiration, and vomiting. Identify precipitating factors or predisposing conditions such as constipation, medications, sickle cell disease, menses, and foods. Determine the functional level of impairment, the anxiety level of the child and family, the family history of functional illness, and the presence of stress in the child's life.

B. Note the site of pain, and document the presence of point tenderness, rigidity of abdominal muscles, and rebound. Do a rectal examination to identify an impaction or mass. Note signs of pneumonia and other extraintestinal manifestations such as arthritis, ascites, hepatosplenomegaly, jaundice, lymphadenopathy, and purpura.

C. Infections which can present with abdominal pain include bacterial enteritis, parasitic disease, urinary tract infections, hepatitis, pelvic inflammatory disease, pneumonia, mononucleosis, and pharyngitis with *S. pyogenes*. Extraintestinal manifestations may suggest Henoch-Schönlein purpura, inflammatory bowel disease, hemolytic uremic syndrome, renal disease, malignancy, collagen vascular disease, or sickle cell disease.

D. With epigastric pain, consider peptic ulcer disease, hiatal hernia, gastroesophageal reflux, esophagitis, and pancreatitis. Right upper quadrant pain suggests hepatitis, liver abscess or tumor, Fitz-Hugh Curtis syndrome, cholecystitis, cholangitis, or choledochal cyst.

E. Patients with a nonspecific pattern may present with mild, chronic diarrhea or constipation. These patients react to stress with excessive rectosigmoid spasm. These children may have associated autonomic symptoms and may exhibit complaint modeling. Their personality profile is often characterized by low self-esteem and insecurity in association with a high level of anxiety in the family. The approach to these patients is outlined on page 190; further diagnostic efforts such as EEG, upper GI series, IVP, CT scans, ultrasonography, or endoscopy are not indicated in these patients. Placebos, antispasmodics, and sedatives are not necessary and may elevate the level of anxiety in the patient and family.

F. Suspect lactose intolerance when abdominal pain is precipitated by foods containing lactose. Consider a lactose tolerance test and/or a lactose-free diet. The frequency of lactose intolerance as an underlying cause of chronic abdominal pain has not been determined.

REFERENCES

Apley J. The Child with Abdominal Pains. London: Blackwell Scientific, 1975.
Bain HW. Chronic vague abdominal pain in children. Ped Clin N Amer 1974; 21:991.
Barbero GB. Recurrent abdominal pain in childhood. Pediatr Rev 1982; 1:29.
Lebenthal E. Marginal comments: recurrent abdominal pain in childhood. Am J Dis Child 1980; 134:347.

CHRONIC ABDOMINAL PAIN

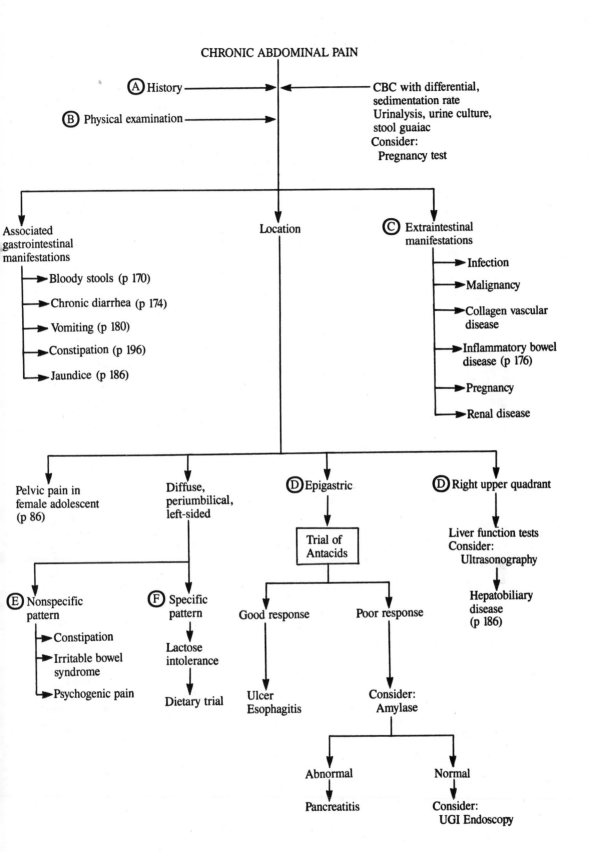

Ⓐ History

Ⓑ Physical examination

CBC with differential,
sedimentation rate
Urinalysis, urine culture,
stool guaiac
Consider:
　Pregnancy test

Associated
gastrointestinal
manifestations

→ Bloody stools (p 170)

→ Chronic diarrhea (p 174)

→ Vomiting (p 180)

→ Constipation (p 196)

→ Jaundice (p 186)

Location

Ⓒ Extraintestinal
manifestations

→ Infection

→ Malignancy

→ Collagen vascular
disease

→ Inflammatory bowel
disease (p 176)

→ Pregnancy

→ Renal disease

Pelvic pain in
female adolescent
(p 86)

Diffuse,
periumbilical,
left-sided

Ⓓ Epigastric

Ⓓ Right upper quadrant

Liver function tests
Consider:
　Ultrasonography

Hepatobiliary
disease
(p 186)

Trial of
Antacids

Good response

Poor response

Ⓔ Nonspecific
pattern

→ Constipation

→ Irritable bowel
syndrome

→ Psychogenic pain

Ⓕ Specific
pattern

Lactose
intolerance

Dietary trial

Ulcer
Esophagitis

Consider:
　Amylase

Abnormal

Pancreatitis

Normal

Consider:
　UGI Endoscopy

BLOODY STOOLS

A. Bloody stools can appear as bright red (hematochezia) or dark, tarry (melena) stools. Hematochezia usually indicates lower intestinal bleeding; however, massive upper intestinal hemorrhage can present with bright red blood. Melena is associated with gastric or small bowel bleeding.

B. Determine the onset, type of bloody stools, and quantity of blood loss. Ask about associated gastrointestinal symptoms such as diarrhea, vomiting, constipation, anorexia, abdominal pain or distention. Note extraintestinal symptoms including fever, weight loss, delayed puberty, arthritis, purpura, rash, or jaundice. Exclude ingestion of substances which may be mistaken for melena or hematochezia, such as iron supplementation, bismuth, chocolate, grape juice, spinach, blue berries, food coloring, beets, jello, or red antibiotics. Identify possible precipitating factors or predisposing conditions such as drug ingestions (maternal or child), current antibiotic use, constipation, bleeding disorders, or milk/soy protein intolerance.

C. Obtain a CBC with differential and platelet count to document an anemia. Consider hemolytic uremic syndrome when thrombocytopenia and a microangiopathic hemolytic anemia are present. Obtain a coagulation screen when hemorrhagic disease of the newborn or other bleeding disorder is suspected. A low serum albumin is associated with a protein-losing enteropathy. An elevated sedimentation rate suggests infection, inflammatory bowel disease, or malignancy. In the newborn period, the Apt-Downey test distinguishes maternal blood from newborn blood. A positive nasogastric aspirate identifies bleeding proximal to the ligament of Treitz.

D. Assess the degree of illness. Severely ill patients appear toxic, have signs of significant blood loss, or appear obstructed. Moderately ill patients have significant blood loss in the stool, associated intestinal findings, or systemic symptoms. Consider a newborn who has blood mixed with stool moderately ill even if asymptomatic. Mildly ill patients have minimal blood loss, with the blood usually being superficial rather than mixed in the stool; they are not anemic, and have mild symptoms.

E. Suspect intussusception when bloody stools are associated with intermittent abdominal pain, abdominal distention, or vomiting. Intussusception usually occurs during the first 2 years of life (61% of patients are between 4 and 10 months of age). A barium enema confirms the diagnosis and, in 80% of cases, results in hydrostatic reduction.

F. Nonspecific colitis related to milk/soy protein intolerance presents in infants under 6 months with loose bloody stools and is often associated with vomiting, abdominal pain and distention. Rarely, it may occur in the newborn period or in infants of breast-feeding mothers who drink large amounts of cow's milk. When diagnosed in infants under 1 month of age, use Pregestimil formula. Consider using a soy formula in older infants, but remember that 30–40% of infants also react to soy formula. Avoid milk products until 12 months of age, then challenge the infant in a controlled setting.

G. Pseudomembranous colitis is frequently associated with antibiotic therapy and a positive assay for *Clostridium difficle* toxin.

H. Most polyps are the juvenile type and do not have malignant potential. In Peutz-Jeghers syndrome, multiple polyps in the small and large bowel are associated with mucocutaneous pigmentation. Multiple large bowel polyps associated with soft tissue tumors or bony abnormalities suggest Gardner's syndrome which is associated with a high risk of malignancy.

I. Suspect a vascular malformation when aortic stenosis, Turner's syndrome, or a mucocutaneous disorder (Osler-Weber-Rendu) is present. Endoscopy (sigmoidoscopy, colonoscopy) is the method most likely to diagnose a lesion. When the bleeding is extensive, arteriography may be necessary to identify the source.

REFERENCES

Feigin RD. Pseudomembranous colitis. Ped Rev 1981; 3:147.

Hillemeir C. Rectal bleeding in childhood. Ped Rev 1983; 5:35.

Lake AM, Whitington PF, Hamilton SR. Dietary protein-induced colitis in breast-fed infants. J Pediatr 1982; 101:906.

Silverman A, Roy CC. Pediatric Clinical Gastroenterology. 3rd ed. St. Louis: CV Mosby, 1983.

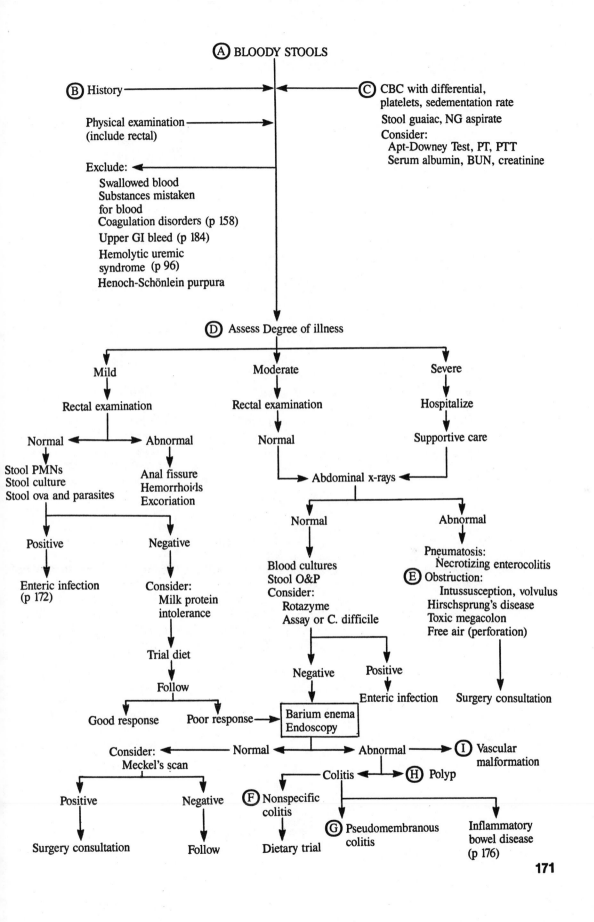

(A) BLOODY STOOLS

(B) History

Physical examination
(include rectal)

(C) CBC with differential,
platelets, sedementation rate

Stool guaiac, NG aspirate

Consider:
  Apt-Downey Test, PT, PTT
  Serum albumin, BUN, creatinine

Exclude:
  Swallowed blood
  Substances mistaken
  for blood
  Coagulation disorders (p 158)
  Upper GI bleed (p 184)
  Hemolytic uremic
  syndrome (p 96)
  Henoch-Schönlein purpura

(D) Assess Degree of illness

Mild

Rectal examination

Normal

Stool PMNs
Stool culture
Stool ova and parasites

Positive

Enteric infection
(p 172)

Abnormal

Anal fissure
Hemorrhoids
Excoriation

Negative

Consider:
  Milk protein
  intolerance

Trial diet

Follow

Good response   Poor response

Moderate

Rectal examination

Normal

Abdominal x-rays

Normal

Blood cultures
Stool O&P
Consider:
  Rotazyme
  Assay or C. difficile

Negative   Positive

Enteric infection

Severe

Hospitalize

Supportive care

Abnormal

Pneumatosis:
  Necrotizing enterocolitis
(E) Obstruction:
  Intussusception, volvulus
  Hirschsprung's disease
  Toxic megacolon
  Free air (perforation)

Surgery consultation

Barium enema
Endoscopy

Consider: Normal   Abnormal   (I) Vascular
Meckel's scan   malformation

Colitis   (H) Polyp

Positive   Negative

Surgery consultation   Follow

(F) Nonspecific
colitis

Dietary trial

(G) Pseudomembranous
colitis

Inflammatory
bowel disease
(p 176)

171

ACUTE DIARRHEA

A. Note the onset, duration, frequency, pattern, and severity of the diarrhea. Ask if the stools contain blood or mucus. Document type and amount of food intake and frequency of urination. Note associated gastrointestinal symptoms such as vomiting, abdominal pain, anorexia. Note systemic symptoms such as fever, cough, coryza, rash, weight loss, mental status, and decreased activity level. Identify precipitating factors such as medications (antibiotics) or ingestions. Ask if other family members have recently experienced diarrhea.

B. Assess the hydration and circulatory status by documenting blood pressure, heart and respiratory rates, skin color and turgor, capillary refill, presence of tears, fullness of the fontanel, and urine output. Assess mental status noting any irritability, lethargy, seizures, or focal neurologic signs. Note extraintestinal manifestations such as rash, hepatomegaly, splenomegaly, lymphadenopathy, and arthritis.

C. Mildly ill patients are alert, active, appear well hydrated and have good urine output. Moderately ill patients may be lethargic and have mild-to-moderate dehydration (decreased tearing, dry skin, decreased urine output, and, possibly, increased pulse). Severely ill patients have an altered mental status and severe dehydration (increased pulse, poor skin color, delayed capillary refill, no tears) with or without hypotension.

D. Admit moderately ill patients with acidosis (pH <7.3, $HCO_3 < 15$), azotemia (BUN >20), or an electrolyte abnormality (Na < 130 or > 150).

E. Give clear fluids for 12 to 24 hours. For infants, recommend an electrolyte solution such as Pedialyte or Lytren or consider an oral rehydration solution to replace mild or moderate fluid deficits. After a period of clear liquids, give half-strength formula for 24 hours, then full strength. The value of using a soy-base lactose-free formula is unclear. When appropriate, recommend ABCs (apple sauce, bananas, cooked carrots) and appropriate constipating solids such as rice, potatoes, or saltine crackers. Avoid juices or sodas which contain large quanitities of sugar and have a high osmotic load. In children over 2 years of age, avoid any foods known to cause loose stools. Avoid prolonged periods of inadequate caloric intake.

F. Calculate and replace deficits of fluids and electrolytes with IV rehydration. For hypertonic dehydration (Na > 150), estimate the fluid deficit at 120 to 170 cc/kg and the Na deficit at 2 to 5 mEq/kg. In isotonic dehydration (Na 130–149), estimate the fluid deficit at 80 to 120 cc/kg and the Na deficit at 7 to 10 mEq/kg. In hypotonic dehydration (Na < 130), estimate the fluid loss at 60 to 80 cc/kg and the Na deficit at 10 to 14 mEq/kg. Stabilize the circulation with 20 cc/kg of isotonic solution given over 1 hour. During the following 8 hours, replace the total estimated fluid deficit as well as significant ongoing losses. Use D/5 ½% isotonic solutions with potassium to replace the deficit of patients with isotonic dehydration and ⅔ to ¾ isotonic solutions with potassium to replace the deficits in hypo- or hypernatremic dehydration. In the 16-hour period following the replacement of extracellular fluid deficits give 24 hours of maintenance fluids.

G. Treat infants and symptomatic older children who have salmonella enteritis with ampicillin or TMP/SMZ. Infants under 6 months are at high risk of developing sequelae. The effect of treatment on the carrier state in children is controversial. Treat Shigella enteritis with TMP/SMZ. Erythromycin decreases the duration of excretion of *Campylobacter* but does not appear to alter the clinical course. Consider an aminoglycoside or tetracycline to treat Yersinia enterocolitis. Treat infections with *Entamoeba histolytica* with metronidazole followed by diloxamide furoate and giardiasis with furazolidone or metronidazole.

REFERENCES

Aperia A. Zetterström R, Gunoz H. Salt and water homeostasis during oral rehydration therapy. J Pediatr 1983; 103:364.

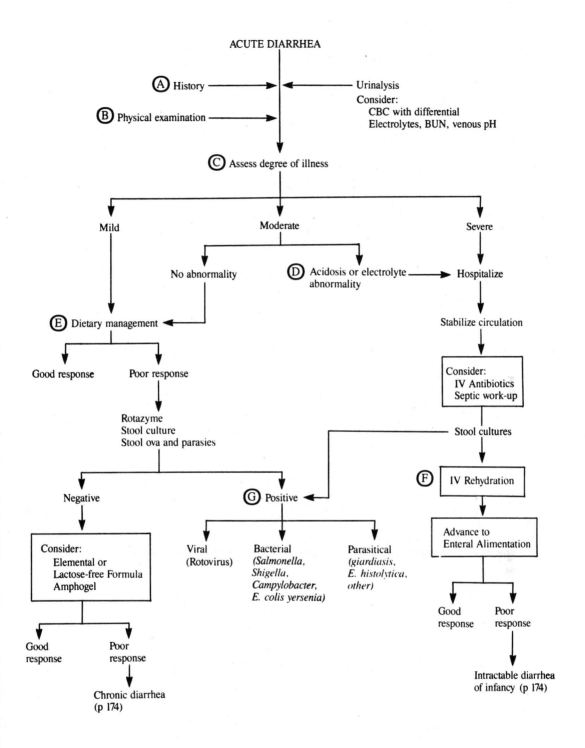

ACUTE DIARRHEA

(A) History

(B) Physical examination

Urinalysis
Consider:
    CBC with differential
    Electrolytes, BUN, venous pH

(C) Assess degree of illness

Mild   Moderate   Severe

No abnormality

(D) Acidosis or electrolyte abnormality → Hospitalize

(E) Dietary management

Stabilize circulation

Good response   Poor response

Consider:
    IV Antibiotics
    Septic work-up

Rotazyme
Stool culture
Stool ova and parasies

Stool cultures

(F) IV Rehydration

Negative   (G) Positive

Advance to
Enteral Alimentation

Consider:
    Elemental or
    Lactose-free Formula
    Amphogel

Viral
(Rotovirus)

Bacterial
*(Salmonella,
Shigella,
Campylobacter,
E. colis yersenia)*

Parasitical
*(giardiasis,
E. histolytica,
other)*

Good
response   Poor
response

Good
response   Poor
response

Chronic diarrhea
(p 174)

Intractable diarrhea
of infancy (p 174)

Finberg L. Treatment of dehydration in infancy. Pediatr Rev 1981; 3:113.

Pal CH, Gillis F, Tuomanen E, et al. Erythromycin in treatment of campylobacter enteritis in children. Am J Dis 1983; 137:286.

Tacket CO, Naram JP, Sattin R et al. A multistate outbreak of infections caused by yersinia enterocolitica transmitted by pasturized milk. JAMA 1984; 251:483.

Winters RW. Principles of Pediatric Fluid Therapy. Boston: Little, Brown, 1982.

CHRONIC DIARRHEA

A. Categorize chronic diarrhea of infancy into 2 syndromes: nonspecific diarrhea (irritable bowel) or intractable diarrhea. Suspect nonspecific diarrhea when the age of onset is 6 to 30 months of age, the patient has 3 to 6 loose stools with mucus per day but has no signs of malabsorption or growth failure. Suspect intractable diarrhea when malabsorption, marked failure to thrive, or severe diarrhea with dehydration is present. Patients with nonspecific diarrhea may have a primary disorder in bowel motility or an acute insult (infection, dietary manipulation, antibiotic therapy) which damages the gastrointestinal epithelial cells causing a decrease in available surface area for the transport of digested nutrients and transient secondary disaccharidase deficiencies. Foods with high osmotic properties or high levels of disaccharides will produce diarrhea. Prolonged treatment with clear liquids and limited caloric intake may prevent adequate repair of the intestinal lining.

B. Ask parents to do a 3-day dietary analysis, listing the total intake for 3 representative 24-hour periods over 2 weeks. A dietitian will calculate the total 24-hour caloric intake for these 3 days. Screen a fresh stool sample for ova and parasites, pH and reducing substances, white blood cells, blood, and fats. If sucrose intolerance is suspected, hydrolyze the stool with hydrochloric acid before testing with a Clinitest tablet. Use a Sudan red stain to identify fat droplets before and after acid hydrolysis of the stool samples.

C. Treat patients with irritable bowel syndrome with a diet modified to increase fat intake to 40% of total calories, using polyunsaturated fats. A low-osmolar formula with corn syrup appears to help in some cases. In older children, avoid frequent feedings of liquids, especially those with high sugar content. Avoid hot, cold, or spicy foods.

D. Treat patients who appear to be recovering from an acute GI insult with adequate calories provided by a low-osmolar formula without lactose. Consider the use of Amphogel (aluminum hydroxide) which binds bile acid and prevents irritation of the colonic mucosa. It may be necessary to tolerate some transient worsening of the diarrhea in patients with starvation stools prior to observing a good response. In difficult cases, consider a more elemental formula such as Pregestimil. Avoid the use of absorbents such as kaolin pectin suspension (Kaopectate), and intestinal paralytic agents such as Lomotil.

E. Hospitalize patients with intractable diarrhea and treat with an elemental formula such as Vivonex and/or parenteral hyperalimentation. Oral elemental formulas contain casein hydrolysates (short-chain polypeptides), medium-chain triglycerides, and sucrose or glucose polymers instead of glucose. Dilute these formulas because of their high osmolality, and begin a slow continuous drip through a nasogastric tube if bolus feedings cannot be tolerated. When severe diarrhea prevents adequate enteroalimentation, use parenteral hyperalimentation. Placement of a central venous catheter for infusion of hypertonic solutions may be necessary in severe cases.

F. Small-bowel biopsy findings such as atrophy, crypt hyperplasia, and a cellular inflammatory response are nonspecific and occur with celiac disease, cow's milk intolerance, soy protein intolerance, eosinophilic gastroenteropathy, immunodeficiency states, bacterial overgrowth, giardiasis, postviral infectious gastroenteritis, and other chronic diarrheal diseases.

REFERENCES

Lo CW, Walker WA. Chronic protracted diarrhea of infancy and nutritional disease. Pediatrics 1983; 72:786.

Silverman A, Roy CC. Pediatric Clinical Gastroenterology. 3rd ed. St. Louis: CV Mosby, 1983.

Sutphen J. Grand RJ, Flores A, et al. Chronic diarrhea associated with *Clostridium difficile* in children. Am J Dis Child 1983; 137:275.

Walker WA. Benign chronic diarrhea of infancy. Pediatr Rev 1981; 3:153.

Weizman Z, Schmuele A, Deckelbaum RJ. Continuous nasogastric drip elemental feeding. Am J Dis Child 1983; 137:253.

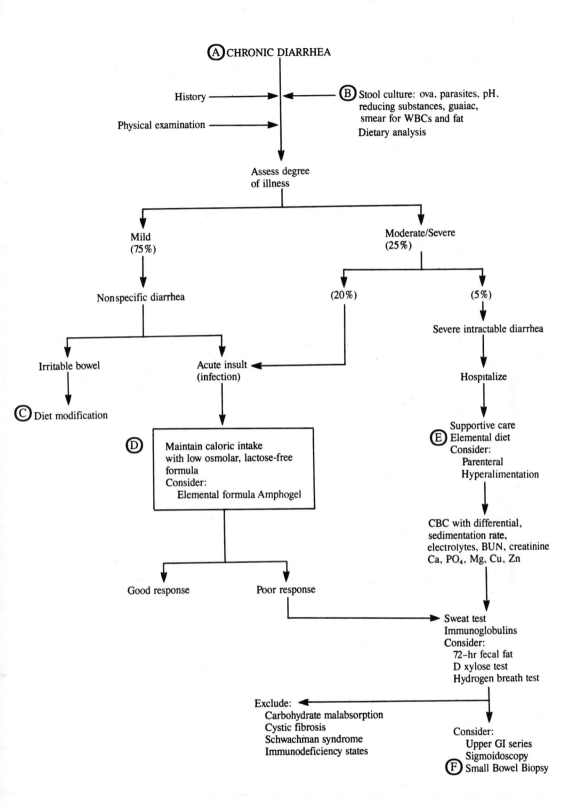

ULCERATIVE COLITIS

A. Note the onset, pattern (nocturnal diarrhea), severity (blood and mucus), and frequency of diarrhea. In ulcerative colitis, stools usually contain blood and mucus. Document associated symptoms including urgency and tenesmus, abdominal pain, fecal incontinence, anorexia, chronic fever, and weight loss. Perianal disease such as fistulas or fissures usually suggests Crohn's disease rather than ulcerative colitis. Extraintestinal manifestations of ulcerative colitis include growth retardation, delayed puberty, mucocutaneous lesions, urethritis, arthritis, arthralgias, conjunctivitis, anemia, chronic active hepatitis, and pericholangitis.

B. Endoscopic findings of ulcerative colitis range from colonic erythema and edema to friable mucosa with ulceration. The barium enema may be unremarkable or show segmental pseudostrictures in the distal colon with the loss of haustral markings and mucosal mottling. When a narrow, short colon without haustral markings is visualized, suspect chronic long-term disease. Patients with pancolitis have more severe disease, a higher incidence of extraintestinal manifestations and an increased risk of toxic megacolon and cancer. Chronic colonic blood loss may lead to hypochromic microcytic anemia. A protein-losing enteropathy results in hypoalbuminemia. Obtain liver function tests to identify cases with hepatic manifestations. Document the presence of *Clostridium difficile* toxin which is associated with pseudomembranous colitis but may also cause an exacerbation in a patient with underlying ulcerative colitis.

C. Mildly ill patients have minimal systemic symptoms, no weight loss, and only slight diarrhea. Moderately ill patients have fever, weight loss, or more than 5 diarrheal stools a day with tenesmus and abdominal pain. Severely ill patients appear toxic and dehydrated.

D. Treat ulcerative colitis with sulfasalazine (Azulfidine) which is split by bacterial action in the colon into sulfapyridine and 5-aminosalicylic salicylate, the active ingredient. Sulfapyridine is absorbed and excreted in the bile. Avoid oral antibiotics which will alter intestinal flora and prevent cleavage of the drug. Give the patient folic acid supplementation. Monitor the patient's blood count weekly for the first month since neutropenia, a Heinz body hemolytic anemia, or a serum sickness reaction can occur. Anorexia, nausea, and headache are common side effects. Consider steroid retention enemas in patients with left-sided colitis or proctitis. Treat patients with unresponsive disease or extraintestinal manifestations with 6–8 weeks of prednisone 1–2 mg/kg/day (maximum 60 mg). Consider azathioprine for patients in whom steroids cannot be weaned after 8 weeks of daily therapy without relapse.

E. Suspect toxic megacolon in a toxic patient with abdominal distention and peritoneal signs. When shock is present, treat toxic megacolon with infusions of salt-poor albumin and blood transfusions. Avoid barium studies and initiate therapy with antibiotics and steroids.

F. Consider surgery when prolonged high-dose steroid therapy is necessary, severe growth retardation is present prior to epiphyseal closure, the colitis has failed to respond after 2 years of medical therapy, or biopsy reveals evidence of a precancerous dysplastic mucosa. The risk of cancer is low during the first 10 years of the disease but increases approximately 1–2% per year thereafter. Yearly follow-up visits and endoscopy are essential to monitor the course of the disease and detect dysplastic changes early.

REFERENCES

Ament M. Inflammatory disease of the colon: Ulcerative colitis and Crohn's colitis. J Pediatr 1975; 86:322.
Devroede G, et al. Cancer risk and life expectancy of children with ulcerative colitis. New Engl J Med 1971; 285:17.
Silverman A, Roy CC. Pediatric Clinical Gastroenterology. 3rd ed. St. Louis: CV Mosby, 1983; 353.

ULCERATIVE COLITIS

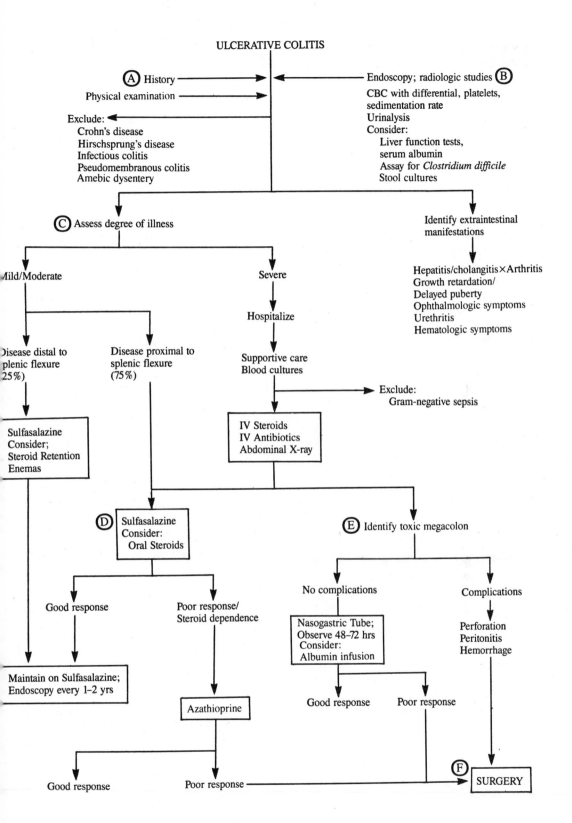

CROHN'S DISEASE

A. Note any anorexia, weight loss, nausea, vomiting, abdominal pain, or diarrhea. Right lower quadrant, crampy abdominal pain may mimic appendicitis. Severe anorexia and protracted vomiting suggest anorexia nervosa or intestinal obstruction. The degree of diarrhea depends on the involvement of the colon. Systemic extraintestinal symptoms include fever, poor growth, aphthous mouth ulcers, delayed puberty, arthritis, conjuctivitis, and rash.

B. Note aphthous ulcers of the mouth and fissures, ulcerations, abscess, fistula, or skin tags in the perianal area. Document signs of chronic malnutrition and hypoalbuminemia, such as muscle wasting, peripheral edema, clubbing of the fingers and toes, and signs of vitamin deficiency. Matted loops of bowel especially in right lower quadrant may present as an abdominal mass. Note extraintestinal signs.

C. Obtain an upper GI series, small bowel follow-through, and barium enema. Characteristic findings include thickened mucosa, ulcerations, pseudopolypoid formation with cobblestoning, and stenotic areas with proximal dilatation. Radiologic findings do not correlate well with clinical symptoms or prognosis. Colonoscopy may show colitis or ulcerations separated by normal mucosa (skip areas). Biopsy shows noncaseating granulomas in less than 25% of cases. The rectum is usually spared. Consider endoscopy with biopsy of the upper GI tract to distinguish gastric Crohn's disease from peptic ulcer disease.

D. Mildly ill patients tolerate oral intake despite abdominal pain and anorexia. Moderately ill patients have severe abdominal pain, often associated with vomiting and other signs of intermittent partial intestinal obstruction. Severely ill patients often suffer from marked malnutrition or appear toxic, with vomiting and dehydration.

E. Manage mild and moderately ill cases with a caloric intake at least 130% over baseline, supplemented with vitamins (fat-soluble folic acid, B_{12}), minerals (calcium, magnesium), and trace metals (zinc, copper, and iron). Supplementation is required because steatorrhea and involvement of the terminal ileum impair absorption of these substances. Iron supplementation is often required because of chronic intestinal blood loss. Consider sulfasalazine in patients with ileocolitis or colitis who have no extraintestinal manifestations. Maintenance sulfasalazine therapy is not indicated. Treat other patients with prednisone, 1 to 2 mg/kg/day for 6 to 8 weeks, followed by an alternate-day regimen and then gradual tapering. Steroid-dependent patients may require a 3 to 6 month trial of 6–mercaptopurine, 1.5 mg/kg/day. Complications of this drug include leukopenia, acute pancreatitis, and renal failure.

F. When necessary, consider enteral alimentation with an elemental formula. Nasogastric feeding for 3 weeks followed by a low residue diet may be required. Elemental diets can effectively treat such GI complications as fistulas and perianal disease. Treat patients with severe disease who cannot tolerate enteral alimentation with an elemental formula with parenteral hyperalimentation.

G. Consider elective surgery for the following: repeated episodes of intestinal obstruction, abscess unresponsive to antibiotic therapy, enterovesicular fistula, toxic megacolon, massive hemorrhage, and progressive disease despite 2 years of adequate steroid therapy. Growth failure is not a clear indication for surgery; surgery is successful in only 20 to 50% of cases. Surgery for colonic disease requires total colectomy and proctectomy since preservation of the rectum is associated with a high incidence of recurrent disease. Adult patients with Crohn's disease have an increased risk of cancer early in the disease, but the risk does not increase linearly with disease duration as it does in ulcerative colitis.

REFERENCES

Crohn BB, Ginsburg L, Oppenheimer GD. Regional ileitis: A pathologic and clinical entity. JAMA 1984; 251:73.

Gryboski JD. Crohn's disease in children. Pediatr Rev 1981; 2:239.

CROHN'S DISEASE

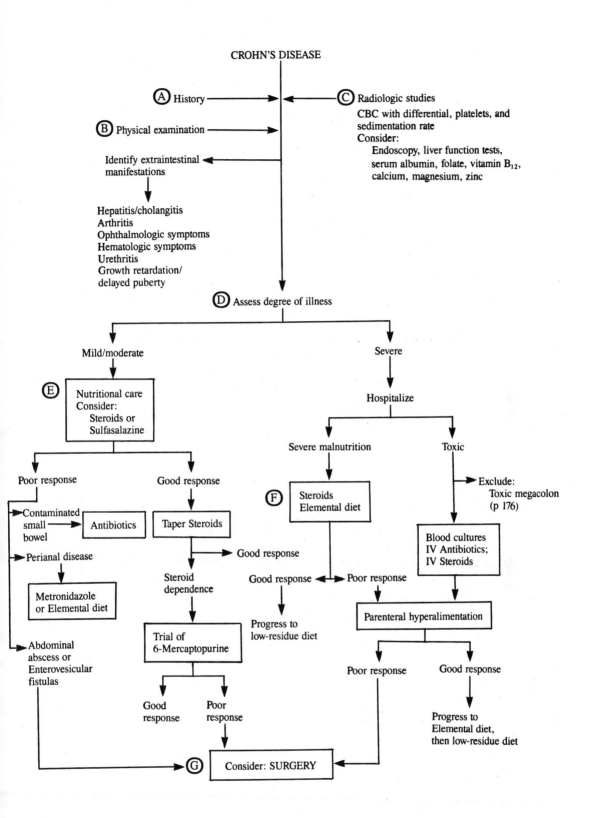

(A) History

(B) Physical examination

(C) Radiologic studies
CBC with differential, platelets, and sedimentation rate
Consider:
    Endoscopy, liver function tests, serum albumin, folate, vitamin B_{12}, calcium, magnesium, zinc

Identify extraintestinal manifestations

Hepatitis/cholangitis
Arthritis
Ophthalmologic symptoms
Hematologic symptoms
Urethritis
Growth retardation/
delayed puberty

(D) Assess degree of illness

Mild/moderate

Severe

(E) Nutritional care
Consider:
    Steroids or
    Sulfasalazine

Hospitalize

Severe malnutrition

Toxic

Poor response

Good response

(F) Steroids
Elemental diet

Exclude:
Toxic megacolon
(p 176)

Contaminated small bowel → Antibiotics

Taper Steroids

Good response

Blood cultures
IV Antibiotics;
IV Steroids

Perianal disease

Good response

Good response ← Poor response

Metronidazole or Elemental diet

Steroid dependence

Progress to low-residue diet

Parenteral hyperalimentation

Abdominal abscess or Enterovesicular fistulas

Trial of 6-Mercaptopurine

Poor response

Good response

Good response

Poor response

Progress to
Elemental diet,
then low-residue diet

(G) Consider: SURGERY

Rosenthal SR, Schnyder JD, Hendricks KN, et al. Growth failure and inflammatory bowel disease: Approach to treatment of a complicated adolescent problem. Pediatrics 1983; 72:481.
Silverman A, Roy CC. Pediatric Clinical Gastroenterology. 3rd ed. St. Louis: CV Mosby, 1983; 353.

VOMITING DURING INFANCY

A. Note the onset, frequency, and severity (quantity, degree of forcefulness, presence of bile) of the vomiting. Determine the type of formula, manner of preparation, the quantity ingested, and the feeding position and technique. Establish the timing of vomiting in relation to the feeding. Spitting up or regurgitation of small amounts of formula during or soon after feeding suggest improper feeding techniques such as bottle propping or mild gastroesophageal reflux. Note associated symptoms such as fever, cough, coryza, respiratory distress, diarrhea, altered mental status, seizures, and failure to thrive. Inquire about perinatal deaths in the family which suggest inborn errors of metabolism and adrenal insufficiency. Identify predisposing conditions such as hydrocephalus or other CNS disorders, adrenal insufficiency, gastroesophageal reflux, peptic ulcer disease, milk protein intolerance, necrotizing enterocolitis, or prior abdominal surgery.

B. Assess hydration and circulatory status by determining blood pressure, pulse, respiratory rate, capillary refill, skin color and turgor, presence of tears, fullness of the fontanel, and urine output. Plot the infant's height, weight, and head circumference on a growth grid to identify cases of failure to thrive or rapid head growth. Assess the mental status. Note the presence of acute otitis media, irritability, lethargy, seizures, or focal neurologic signs. Observe a feeding and note the presence of peristaltic waves. An abdominal mass (olive) suggests pyloric stenosis.

C. Mildly ill infants have vomiting closely associated with feeding but no failure to thrive or signs of systemic infection or disease. An error in feeding technique or preparation of formula is frequently identified in these cases. Moderately ill patients appear dehydrated or have signs which suggest intestinal obstruction or pyloric stenosis. Any infant with a past history of necrotizing enterocolitis or bilious vomiting should be considered moderately or severely ill with possible intestinal obstruction. Severely ill children appear toxic with alterations in mental status or have significant circulatory compromise.

D. When chalasia (gastroesophageal reflux) is suspected, change the infant's feeding schedule. Small volumes of formula given more frequently reduce gastric distention. Consider adding cereal to the formula; attempt to position the infant's body prone at a 30° incline throughout most of the day. This can best be accomplished when the infant straddles a padded post or uses a chalasia harness. When severe symptoms are associated with failure to thrive, consider the use of bethanecol which decreases vomiting by increasing esophageal sphincter pressure or metoclopramide (Reglan) which increases gastric emptying. If esophagitis is present, consider using antacids and/or cimetidine. Consider surgery (Nissen fundoplication) if severe symptoms fail to resolve after 2 months of therapy or if an esophageal stricture develops.

E. The most useful radiologic procedure is the upper GI series. This procedure identifies causes of bowel obstruction as well as gastrointestinal reflux. The value of other procedures or tests for gastroesophageal reflux such as the gastric scintiscan, esophageal manometry, and the measurement of esophageal PH (Tuttle test) are unclear.

F. Protracted vomiting may result in significant loss of stomach acid causing hypochloremic alkalosis. Hypochloremic alkalosis is often associated with a paradoxically acid urine because of intracellular potassium deficits. Treat these patients with normal saline and replace the potassium deficit; alkalinization of the urine indicates that the potassium has been replaced. Acidosis, vomiting, and failure to thrive suggest the possibility of an endocrine or metabolic disorder such as diabetic ketoacidosis, adrenal insufficiency, adrenogenital syndrome, aminoaciduria, galactosemia, glycogen storage disease, lysosomal disease, and fructose intolerance.

REFERENCES

Herbst JJ. Diagnosis and treatment of gastroesophageal reflux in children. Pediatr Rev 1983; 5:75.
Orenstein S, Whitington PF. Positioning for prevention of infant gastroesophageal reflux. J Pediatr 1983; 103:534.

PERSISTENT VOMITING DURING INFANCY

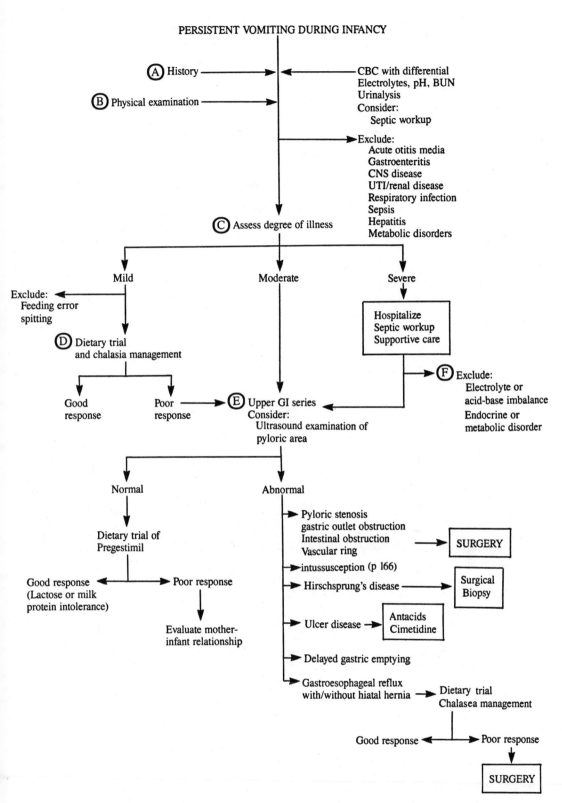

Silverman A, Roy CC. Pediatric Clinical Gastroenterology. 3rd ed. St. Louis: CV Mosby, 1983.
Strickland AD, Chang JHT. Results of treatment of gastroesophageal reflux with bethanechol. J Pediatr 1983;
103:311.

PERSISTENT VOMITING AFTER INFANCY

A. Note the onset, frequency, severity (quantity and forcefulness), and timing of vomiting. Identify precipitating factors such as feeding, cough, or activity. Note associated symptoms such as fever, diarrhea, cough, coryza, abdominal pain, dysuria, frequency, polydypsia, jaundice, bloody stools, headache, alterations in mental status, and failure to thrive. A recent history of chicken pox or influenza syndrome suggests the possibility of Reye's syndrome. Vomiting associated with bloody stools and intermittent abdominal pain suggests intussusception. Nighttime vomiting suggests a CNS disorder. Identify predisposing conditions such as sickle cell disease, pregnancy, prior abdominal surgery, prior alkali ingestion, necrotizing enterocolitis, or inflammatory bowel disease. Precipitating factors include current medications, ingestions (salicylate), and exposure to hepatitis. In adolescence, suspect bulimia or superior mesenteric artery syndrome when vomiting is associated with marked weight loss.

B. Assess the circulatory and hydration status by ascertaining blood pressure, pulse, respiratory rate, capillary refill, skin color and turgor, presence of tears, fullness of the fontanel, and urine output. Plot the child's height, weight, and head circumference on a growth grid to identify cases with failure to thrive or rapid head growth. Assess the mental status and note the presence of irritability, lethargy, seizures, papilledema, retinal hemorrhage, ataxia, or focal neurologic signs. Document the presence of extraintestinal manifestations such as rash, arthritis, lymphadenopathy, or hepatosplenomegaly.

C. Mildly ill patients appear well and have no signs of dehydration or systemic disease. Moderately ill patients have mild to moderate dehydration or a prolonged history of vomiting often associated with failure to thrive. Severely ill patients have moderate to severe dehydration, appear toxic, or have an altered mental status.

D. Peptic ulcer disease may present with persistent vomiting rather than epigastric pain. Consider a trial of antacids in these patients.

E. Suspect Reye's syndrome when the patient presents with persistent vomiting, hyperventilation, and altered mental status (confusion, combativeness, disorientation, stupor, coma) in association with hepatic dysfunction (elevated serum transaminases and ammonia). Stage the patient according to the following criteria: stage 1—vomiting and lethargy but responsive to commands; stage 2—disorientation, confusion or combativeness with purposeful motor responses and no abnormal posturing; stage 3—comatose (unresponsive to commands), periodic irregular breathing pattern, decorticate posturing, and doll's eyes (oculocephalic) reflexes; stage 4—comatose with decerebrate posturing and disconjugate gaze; stage 5—comatose, areflexic, flaccid paralysis, and fixed dilated pupils. Associated metabolic disturbances in these patients include hyperuricemia, hypophosphatemia, hypoglycemia, and azotemia. Treat patients who have reached stage 3 with elective nasotracheal or oral intubation, a central venous pressure line, an arterial line, a Foley catheter, and an intracranial pressure monitor. Institute osmotherapy with mannitol 0.25–1 g/kg IV and controlled ventilation to maintain the PCO_2 between 25 and 30 torr. If these measures fail to control intracranial pressure, consider paralysis with pavulon, steroids, and pentobarbital-induced coma.

REFERENCES

Frewen TC, Swedlow DB, Watcha N et al. Outcome in severe Reye's syndrome with early pentobarbital coma and hypothermia. J Pediatr 1982; 100:663.

Henretig FN. Vomiting. In: Fleicher, Ludwig, eds. Textbook of Pediatric Emergency Medicine. Baltimore: Williams & Wilkins, 1983.

Holmberg SD, Blake PA. Staphylococcal food poisoning in the United States. New facts and old misconceptions. JAMA 1984; 251:487.

VOMITING AFTER INFANCY

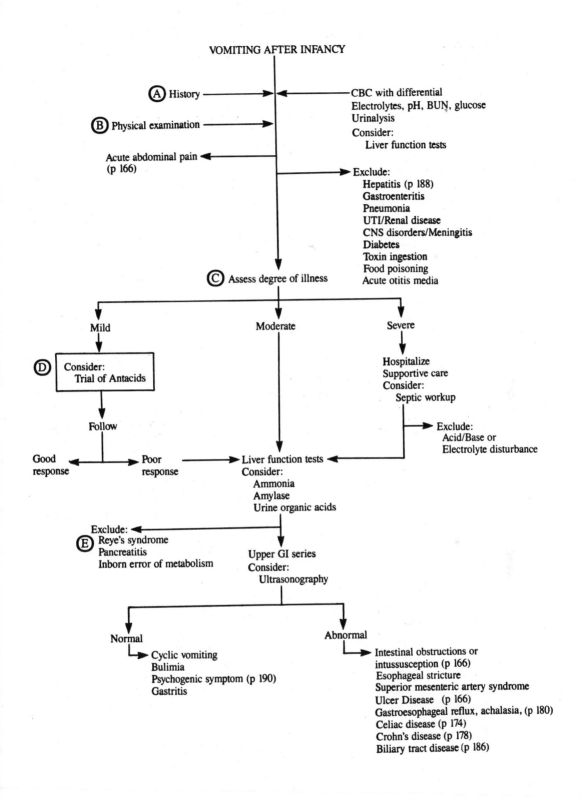

Lichtenstein PK, Henke JE, Dougherty CC et al. Grade I Reyes syndrome. A frequent cause of vomiting and liver dysfunction after varicella and upper respiratory tract infection. N Engl J Med 1983; 309:133.

Silverman A, Roy CC. Pediatric Clinical Gastroenterology. 3rd ed. St. Louis: CV Mosby, 1983.

HEMATEMESIS

A. Gastrointestinal bleeding above the ligament of Treitz may present with hematemesis. The most common causes of upper GI bleeding are duodenal ulcers, gastric ulcers, esophagitis, gastritis, and esophageal varices. A large quantity (cupful) of bright red blood suggests extensive hemorrhage. Blood which has been in prolonged contact with stomach acid is dark brown or black (like coffee grounds). Vomited material which can be mistaken for blood includes jello, Koolaid, food dyes, red candy, and some antibiotic syrups.

B. In the history, note the onset of hematemesis and the volume of blood loss. Identify possible precipitating factors and predisposing conditions such as protracted vomiting, peptic ulcer disease, chronic liver disease, current medications (aspirin, steroid, or anticoagulants), corrosive ingestions, bleeding disorders, or recent major stress (difficult delivery, burns, surgery, traumatic injury, dehydration, shock, serious infection). Ask about recent possible oral pharyngeal sites of bleeding (epistaxis, dental work, tonsillectomy, sore throat) or ingestion of a foreign body which may have lodged in the esophagus or stomach.

C. On physical examination, evaluate the circulatory status and document the presence of orthostatic blood pressure changes. Examine the mouth and oropharynx to identify possible sites of bleeding. Note signs of a generalized coagulation disorder such as petechiae, bruising, or ecchymosis. Note signs of liver disease and portal hypertension such as hepatomegaly, splenomegaly, and ascites.

D. Systemic diseases associated with upper GI bleeding include immunodeficiency disorders, pulmonary or GI infections, malignancy, collagen vascular disease, CNS disease, renal failure, and congenital heart disease.

E. Mildly ill infants are stable, have no evidence of anemia, and vomit small amounts of coffee grounds material. The history often suggests swallowed blood, aspirin-associated gastritis, or a Mallory-Weiss tear caused by vomiting. In the newborn period, an Apt-Downey test distinguishes swallowed mother's blood from the newborn's blood. Moderately ill patients are anemic, have a significant history of blood loss, or active evidence of hemorrhage documented with gastric lavage. Severely ill children have signs of circulatory compromise or shock and ongoing significant blood loss. Factors indicating a poor prognosis in severely ill patients include an initial hematocrit <20% or hemoglobin level <7, transfusion requirements which exceed 85 cc/kg of blood without surgical intervention, failure to identify an active source of bleeding, the presence of a coexisting coagulation disorder, and the presence of associated systemic disease.

F. Institute ice saline lavage when active bleeding is documented. Treat patients with suspected gastritis or peptic ulcer disease with antacids and/or cimetidine. Patients older than 5 years of age should be treated with magnesium and aluminum hydroxide preparations, 30 cc/hour for the initial 48 hours, then at 1 and 3 hours after meals. In patients with known esophageal varices and severe hemorrhage, consider tamponade with an esophageal or gastric balloon or endosclerosis. Inability to control hemorrhage is an indication for portocaval shunt surgery.

G. Endoscopy will identify the cause of hemorrhage in approximately 90% of patients and upper GI examination identifies the underlying causes in approximately ⅔ of cases. Causes of gastritis or esophagitis include hiatal hernia, gastric outlet obstruction secondary to pyloric stenosis web or diaphragm, or gastroesophageal reflux. Consider angiography which will diagnose possible aneurysms of the hepatic artery or gastropancreatic duplication cyst when bleeding is massive, or when endoscopy and upper GI series have failed to reveal the cause in recurrent bleeding.

REFERENCES

Boyle JT. Gastrointestinal bleeding. In: Textbook of Emergency Medicine. Fleisher G, Ludwig S, eds. Baltimore: Williams & Wilkins, 1983.

Cox K, Ament NE. Upper gastrointestinal bleeding in children and adolescents. Pediatrics 1979; 63:408.

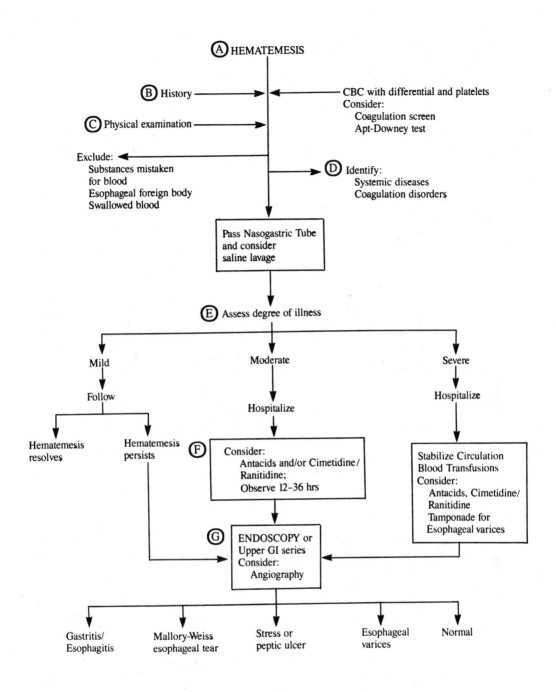

Hillemeier C. Rectal bleeding in childhood. Pediatr Rev 1983; 5:35.
Silverman A, Roy CC. Pediatric Clinical Gastroenterology. 3rd ed. St. Louis: CV Mosby, 1983.
Zeldis JB, Friedman LS, Isselbacher KJ. Ranitidine: a new H2 receptor antagonist. N Engl J Med 1983; 309:1368.

JAUNDICE AFTER
6 MONTHS OF AGE

A. Note the feeding pattern, color of stools, and presence of fever, malaise, vomiting, abdominal pain, jaundice, pruritis, and dark urine. Document exposure to a hepatitis carrier or person with acute hepatitis, blood products, medications, or illicit drugs. Note if the child attends a large day-care or residential facility. Identify hematologic abnormalities such as hemolytic anemia, sickle cell disease, or thalassemia. Identify preexisting liver disease which causes elevations in indirect bilirubin (hepatitis, Gilbert's disease, Crigler-Najjar syndrome) and direct bilirubin (Rotor's syndrome, Dubin-Johnson syndrome, hepatitis). Note extrahepatic symptoms such as arthritis, polyarthralgia, amenorrhea, colitis, thyroiditis, glomerulonephritis, pleurisy, or rash.

B. Note any right upper quadrant abdominal mass or tender hepatomegaly. Exudative tonsillitis, adenopathy, or splenomegaly suggests mononucleosis. Signs of chronic liver disease include acne, ascites, cushingoid facies, digital clubbing, and gynecomastia.

C. The degree of cholestasis and obstructive jaundice is reflected by the level of direct bilirubin, the degree of elevation of alkaline phosphatase and gamma glutamyltranspeptidase (GGT). Hepatocyte membrane disruption is correlated with the levels of the serum transaminases (SGOT, SGPT). With extensive hepatocyte damage, serum albumin is depressed and the prothrombin time prolonged. Anemia associated with burr cells or severe thrombocytopenia suggests severe liver disease. A Coombs-positive hemolytic anemia, aplastic anemia, or pancytopenia may complicate hepatitis.

D. Choledochus cyst is a congenital dilatation of the common bile duct. The degree of jaundice, abdominal pain, vomiting, and alteration in stool color are variable. The scintiscan documents continuity of the cyst with the biliary tree. Suspect acute hydrops of the bladder in children with Kawasaki's disease when ultrasound demonstrates distention of the gall bladder without calculi and with normal extrahepatic bile ducts. Attempt treatment with supportive care (IV fluids) followed by a low-fat diet before considering surgery in the latter condition.

E. Acute cholecystitis can be caused by bacterial infections (*Salmonella, Shigella, E. coli*), viruses, or parasites (*Giardia* and *Ascaris*). Sclerosing cholangitis usually associated with inflammatory bowel disease is a rare progressive disease which causes stenosis of the extrahepatic bile ducts; when suspected obtain an endoscopic retrograde cholangiogram. No effective therapy is available for sclerosing cholangitis.

F. The presence of a Kayser Fleischer ring on slit-lamp examination, reduced serum copper and ceruloplasmin, and elevated urine and liver tissue copper identify patients with Wilson's disease, an autosomal recessive disorder associated with excessive copper in the liver, brain, kidneys, and cornea. Galactosemia presents with vomiting, diarrhea, failure to thrive, hypoglycemia, cataracts, development delays, and seizures. It is associated with a deficiency of galactose-1-phosphate uridyl transferase. Alpha-1-antitrypsin deficiency presents with neonatal cholestatic jaundice and hepatomegaly in association with elevated transaminases. In hereditary fructose intolerance, the child is deficient in fructose-1-phosphate aldolase or fructose-1-6-diphosphatase. Test urine for amino and organic acids to identify cases of hereditary tyrosinenemia, an autosomal recessive disorder. The chronic form is characterized by cirrhosis, vitamin D-resistant rickets, failure to thrive, and Fanconi's syndrome. Obtain a sweat test to identify cases of cystic fibrosis.

REFERENCES

Ghishan FK. Trimethoprim-sulfamethoxazole-induced intrahepatic cholestasis. Clin Pediatrics 1983; 22:212.

Hadide A. Types I and III choledochal cyst. Preoperative diagnosis by ultrasound. Am J Dis Child 1983; 137:663.

Komrower GM. Inborn errors of metabolism. Pediatr Rev 1980; 2:175.

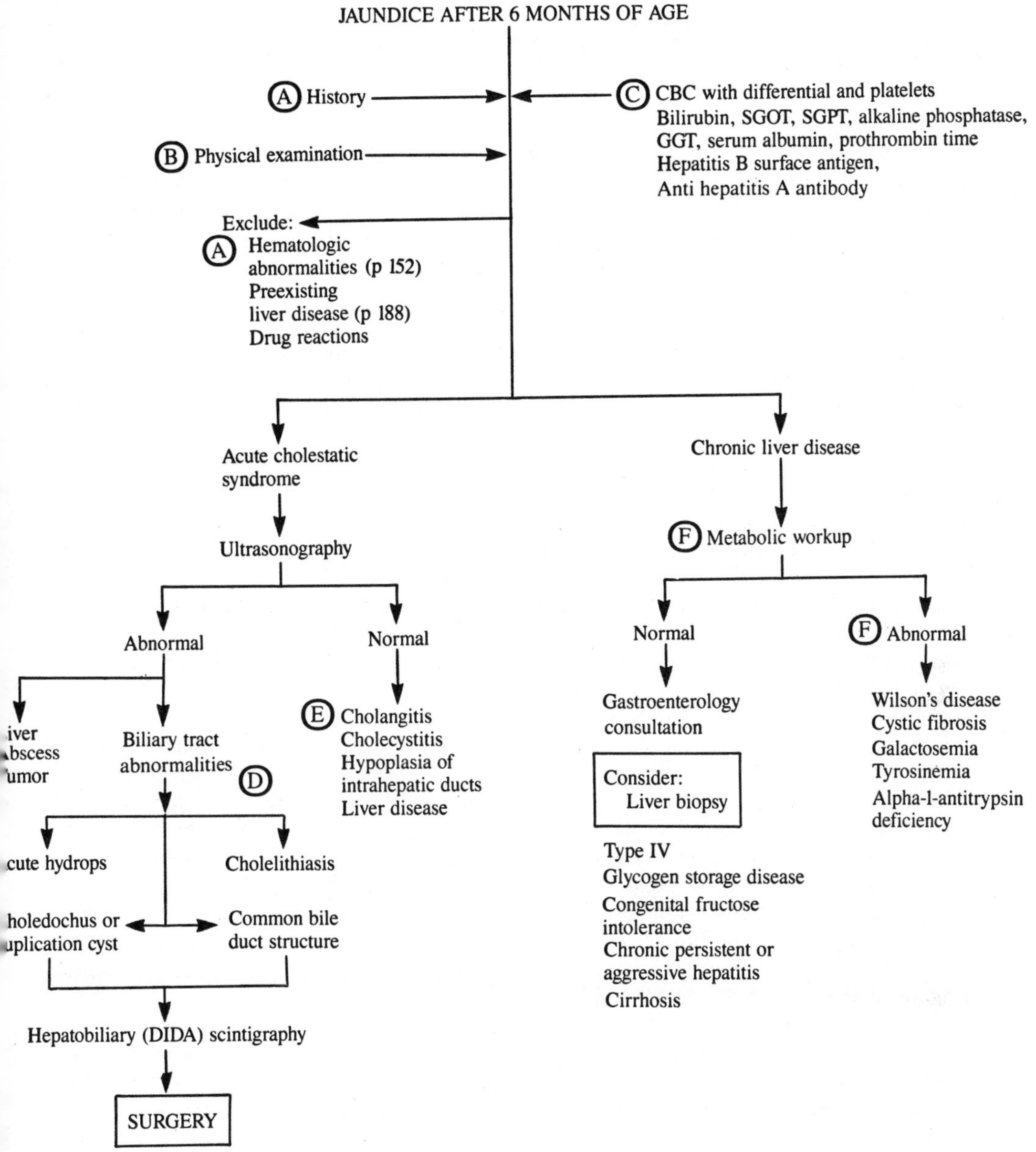

JAUNDICE AFTER 6 MONTHS OF AGE

(A) History

(B) Physical examination

(C) CBC with differential and platelets
Bilirubin, SGOT, SGPT, alkaline phosphatase,
GGT, serum albumin, prothrombin time
Hepatitis B surface antigen,
Anti hepatitis A antibody

Exclude:
(A) Hematologic
abnormalities (p 152)
Preexisting
liver disease (p 188)
Drug reactions

Acute cholestatic
syndrome

Ultrasonography

Abnormal

Normal

iver
Abscess
umor

Biliary tract
abnormalities (D)

(E) Cholangitis
Cholecystitis
Hypoplasia of
intrahepatic ducts
Liver disease

cute hydrops

Cholelithiasis

holedochus or
uplication cyst

Common bile
duct structure

Hepatobiliary (DIDA) scintigraphy

SURGERY

Chronic liver disease

(F) Metabolic workup

Normal

(F) Abnormal

Gastroenterology
consultation

Consider:
Liver biopsy

Type IV
Glycogen storage disease
Congenital fructose
intolerance
Chronic persistent or
aggressive hepatitis
Cirrhosis

Wilson's disease
Cystic fibrosis
Galactosemia
Tyrosinemia
Alpha-1-antitrypsin
deficiency

Scharschmidt BF, Goldberg HI, Schmid R. Current concepts in diagnosis: approach to the patient with cholestatic jaundice. N Engl J Med 1983; 308:1515.

Silverman A, Roy CC. Pediatric Clinical Gastroenterology. St. Louis: CV Mosby, 1983.

ACUTE HEPATITIS

A. Causes of hepatitis include viral infections (hepatitis A, B, nonA nonB, EB virus, CMV), bacterial infections (leptospirosis, syphilis, gonorrhea, chlamydia), and parasitic infections (malaria, amoeba). Drug or toxic hepatitis can be associated with phenothiazines, oral contraceptives, valproic acid, erythromycin estolate, indomethacin, and gold. Severe hypoxia, hypotension, right heart failure, and mushroom and acetominophen intoxications may result in fulminant hepatic necrosis.

B. Note any fever, anorexia, malaise, vomiting, abdominal pain, jaundice, dark urine, or clay-colored stools. Inquire if the child has begun to feel better when the jaundice increases. If symptoms fail to improve after the onset of jaundice, this is a poor prognostic sign.

C. Note any jaundice, tender hepatomegaly, splenomegaly, or abdominal mass. Suspect infectious mononucleosis when exudative tonsillitis, adenopathy, or splenomegaly is present. Signs of chronic liver disease include acne, ascites, cushingoid facies, digital clubbing, and gynecomastia. Note signs of chronic active disease such as arthritis, polyarthralgia, amenorrhea, colitis, thyroiditis, glomerulonephritis, diabetes, or pleurisy.

D. Viral hepatitis is typically characterized by clinical improvement with the onset of jaundice and a normalization of bilirubin and transaminases within 4–6 weeks. Slight elevation of unconjugated bilirubin and serum transaminases may presist for up to 3 months. A mild relapse often occurs after 10–12 weeks.

E. Acute hepatitis associated with hepatitis A virus rarely has a complicated course. Persistence of clinical symptoms and markedly elevated serum transaminases and bilirubin after 4 weeks suggests persistent hepatitis. Approximately 10% of children with hepatitis B or nonA nonB infections may experience persistent hepatitis. Ongoing liver damage is indicated by a depressed serum albumin <3.5 mg% and a prolonged prothrombin time. Consider early liver biopsy when the clinical presentation is atypical for benign viral hepatitis or includes a positive ANA, an elevated IgG associated with a reduced serum albumin, a Coombs-positive hemolytic anemia, or the presence of extrahepatic manifestations. When signs of inflammation (elevated serum transaminases and bilirubin) persist beyond 3–6 months, biopsy may also be indicated.

F. In chronic persistent hepatitis the biopsy is characterized by inflammation involving the portal tract with minimal or no fibrosis. The lesion may be related to a persistent hepatitis B surface antigen carrier state, a metabolic disease, or exposure to a drug or toxin. While the majority of cases resolve spontaneously, careful follow-up is required to identify the small number of cases that deteriorate. In subacute hepatic necrosis or bridging necrosis the liver biopsy is characterized by bands of necrosis which connect portal zones to central veins. This lesion may progress to cirrhosis or fulminant hepatic necrosis. Treatment is unclear. Steroid therapy is contraindicated in cases of persistent hepatitis B virus infection. In chronic aggressive hepatitis, the biopsy is characterized by severe and diffuse inflammation with involvement of the lobular architecture. Initiate therapy in these patients with prednisone 2 mg/kg/day (maximum dose 60 mg) in order to achieve a remission. When the patient is in remission, consider adding azothiaprine (Imuran 1 mg/kg/day) in order to reduce the steroid dose.

G. Suspect acute fulminant hepatic necrosis when the bilirubin is >20 mg/ml, serum transaminases are >3000, prothrombin time is markedly prolonged, and serum albumin is depressed. A rapidly shrinking liver in association with altered mental status, ascites, thrombocytopenia, and hypoglycemia indicates the development of liver failure.

REFERENCES

Chilton L. Viral hepatitis in school age children. Pediatr Rev 1981; 4:105.
Krugman S. The newly licensed hepatitis B vaccine: characteristics and indications for use. JAMA 1982; 247:2012.
Silverman A, Roy CC. Pediatric Gastoenterology. St. Louis: CV Mosby, 1983.

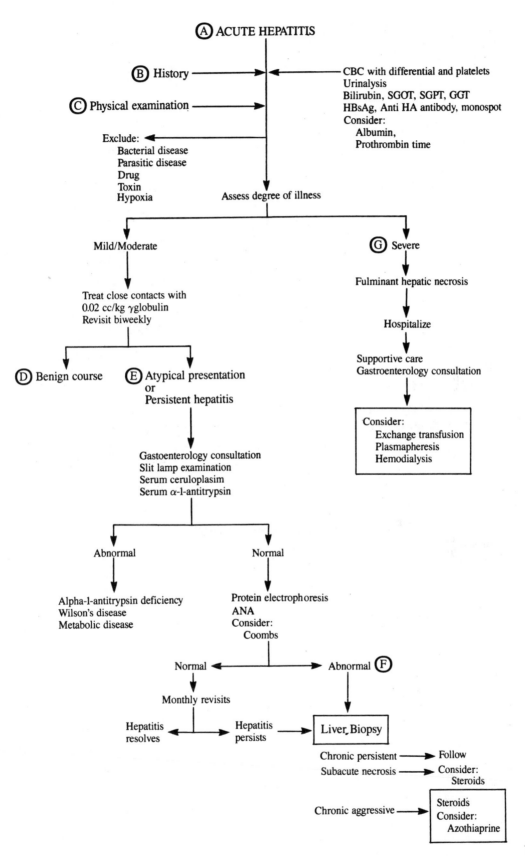

(A) ACUTE HEPATITIS

(B) History ────────────→ ←──────── CBC with differential and platelets
                                      Urinalysis
(C) Physical examination ──→   Bilirubin, SGOT, SGPT, GGT
                                      HBsAg, Anti HA antibody, monospot
                                      Consider:
          Exclude: ←   Albumin,
              Bacterial disease   Prothrombin time
              Parasitic disease
              Drug
              Toxin
              Hypoxia   Assess degree of illness

     Mild/Moderate   (G) Severe

                                            Fulminant hepatic necrosis

Treat close contacts with   Hospitalize
0.02 cc/kg γglobulin
Revisit biweekly   Supportive care
                                            Gastroenterology consultation

(D) Benign course   (E) Atypical presentation   Consider:
                        or   Exchange transfusion
                        Persistent hepatitis   Plasmapheresis
                                                     Hemodialysis

                    Gastoenterology consultation
                    Slit lamp examination
                    Serum ceruloplasim
                    Serum α-1-antitrypsin

         Abnormal   Normal

Alpha-1-antitrypsin deficiency   Protein electrophoresis
Wilson's disease   ANA
Metabolic disease   Consider:
                                     Coombs

              Normal ←──────────────→ Abnormal (F)

          Monthly revisits

Hepatitis ←──────────→ Hepatitis ──→ Liver Biopsy
resolves   persists
                              Chronic persistent ──────→ Follow
                              Subacute necrosis ──────→ Consider:
                                                            Steroids

                                                        Steroids
                              Chronic aggressive ─────→ Consider:
                                                            Azothiaprine

189

EVALUATION OF PSYCHOGENIC SYMPTOMS

A. Common psychogenic symptoms include recurrent or chronic abdominal pain, limb pain, vomiting, headache, chest pain, dizziness, syncope, hyperventilation, night terrors, enuresis, fighting, and phobias. Identify any evidence of psychosis as suggested by an altered sense of reality, delusions or hallucinations. Serious psychiatric problems include autistic behavior, antisocial behavior, anorexia nervosa, severe depression, suicidal ideation, sexual identity disturbances, and substance abuse. Assess the patient's degree of self-esteem, self-confidence, anxiety level, and sense of security. Question the patient and family to learn how they deal with stressful situations and identify the source of stress, including possible sexual abuse, recent serious illness or death of family members or friends, recent divorce or separation, change of residence, new school or teachers, recent financial reverses, including unemployment. Assess family life for sustained mistreatment or unusual lifestyle. Obtain a family history of psychogenic illnesses such as headache, irritable bowel syndrome, peptic ulcer disease, or chronic abdominal pain and psychiatric illness such as schizophrenia, depressive disorders, sociopathy, and substance abuse.

B. Perform a mental status examination and note orientation, memory, affect, and quality of thinking. Perform a careful, complete physical examination to identify any signs of underlying non-functional disease.

C. Severely affected patients have evidence of psychopathology. Moderately affected patients have symptoms which compromise their life style, for example, by resulting in school absences or failure, or limitation of activity. Mildly affected patients experience minimal disruption of normal activities.

D. Consider school phobia as a common cause of pain in grade-school children, especially if the youngster has missed 5 or more days because of vague symptoms. Contact the child's teachers and school nurse. Identify any precipitating events in school, provide the child and family with reassurance regarding the child's physical health, and have the child return to school immediately. Ask that the family contact you whenever the child misses any school day. High-school students who have school phobia are often either reacting to a significant life stress or have underlying psychopathology. When counseling and reassurance are not sufficient, refer these patients for family or individual therapy.

E. Counsel the child and family by explaining the mechanism of stress-related functional pain. Provide reassurance that the pain, while real, is not due to physical illness. When appropriate, suggest relaxation techniques such as deep, slow breathing, imagery, or self-induced hypnosis. When counseling fails to improve symptoms after 2–4 visits, refer to a psychiatrist or psychologist for individual and/or family therapy.

REFERENCES

Schmitt BD. School phobia. The great imitator: A pediatric viewpoint. Pediatrics 1971; 48:433.

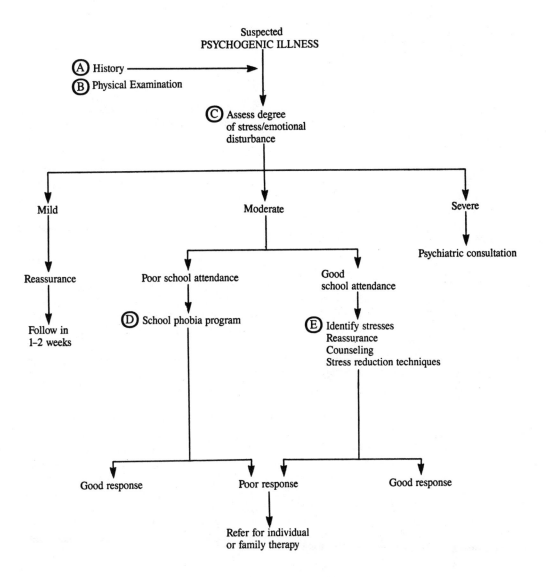

Suspected
PSYCHOGENIC ILLNESS

(A) History
(B) Physical Examination

(C) Assess degree
of stress/emotional
disturbance

Mild

Moderate

Severe

Psychiatric consultation

Reassurance

Poor school attendance

Good
school attendance

Follow in
1–2 weeks

(D) School phobia program

(E) Identify stresses
Reassurance
Counseling
Stress reduction techniques

Good response

Poor response

Good response

Refer for individual
or family therapy

CHEST PAIN

A. Separate musculoskeletal pain into traumatic and nontraumatic categories. Traumatic pain is frequently caused by a bruised or fractured rib. Nontraumatic pain is most often the result of costrochondritis or anterior chest wall syndrome. Palpate each rib cartilage with only one finger; two or more fingers may splint the affected cartilage and not reproduce the pain. Costochondritis presents with tenderness over the costochondral or costosternal junctions. Anterior chest wall syndrome (xiphoidalgia, intercostal neuritis, myodynea, fibrocystitis, precordial catch syndrome, slipping rib syndrome, or Tietze's syndrome) presents with chest wall pain at rest and is exacerbated by trunk or shoulder movements. The pain can often be precipitated by isometric exercises.

B. A breast mass or the presence of gynecomastia in the male results in chest pain secondary to a high level of anxiety related to either appearance or concern about malignancy.

C. Gastrointestinal disorders causing chest pain include peptic ulcer disease, esophagitis or esophageal spasm, odynophagia, and referred pain from the abdomen.

D. Hyperventilation results in a reduction in carbon dioxide tension, alkalosis, a decreased ionized-calcium level, and carpal pedal spasm. Hyperventilation produces chest pain as a result of stomach dilatation, aerophagia, spasm of the left diaphragm, or the induction of a transient cardiac arrythmia. A high level of anxiety can be identified in most cases, related to either life stress of underlying psychopathology.

E. Pulmonary diseases produce pain because of muscle strain, pleural irritation, diaphragmatic irritation, or acute anxiety. Consider birth control pills a risk factor predisposing to pulmonary embolus. Other entities causing chest pain are acute respiratory infections, pleurisy, pneumothorax, and asthma.

F. Risk factors for cardiac disease include a family history of early myocardial infarction or hypercholesterolemia, a history of Kawasaki disease, hypertension, or congenital disease. Findings which suggest cardiac disease are heart murmurs, increased intensity of the second heart sound, clicks, gallop rhythm, friction rub, hypertension, and decreased femoral pulses. Findings on chest x-ray and ECG may suggest cardiac disease. Pericarditis and myocarditis related to an infection or vasculitis will present with cardiomegaly and ST-T wave changes. Aortic stenosis and idiopathic hypertrophic subaortic stenosis present with a systolic heart murmur and left-ventricular hypertrophy. Primary pulmonary hypertension and pulmonary stenosis produce right-ventricular hypertrophy. Coronary artery disease related to Kawasaki disease, hypercholesterolemia, aberrant left coronary artery, and lesions associated with decreased coronary artery blood flow such as severe aortic stenosis or IHSS produce ischemic ST-T wave changes. Arrhythmias such as AV block, sick sinus syndrome, or supraventricular tachycardia are associated with ECG findings of abnormal conduction patterns.

REFERENCES

Agnes RS, Santulle R, Bemoporad JF. Psychogenic chest pain in children. Clin Pediatr 1981; 20:788.

Brown RT. Costochondritis in adolescents. J Adolesc Health Care 1981; 1:198.

Driscoll OJ, Clinklish LB, Ballen WJ. Chest pain in children: a perspective study. Pediatrics 1976; 57:648.

Herman SP, Stickler GB, Lucas AR et al. Hyperventilation syndrome in children and adolescents. Pediatrics 1981; 67:183.

Pantell, RH, Goodman BW Jr. Adolescent chest pain: a prospective study. Pediatrics 1983; 71:881.

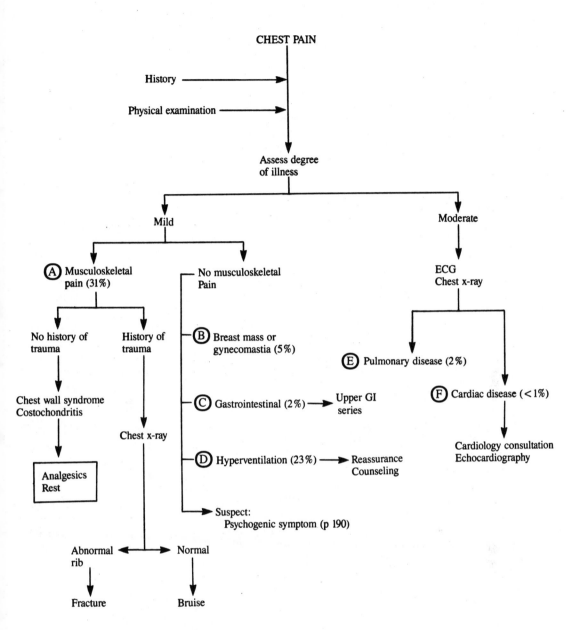

CHEST PAIN

History

Physical examination

Assess degree
of illness

Mild   Moderate

(A) Musculoskeletal   No musculoskeletal   ECG
pain (31%)   Pain   Chest x-ray

No history of   History of
trauma   trauma   (E) Pulmonary disease (2%)

                                      (B) Breast mass or
                                          gynecomastia (5%)
Chest wall syndrome
Costochondritis   Chest x-ray   (C) Gastrointestinal (2%) → Upper GI   (F) Cardiac disease (<1%)
                                                                            series

Analgesics   (D) Hyperventilation (23%) → Reassurance   Cardiology consultation
Rest   Counseling   Echocardiography

                                      → Suspect:
                                        Psychogenic symptom (p 190)

Abnormal ◄──────► Normal
rib

Fracture   Bruise

SYNCOPE

A. The history should clarify predisposing conditions and any precipitating events such as prolonged or sudden standing, prolonged fasting, micturation, paroxysm of coughing, physical exercise, recent closed head trauma, or a sudden, strong emotion.

B. Orthostatic syncope is associated with a fall in blood pressure upon standing. Rarely, syncope may follow micturation, when rapid bladder decompression produces postural hypotension and decreased cardiac return.

C. Vasovagal syncope is caused by a sudden decrease in peripheral vascular resistance. It is usually precipitated by sudden fear, anger, or other strong emotions.

D. Breath-holding occurs in children under 6 years of age and is precipitated by crying, sudden pain, or fear. Loss of tone and consciousness is followed by stiffening and clonus. Cyanosis, if present, should precede any abnormal movements. No postictal or confusional state occurs. The prognosis is excellent; spells of breath-holding usually are discontinued by 6 years of age. Treatment involves reassuring the parents of the benign nature of the problem.

E. Hyperventilation produces reduction in carbon dioxide tension with alkalosis, decreased ionized-calcium, and tetany. This syndrome is frequently associated with light-headedness, giddiness, dizziness, parasthesias, and chest pain. In most cases, a high level of anxiety is identified, related to life stress or underlying psychopathology.

F. Seizure activity is suggessted when a syncopal episode lasts longer than 2 minutes, is followed by confusion or impaired mental status (postictal state), or is associated with incontinence, muscle jerks, or cyanosis. Frequent recurrent episodes also suggest seizures. Signs of CNS disease include an altered mental status, focal neurologic signs, weakness, abnormal tone and reflexes, and abnormal growth and development.

G. Paroxysmal coughing produced by *B. pertussis* or asthma may decrease cardiac output and cause hypoxia resulting in syncope. Signs of respiratory distress are tachypnea, retractions, decreased breath sounds, wheezing, rales, and cyanosis.

H. Risk factors for cardiac disease include a family history of early myocardial infarction or hypercholesterolemia, a history of Kawasaki disease, hypertension, and congenital heart disease. Findings which suggest cardiac disease are heart murmurs, increased intensity of the second heart sound, clicks, gallop rhythm, friction rub, hypertension, and decreased femoral pulses. Findings on chest x-ray and ECG may suggest cardiac disease. Pericarditis and myocarditis related to an infection or vasculitis will present with cardiomegaly and ST-T wave changes. Aortic stenosis and idiopathic hypertrophic subaortic stenosis present with a systolic heart murmur and left-ventricular hypertrophy. Coarctation syndromes present with decreased femoral pulses and left-ventricular hypertrophy. Primary pulmonary hypertension and pulmonary stenosis produce right-ventricular hypertrophy. Coronary artery disease related to Kawasaki disease, hypercholesterolemia, aberrant left coronary artery, and lesions associated with decreased coronary artery blood flow, such as severe aortic stenosis or IHSS, produce ischemic ST-T wave changes. Arrhythmias such as AV block, sick sinus syndrome, or supraventricular tachycardia are associated with ECG findings of abnormal conduction patterns.

REFERENCES

Herman SP, Stickler GB, Lucas AR. Hyperventilation syndrome in children and adolescents. Pediatrics 1981; 67:183.

Katz RM. Cough syncope in children with asthma. J Pediatr 1979; 77:48.

Lombroso CT, Lerman P. Breathholding spells. Pediatrics 1967; 39:563.

SYNCOPE

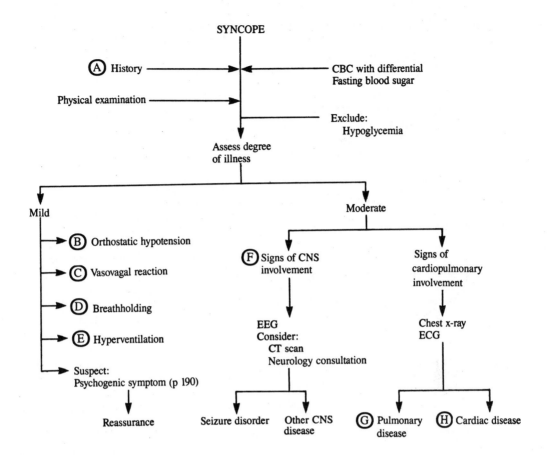

ENCOPRESIS OR SOILING

Barton D. Schmitt, M.D.

A. Encopresis or soiling is the voluntary or involuntary passing of feces into the underwear or other inappropriate site.

B. Over half of these children have no primary emotional problem and become impacted to avoid the passage of painful bowel movements. The impacted children periodically have pain with bowel movements, blood on toilet tissue, and a huge stool that clogs the toilet. Since psychogenic factors are common, perform a thorough psychosocial evaluation on all children with encopresis. Many have experienced coercive and punitive toilet training. Others have mild resistance as a result of too much punishment, lectures, or nagging. Refer patients who are depressed, acting out, or over the age of 8 to a child psychologist or psychiatrist for therapy.

C. Differentiate retentive from nonretentive encopresis on the basis of impacted stool in the rectum. In impacted children, the rectum is distended and packed with clay-like stool and a midline suprapubic mass is usually palpable. Leakage of loose stool around the impaction may occur several times per day (overflow diarrhea). Suspect nonretentive encopresis when a normal bowel movement is passed into the underwear once or twice a day without any history of constipation. A barium enema is only indicated if the anal canal won't admit a finger or if the rectum is empty on repeated examination.

D. Remove the impaction with 2 or 3 hyperphosphate enemas. Treat the child with a stool softener such as mineral oil or milk of magnesia for 3 months until the diameter and tone of the bowel return to normal. Recommend a diet that includes increased bran, salads, and fresh fruits and vegetables. Instruct the parents that the child should also sit on the toilet 3 times a day or the program will fail. The physician's continued involvement is critical even if the child needs referral to a psychologist or psychiatrist.

E. Pediatric counseling, especially for nonretentive soiling, involves advising the parents to discontinue any coercive child-rearing practices, increasing positive contact with the parents, setting up a new toileting program with the child's active participation, using a calendar and rewards, and stopping any reminders to sit on the toilet. The parents' main job is to detect any accidents and help the child change as soon as possible. Enemas and medications are not needed in nonretentive encopresis. Refer severely emotionally disturbed children for therapy.

REFERENCES

Fleisher DR. Diagnosis and treatment of disorders of defecation in children. Pediatr Ann 1976; 5:701.
Levine MD. The schoolchild with encopresis. Pediatr Rev 1981; 2:285.

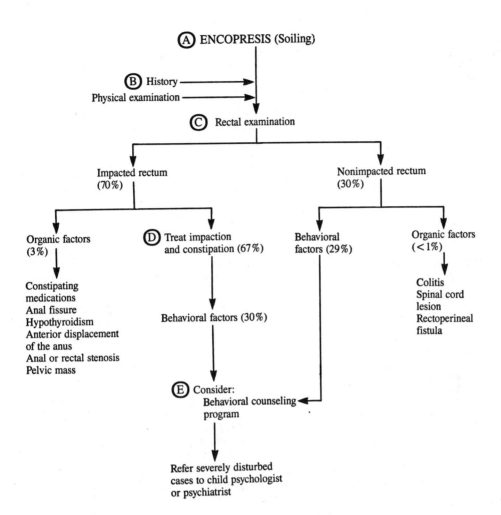

(A) ENCOPRESIS (Soiling)

(B) History ⟶
Physical examination ⟶

(C) Rectal examination

Impacted rectum
(70%)

Nonimpacted rectum
(30%)

Organic factors
(3%)

(D) Treat impaction
and constipation (67%)

Behavioral
factors (29%)

Organic factors
(<1%)

Constipating
medications
Anal fissure
Hypothyroidism
Anterior displacement
of the anus
Anal or rectal stenosis
Pelvic mass

Behavioral factors (30%)

Colitis
Spinal cord
lesion
Rectoperineal
fistula

(E) Consider:
Behavioral counseling ⟵
program

Refer severely disturbed
cases to child psychologist
or psychiatrist

ENURESIS

Barton D. Schmitt, M.D.

A. Determine the onset, pattern (daytime vs nighttime), and frequency of wetting. Note the presence of dysuria, an abnormal urine stream (dribbling), hematuria, abdominal pain, constipation, polydipsia, and polyuria. Identify predisposing conditions such as frequent urinary tract infections, fecal impaction, diabetes mellitus, CNS disease or trauma (diabetes insipidus), and severe emotional disturbance (psychogenic polydipsia). Obtain a complete psychosocial history (p 190) and identify children who appear severely disturbed.

B. Note the presence of a distended bladder or fecal impaction. Assess the anal sphincter wink, the child's gait, and the ankle deep tendon reflexes. Observe the urine stream. Perform a urinalysis in all patients with special emphasis on the specific gravity and urine glucose.

C. Suspect an associated urinary tract malformation when an abnormal urine stream, constant wetness (dampness), or recurrent urinary tract infections are present. Radiologic studies including an IVP and voiding cystourethrogram (VCUG) will identify ectopic ureters, a lower urinary tract obstruction, or a neurogenic bladder.

D. Categorize patients according to the pattern of enuresis. Nocturnal enuresis is common (> 10% of 5-year-olds wet their beds); diurnal enuresis is far less common. Nocturnal enuresis is involuntary; diurnal enuresis is commonly voluntary. When both forms of enuresis are present, treat diurnal enuresis first.

E. Approximately ⅓ of daytime wetters have urgency incontinence. These children wet themselves while running to the toilet or while trying to undress; they do use the toilet, unlike those with behavior problems; they are usually female and may have a long history of intense bladder spasms; they are embarrassed by their problem; and the family history is commonly positive. Treat these children with stream-interruption exercises (counting to 10 before initiating the stream and at midstream); they should work up to interrupting for 3 minutes (use an egg timer). Bladder-stretching exercises are contraindicated; they lead to increased wetting.

F. Many daytime wetters deliberately wet themselves to retaliate for the pressures of toilet training. Some have been physically punished; others have been endlessly nagged and reminded. Most have mild problems and can be treated by the primary physician. Refer to the child psychiatrist or psychologist those who are depressed, overtly angry, or more than 8 years old. Also refer children with pervasive emotional problems. Treat daytime wetters who have minimal psychopathology by instructing the parents to discontinue any coercive child-raising practices and to increase positive contact time at home. Set up a new toilet-training program with the child's active participation using a calendar and reward system. Have the parents discontinue any reminders to use the toilet but continue to remind the youngster to change to dry clothing when wet. Stream-interruption and bladder-stretching exercises are both counterproductive as the child considers them an intrusion.

G. Over 75% of nighttime bed wetters have a small bladder capacity. Normal bladder capacity is 1 ounce per year of age or 10 ml/kg. Children with small bladders need to learn to awaken at night. Self-awakening programs are helpful as are the new portable, transistorized enuresis alarms (Wet Stop, Nytone, or Night Trainer). Bladder-stretching exercises can be used, but they only cure 35% of children and yield slow progress. No effective, safe drug is currently available.

H. Children with an increased or normal bladder capacity respond to a program that helps them take responsibility for their symptoms. Have the family discontinue all punishment. Dry mornings should result in positive recognition (praise, a calendar, treats). Fluids are decreased during the 3 hours prior to bedtime and the bladder is emptied at bedtime.

REFERENCES

Azrin NH, Thienes PM. Rapid elimination of enuresis in intensive learning without a conditioning apparatus. Behavior Ther 1978; 9:342.

Blackwell B, Currah J. The psychopharmacology of nocturnal enuresis. In: Kolvin I, MacKeith RC, Meadow SR, eds. Bladder Control and Enuresis. London: Wm Heinemann Med Books, 1973: 231.

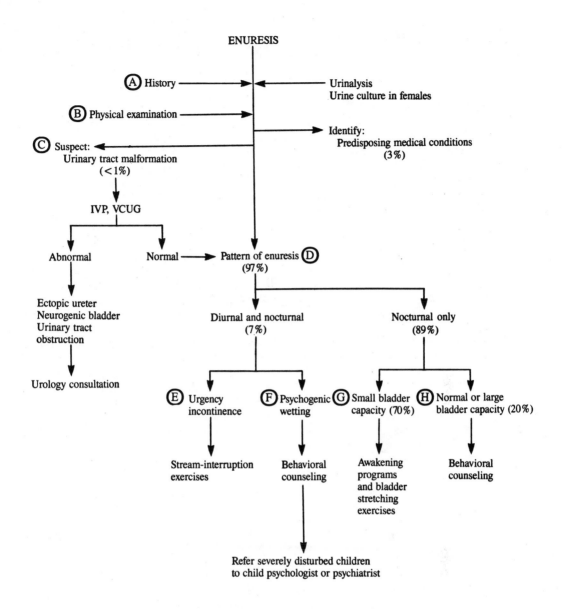

ENURESIS

Ⓐ History ⟶ ⟵ Urinalysis
Urine culture in females

Ⓑ Physical examination ⟶

⟶ Identify:
Predisposing medical conditions
(3%)

Ⓒ Suspect: ⟵
Urinary tract malformation
(<1%)

IVP, VCUG

Abnormal ⟶ Normal ⟶ Pattern of enuresis Ⓓ
(97%)

Ectopic ureter
Neurogenic bladder
Urinary tract
obstruction

Urology consultation

Diurnal and nocturnal
(7%)

Nocturnal only
(89%)

Ⓔ Urgency
incontinence

Ⓕ Psychogenic
wetting

Ⓖ Small bladder
capacity (70%)

Ⓗ Normal or large
bladder capacity (20%)

Stream-interruption
exercises

Behavioral
counseling

Awakening
programs
and bladder
stretching
exercises

Behavioral
counseling

Refer severely disturbed children
to child psychologist or psychiatrist

Schmitt BD. Daytime wetting (Diurnal enuresis). Pediatr Clin North Am 1982; 29:9.
Schmitt BD. Nocturnal enuresis: An update on treatment. Pediatr Clin North Am 1982; 29:21.

FAILURE TO THRIVE IN INFANCY

A. Obtain a detailed history of diet and feeding. Determine family composition; assess employment and financial status, degree of social isolation, and level of family stress. Determine infant's immunization history, missed appointment rate, and accessibility of medical care. Note predisposing conditions such as intrauterine/growth retardation, perinatal stress, prematurity, or chronic diseases. Note the frequency of intercurrent acute illnesses such as acute otitis media, vomiting, diarrhea, respiratory infections, or urinary tract infections.

B. Assess the mother-child interaction. Note signs of neglect or abuse such as bruises, burns, dirty unkempt appearance, severe diaper rash, impetigo, flat occiput, or bald spot. Assess infant's developmental status with a full DDST. Note any dysmorphic features or signs of CNS, pulmonary, or cardiac disase. Determine the median age for the patient's height (height age), median age for the patient's weight (weight age), and median age for the patient's head circumference (head circumference age). Suspect nutritional causes when the weight age is disproportionate to the height and head circumference ages. Suspect CNS disease and intrauterine growth retardation when weight, height and head circumference ages are all reduced proportionately. Suspect dystrophies, dwarfism, and endocrinopathies when weight is reduced in proportion to height, while head circumference is either normal or enlarged.

C. Assess the degree of illness. Severely ill infants have findings of marasmus or kwashiorkor. Moderately ill infants fail to regain birth weight by age 1 month, have a flat weight curve for more than 2 months, have a height well above the third percentile with a weight below the third percentile. These infants may also present with deprivational behaviors such as rumination or head banging. Mildly ill patients fail to regain birth weight by age 2 weeks, have a flat weight curve for 1–2 months, or present with a height: weight discrepancy.

D. Attempt to document rapid weight gain (>2 oz/day for 1 week or >1.5 oz/day for 2 weeks) during the patient's hospital stay. Initially, institute unlimited feelings of regular diet for age using the same formula as home. Obtain a developmental assessment on the day of admission and institute an infant stimulation program if deprivational behavior is observed. When neglect is suspected, obtain a social service evaluation of the family, and assess the parent-child interaction.

E. If nutritional deprivation is diagnosed, report the case to child protective services. If nonaccidental trauma is suspected, obtain a skeletal bone series to identify fractures. Disposition options to be considered include home placement with support services, close medical follow-up visits, temporary foster placement while a parent receives therapy, or long-term foster placement.

F. When poor weight gain is associated with diarrhea or malabsorption, consider cystic fibrosis, celiac disease, milk protein intolerance, disaccharidase deficiencies, parasites, pancreatic insufficiency, short bowel syndrome, and inflammatory bowel disease. When poor weight gain is associated with vomiting or rumination, consider gastroesophageal reflux, pyloric stenosis, duodenal stenosis or atresia, vascular rings, metabolic disease, renal disease, adrenal disease, or CNS disease (mass lesion, hydrocephalus, cerebral atrophy, subdural hematoma, CNS infection).

G. Suspect a hypermetabolic state when adequate caloric intake does not result in weight gain. Possible causes include hyperthyroidism, chronic infection, malignancy, inflammatory bowel disease, collagen vascular disease, and diencephalic syndrome.

REFERENCES

Berwick DM: Non-organic failure to thrive. Pediatr Rev 1980; 1:265.
Hannaway PJ. Failure to thrive: A study of 100 infants and children. Clin Pediatr 1970; 9:96.
Sills RH. Failure to thrive: The role of clinical and laboratory evaluation. Am J Dis Child 1978; 132:967.

FAILURE TO THRIVE IN INFANCY

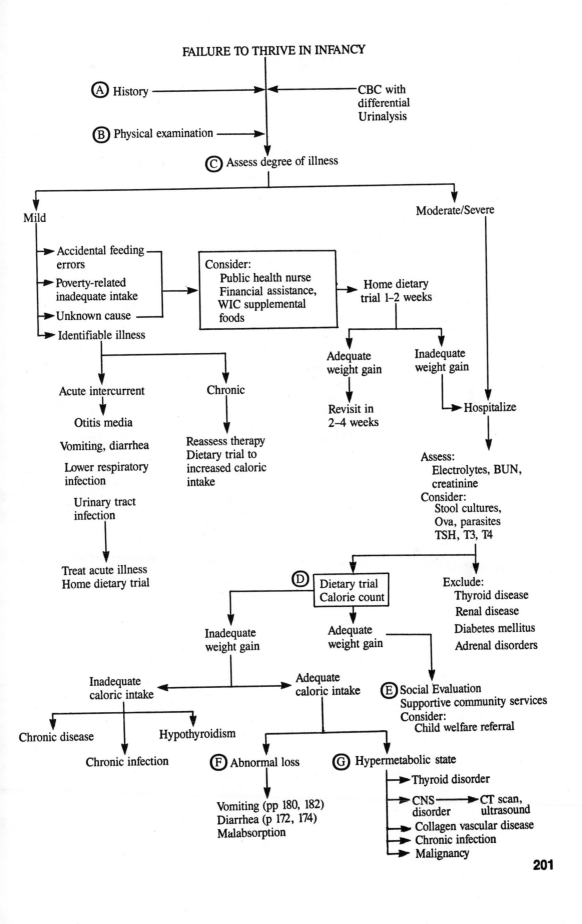

PHYSICAL ABUSE

Barton D. Schmitt, M.D.

A. Obtain detailed history of how the injury allegedly happened, including sequence of events, people present, and time lag before medical attention sought. The parent's explanation for each positive physical finding should be recorded. If the child is over age 3, the history should be elicited in a private setting and compared to the parent's version.

B. List all bruises by site, size, shape, and color; note their resemblance to any identifiable object. Pay special attention to the retina, eardrums, oral cavity, and genitals for signs of occult trauma. In severe cases, color photographs are helpful records. Palpate all bones for tenderness and test joints for full range of motion.

C. Treat the child's medical and surgical problems appropriately, regardless of cause. Hospitalize children with severe injuries.

D. Many cases of physical abuse are first suspected because the injury is unexplained or the explanation is implausible and incompatible with the physical findings. A child over 3 or 4 years will often confirm that a particular adult hurt him. Note accusations of one parent by the other. Most diagnoses of physical abuse (nonaccidental trauma) can be based solely on the physical findings. Many bruises, burns, and scars are pathognomonic. Bruises on the buttocks and lower back are almost always related to punishment; finger- and thumbprints are found where a child has been forcefully grabbed; hard pinching leaves curvilinear bruises; slapping leaves a bruise with parallel lines running through it; attempts to silence a screaming child may bruise the upper lip and frenulum; human bite marks are distinctive, paired, crescent-shaped bruises facing each other; a bruise or welt often resembles the blunt instrument used. The most common sites of *accidental* bruises are the forehead, anterior tibia, and bony prominences.

E. Some cases are obvious, others are confusing. If you are unable to decide whether the injuries are accidental or inflicted, seek immediate consultation. When in doubt, report suspicious injuries to CPS for investigation and follow-up observation.

F. Make a report to local child protection services (CPS) *immediately*. Reporting should secure evaluation, treatment, protection of the child, follow-up, and access to the juvenile court when necessary.

G. Order a bleeding disorder screen in children with bruises if you suspect a bleeding disorder, if the case is expected to go to court, or if the parents deny inflicting the injuries and claim "easy bruising". A bleeding disorder screen includes a platelet count, bleeding time, partial thromboplastin time, prothrombin time, thrombin time, and fibrinogen level (the last two may be optional).

H. In suspicious cases, order bone survey x-rays on every child under 2 years of age; between 2 and 5 years, most children should receive a bone survey unless the child has very mild injuries or is in a supervised setting (e.g., preschool); over age 5, obtain x-rays only if there is bone tenderness or limited range of motion. Ask the radiologist to date positive x-ray findings. Bone trauma is found in 10–20% of physically abused children; metaphyseal chip fractures or multiple bony injuries at different stages of healing are diagnostic.

REFERENCES

Bittner S, Newberger EH. Pediatric understanding of child abuse and neglect. Pediatr Rev 1981; 2:209.

Caffey, J. The whiplash shaken-infant syndrome. Pediatrics 1974; 54:396.

Feldman KW, Schaller RT, Feldman JA, McMillon M. Tap-water scald burns in children. Pediatrics 1978; 62:1.

McNeese MC, Hebeler JR. The abused child. CIBA Clin Symp 1977; 29(5):1.

Schmitt, BD. The child with non-accidental trauma. In: Kempe CH, Helfer RE, eds. The Battered Child. 3rd ed. Chicago: University of Chicago Press, 1980:128.

PHYSICAL INJURY
(Bruises, burns, fractures, subdural hematoma)

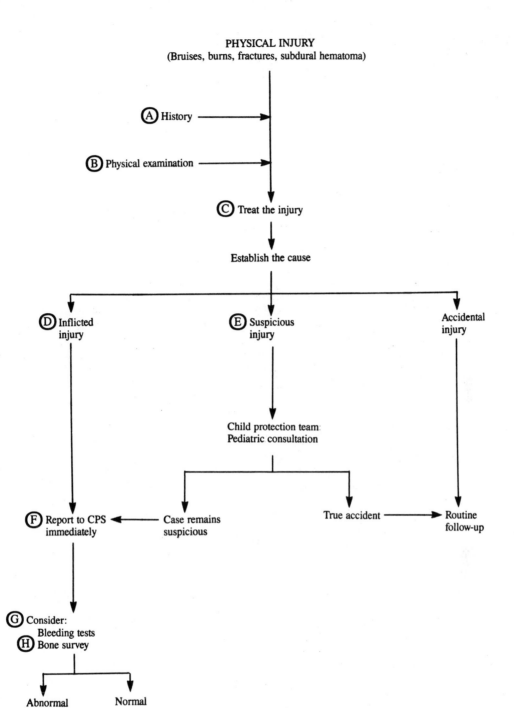

(A) History

(B) Physical examination

(C) Treat the injury

Establish the cause

(D) Inflicted injury

(E) Suspicious injury

Accidental injury

Child protection team:
Pediatric consultation

(F) Report to CPS immediately ← Case remains suspicious

True accident → Routine follow-up

(G) Consider:
    Bleeding tests
(H) Bone survey

Abnormal   Normal

Bleeding disorders
Fractures/bone trauma

SEXUAL ABUSE
Barton D. Schmitt, M.D.

A Sexual mistreatment of children is most commonly family-related (incest). Sexual abuse by friends and acquaintances of the family is the second most common type and the least common is sexual abuse by strangers. Suspicion should be aroused when a prepubertal child presents with vaginal bleeding or other unexplained genital symptoms, compulsive masturbation, precocious sexual behaviors, sexually transmitted disease, a rectal or vaginal foreign body, proctitis, or recurrent urinary tract infections.

B. Take a careful history; fewer than 50% of abuse victims have physical or laboratory findings. A detailed account of sexual experiences by a prepubertal child should be considered hard evidence of abuse. Children older than 2½ years of age can usually provide an accurate description to a skillful interviewer. Encourage the patient by appropriate questioning to reveal all details concerning types and frequency of sexual activities. Note the child's special names for body parts. In addition to facts regarding date, time, place and person, document sites of sexual abuse, menstrual history, whether or not force was involved, the patient's concept of intercourse, and whether or not penetration and ejaculation occurred.

C. Medication to prevent pregnancy can be given to girls who are postmenarchal, midcycle, and have experienced vaginal intercourse within 72 hours. If the pregnancy test is negative, the drug of choice is Ovral, 2 tablets immediately, repeated once in 12 hours. Treat selected victims with antibiotics to prevent sexually transmitted disease (p 88).

D. Conduct a body surface examination for any signs of nongenital trauma. Assess the possibility of pregnancy. Examine the mouth and rectum for signs of acute trauma. Visually examine the external genitals for signs of trauma, laxity, or vaginal discharge. Speculum examination of the vagina is rarely needed. Most acute genital injuries occur between the 4 and 8 o'clock positions. The labia minora and posterior fourchette are damaged first, followed by tears of the posterior hymenal ring. Acute trauma of the genitals, rectum, or mouth usually heals in 4–7 days. Laxity of the anal sphincters is usually temporary and changes to spasm within a few hours of penetration. In prepubertal girls, a hymenal ring ≥ 5 mm is abnormal. After puberty, hymenal laxity must usually be assessed by palpation. There are 3 types of sexual abuse: (1) molestation, (viewing or fondling the child's genitals, asking the child to fondle or masturbate the adult's genitals, and exposure to pornography); (2) sexual intercourse (including attempted and actual vaginal, oral, or rectal penetration on a nonassaultive basis); and (3) rape.

E. Test for sperm from site penetrated. Take cultures for gonorrhea from the throat, vagina, and anal canal.

F. Collect specimens that help to determine the identity of the rapist (pubic hair, scalp hair, fingernail scrapings, blood samples, sperm type).

REFERENCES

Cowell CA. The gynecologic examination of infants, children and young adolescents. Pediatr Clin North Am 1981; 28:247.

Orr DP, Prietto SV. Emergency management of sexually abused children. Am J Dis Child 1979; 133:628.

Rimsza ME, Niggemann EH. Medical evaluation of sexually abused children: A review of 311 cases. Pediatrics 1982; 69:8.

Schmitt, BD. Sexual abuse (incest). In: Green M, Haggerty RJ. Ambulatory Publications. 3rd ed. Philadelphia: WB Saunders, 1984:317.

Woodling BA, Kossoris PD. Sexual misuse: Rape, molestation, and incest. Pediatr Clin North Am 1981; 28:481.

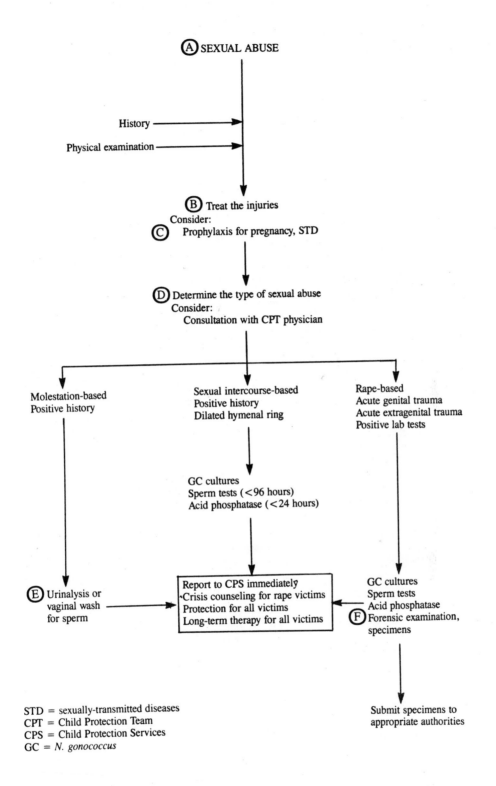

(A) SEXUAL ABUSE

History ──────────▶

Physical examination ──────▶

(B) Treat the injuries
Consider:
(C) Prophylaxis for pregnancy, STD

(D) Determine the type of sexual abuse
Consider:
Consultation with CPT physician

Molestation-based
Positive history

Sexual intercourse-based
Positive history
Dilated hymenal ring

Rape-based
Acute genital trauma
Acute extragenital trauma
Positive lab tests

GC cultures
Sperm tests (<96 hours)
Acid phosphatase (<24 hours)

(E) Urinalysis or
vaginal wash
for sperm

Report to CPS immediately
Crisis counseling for rape victims
Protection for all victims
Long-term therapy for all victims

GC cultures
Sperm tests
Acid phosphatase
(F) Forensic examination,
specimens

Submit specimens to
appropriate authorities

STD = sexually-transmitted diseases
CPT = Child Protection Team
CPS = Child Protection Services
GC = *N. gonococcus*

205

ANEMIA IN THE NEWBORN
Peter A. Lane, M.D.

A. Document the presence or absence of prenatal infections or drug use. Also note any history of maternal vaginal bleeding, placenta previa, abruptio placenta umbilical cord rupture, constriction or velamentous insertion, as well as cesarean, breech, or traumatic delivery. Obtain a family history of neonatal jaundice, anemia, splenomegaly, or unexplained gallstones.

B. Note tachypnea, tachycardia, and peripheral vasoconstriction (acute blood loss) or hepatosplenomegaly (chronic anemia, intrauterine infection, congenital malignancy). Jaundice appearing before 24 hours of age suggests significant hemolysis.

C. A hematocrit <45% during the first 3 days of life is abnormal and requires explanation. Except in an emergency, no anemic newborn should receive a blood transfusion prior to obtaining adequate diagnostic studies.

D. Normal reticulocyte values are 3 to 7% during the first day of life and 1 to 3% during the second and third day. A low reticulocyte count in the face of significant anemia suggests bone marrow failure.

E. An indirect hyperbilirubinemia (p 208), an abnormal peripheral blood smear, or an ABO or Rh blood group incompatibility between the mother and infant suggests the possibility of hemolysis.

F. Perform both a direct and an indirect Coombs test. ABO isoimmunization is usually associated with a negative direct and a positive indirect Coombs test.

G. Infants with immune hemolysis have variable degrees of hemolysis which may continue for 3 months.

H. A low MCV on the initial CBC suggests α or γ thalassemia or hereditary elliptocytosis or pyropoikilocytosis. *Microcytosis without hemolysis suggests chronic blood loss in utero.* A hemoglobin electrophoresis positive for Bart's hemoglobin (α thalassemia) or the finding of microcytosis or elliptocytosis in other family members helps confirm the correct diagnosis.

I. Examine the peripheral blood smear. Spherocytes suggest ABO isoimmunization, hereditary spherocytosis, or infection (i.e., CMV). Red cell fragmentation suggests intravascular hemolysis (infection, disseminated intravascular coagulation). Consider the possibility of infection and/or DIC in any ill newborn with hemolysis, particularly if thrombocytopenia is also present.

J. Review the obstetrical history and examine the placenta for clues to the etiology of fetal blood loss.

K. Perform a Kleihauer test to detect the presence of fetal red cells in the maternal circulation. False negatives occur when an ABO incompatibility results in the rapid clearance of the infant's red cells from the maternal circulation.

L. Any newborn with significant prenatal or perinatal blood loss is at risk for the development of iron deficiency during the first 6 months of life.

REFERENCES

Glader BE, Platt O. Haemolytic disorders of infancy. Clin Haematol 1978; 7:35.

Oski FA. Anemia in the neonatal period. In: Oski FA, Naiman JL. Hematologic Problems in the Newborn. 3rd ed. Philadelphia: WB Saunders, 1982; 56.

ANEMIA IN THE NEWBORN

(A) History ——————————→←—————————— CBC (C)

(B) Physical ——————————→
    examination

(D) Reticulocyte count

Low   Normal or high

Under production   (E) Smear, bilirubin
                                           Mother/baby blood types

Hematology consultation
Consider:
    Bone marrow test

Hemolysis ←——————————   No hemolysis

(F) Coombs tests   (J) Identify
                                           blood loss

Positive   Negative   Obvious   No obvious
                                       cause   cause

→Isoimmune   →Obstetrical   (K) Maternal
  ABO, Rh, other   accidents   Kleihauer test
                                       →Twin-twin
→Maternal autoimmune   transfusion

Treat jaundice   MCV   Negative   Positive
Follow hematocrit 3 mos
                                                            Observe for
                                                            internal hemorrhage,
                                                            jaundice

<95   >95   Fetal-Maternal
                                                                           Transfusion

(I) Hemoglobin electrophoresis   (I) Smear
    Family studies   Exclude:
    Consider: Infection
        Hematology consultation   DIC
                                      Consider:
                                          Hematology consultation

→α thalassemia   →Infections   (L) Consider:
                                                               Early Iron
→γ thalassemia   →Hereditary spherocytosis   Supplementation

→Hereditary elliptocytosis,   →Infantile pyknocytosis
  pyropoikilocytosis
                                  →RBC enzyme deficiency

207

NEONATAL JAUNDICE

A. Identify predisposing conditions such as maternal infection or chronic illness (diabetes). Inquire as to medications taken during pregnancy, especially sulfonamides, nitrofurantoins, or antimalarials. In the labor and delivery history, note the use of forceps or vacuum extraction (cephalohematoma), delayed cord clamping, and Apgar score. Note family history of anemia, jaundice, or liver disease, especially in siblings. Note associated symptoms such as fever or temperature instability, abdominal distention, vomiting, seizures, and failure to thrive.

B. Determine if the infant is premature or small for gestational age. Document presence of a right upper quadrant mass (choledochal cyst). The presence of microcephaly, petechiae, hepatosplenomegaly, or chorioretinitis suggests intrauterine infection. Pallor and hepatosplenomegaly suggest severe hemolytic anemia. Note signs of extravascular bleeding such as cephalohematoma or bruising.

C. Elevations in bilirubin above 12.9 mg% in a term newborn and 15 mg% in a premature, a rate of rise of bilirubin >5 mg%/day or a direct bilirubin >1.5 mg% are abnormal findings that suggest an underlying disease process. Hemolytic disease or acute blood loss may present with or without an associated anemia.

D. A positive direct and/or indirect Coombs test will identify isoimmunization related to Rh, ABO, or minor blood group antigens or maternal autoimmune hemolytic anemia. Guidelines for phototherapy and exchange transfusion are unclear. Patients with a positive Coombs test, especially when associated with Rh incompatibility, should be followed carefully for 3 months to identify anemia.

E. An abnormal peripheral smear showing red-cell fragments, spherocytes, or abnormal red cell shape with or without elevation in the reticulocyte count (day 1 >7%; day 2–3 >3%) suggests hemolytic anemia. Such disorders include spherocytosis, elliptocytosis, infantile pyknocytosis, enzyme deficiencies (G6PD, pyruvate kinase deficiency), congenital viral infections (CMV), disseminated intravascular coagulation, and α and γ thalassemia.

F. Extravascular bleeding often presents as a cephalohematoma or facial bruising. Pyloric stenosis, small- or large-bowel obstruction, and swallowed blood will increase the enterohepatic circulation of bilirubin. Galactosemia, hypothyroidism, hypopituitarism, and Crigler-Najjar syndrome are endocrine or metabolic disorders which present with jaundice. Jaundice may be associated with polycythemia (idiopathic twin-twin transfusion or delayed cord clamping).

G. It is often difficult to distinguish neonatal hepatitis from biliary atresia. Perform hepatobiliary scintigraphy with isopropylacetanilido-iminodiacetic acid (PIPIDA) which provides better imaging of the biliary tree than rose bengal I[131]. When the continuity between the biliary track and gut is in doubt, surgery and operative cholangiogram are indicated. Hepatic portoenterostomy (Kasai procedure) should be performed in the first 8 to 10 weeks of life. When neonatal hepatitis is suspected, perform a hepatitis workup which includes hepatitis B surface antigen, alpha-1-antitrypsin screen, sweat teest for cystic fibrosis, urine for reducing substances, amino and organic acids, galactose-1-phosphate uridyl transferase (galactosemia), and tests for congenital infections.

REFERENCES

Gartner LM. Cholestasis of the newborn. Pediatr Rev 1983; 5:163.
Maisels MJ. Jaundice in the newborn. Pediatr Rev 1982; 3:305.
Watson S, Giacoia GP. Cholestasis in infancy: a review. Clin Pediatr 1983; 22:30.

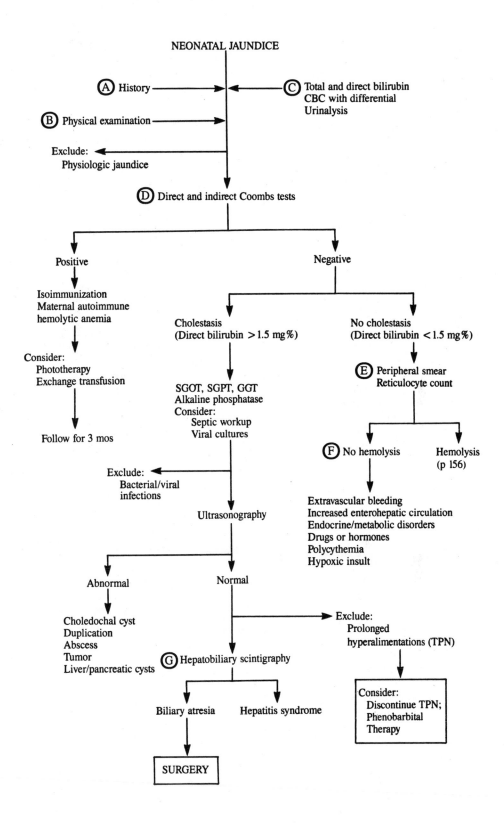

NEONATAL JAUNDICE

(A) History

(B) Physical examination

(C) Total and direct bilirubin
CBC with differential
Urinalysis

Exclude:
Physiologic jaundice

(D) Direct and indirect Coombs tests

Positive

Isoimmunization
Maternal autoimmune
hemolytic anemia

Consider:
Photometherapy
Exchange transfusion

Follow for 3 mos

Negative

Cholestasis
(Direct bilirubin > 1.5 mg%)

SGOT, SGPT, GGT
Alkaline phosphatase
Consider:
Septic workup
Viral cultures

Exclude:
Bacterial/viral
infections

Ultrasonography

No cholestasis
(Direct bilirubin < 1.5 mg%)

(E) Peripheral smear
Reticulocyte count

(F) No hemolysis   Hemolysis
                          (p 156)

Extravascular bleeding
Increased enterohepatic circulation
Endocrine/metabolic disorders
Drugs or hormones
Polycythemia
Hypoxic insult

Abnormal

Choledochal cyst
Duplication
Abscess
Tumor
Liver/pancreatic cysts

Normal

Exclude:
Prolonged
hyperalimentations (TPN)

(G) Hepatobiliary scintigraphy

Biliary atresia   Hepatitis syndrome

SURGERY

Consider:
Discontinue TPN;
Phenobarbital
Therapy

209

BLEEDING IN THE NEWBORN
Peter A. Lane, M.D.

A. Note significant maternal illnesses such as epilepsy (vitamin K deficiency), diabetes (renal vein thrombosis), hypertension, or autoimmune disease (thrombocytopenia). Identify drugs ingested during pregnancy associated with platelet dysfunction (salicylates), Vitamin K deficiency (anticonvulsants, antituberculous chemotherapy, warfarin) or thrombocytopenia (antihypertensives). Note gestational history, method of delivery, and Apgar scores. Consider risk factors for bacterial infection such as prematurity, prolonged rupture of membranes, maternal amnionitis, or fetal distress during labor. Take a detailed family history for bleeding. Finally, *document with certainty the administration of vitamin K at birth.*

B. Note the extent and type of bleeding. Assess the cardiovascular status for signs of intravascular volume depletion (rapid blood loss or sepsis). Severe jaundice, hepatosplenomegaly, respiratory distress, or signs of sepsis suggests a generalized, acquired bleeding disorder. Congenital hemostatic defects present most typically in a well-appearing child with "unexplained" bleeding. Look carefully for a cavernous hemangioma, and consider the possibility of intracranial hemorrhage.

C. Perform a CBC, and review the peripheral smear. Leukocytosis or neutropenia suggests sepsis. Significant red-cell fragmentation with decreased platelets suggests a consumptive coagulopathy (DIC, NEC, large vessel thrombosis, cavernous hemangioma). In sick newborns, consider cultures, antibiotics, an arterial blood gas assessment, chest and abdominal x-rays, and urinalysis.

D. Perform a prothrombin time (PT), partial thromboplastin time (PTT), and platelet count. The PT and PTT are physiologically prolonged in normal newborns, so values obtained in a bleeding newborn should be compared with newborn norms in a given laboratory.

E. A normal coagulation screen does *not* exclude a coagulopathy. A newborn with unexplained bleeding and a normal PT, PTT, and platelet count should be evaluated with a bleeding time and a hematology consultation.

F. Prolongation of both the PT and PTT with thrombocytopenia suggests a consumptive coagulopathy. Identify the etiology of the coagulopathy, and order fibrinogen level and fibrin split products (FSP). Treat serious bleeding with fresh frozen plasma and platelet transfusion. Heparin therapy is indicated in the treatment of major vessel thrombosis in the newborn, but not for disseminated intravascular coagulation. Consider liver function tests and viral cultures if the etiology of the coagulopathy is uncertain. In the newborn, liver disease may be associated with thrombocytopenia as well as a prolonged PT and PTT.

G. Obtain fibrinogen level, fibrin split products (abnormal with consumptive coagulopathy or severe liver disease), and liver function tests. Treat serious bleeding with fresh frozen plasma. If vitamin K has not been given, it should be ordered immediately with a repeat PT and PTT 4 to 6 hours later; a marked improvement strongly suggests vitamin K deficiency. DIC may occur without thrombocytopenia in the asphyxiated newborn. Congenital deficiencies of factors I, II, V, or X are very rare.

H. An isolated prolongation of the PTT suggests a congenital defect in hemostasis or heparin effect. Order clotting assays for factors VIII, IX, XI. Treat serious bleeding with fresh frozen plasma (or cryoprecipitate for confirmed factor VIII deficiency), and consider obtaining a hematology consultation.

REFERENCES

Glader BE, Buchanan GR. The bleeding neonate. Pediatrics 1976; 58:548.
Hathaway WE, Bonnar J. Perinatal Coagulation. New York: Grune and Stratton, 1978.
McDonald MM, Hathaway WE. Neonatal hemorrhage and thrombosis. Semi Perinatol 1983; 7:213.
Oski FA. Blood coagulation and its disorders in the newborn. In: Oski FA, Naiman JL. Hematologic Problems in the Newborn. 3rd ed. Philadelphia: WB Saunders, 1982:137.

NEONATAL BLEEDING

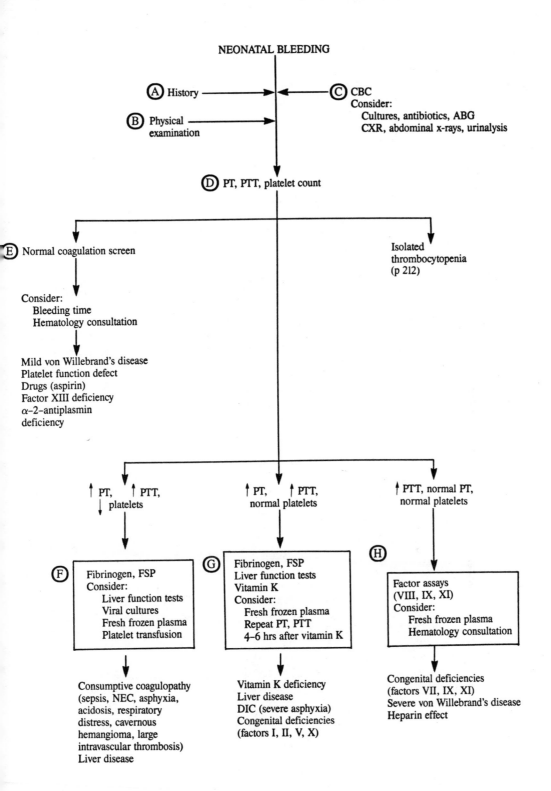

THROMBOCYTOPENIA IN THE NEWBORN

Peter A. Lane, M.D.

A. Note any maternal illnesses that might suggest maternal autoimmune thrombocytopenia (ITP, SLE). Inquire about drug use, hypertension, or preeclampsia during pregnancy. Document a history of rubella immunization; obtain the maternal rubella titer, a serologic test for syphilis, and a maternal red cell antibody screen. Consider risk factors for bacterial infection such as prematurity, prolonged rupture of membranes, maternal amnionitis, or fetal distress during labor. Finally, note any family history of bleeding disorders.

B. Note any growth retardation, rash, jaundice, or hepatosplenomegaly (congenital infection, severe hemolysis), congenital anomalies (trisomy syndromes, congenital rubella, thrombocytopenia with absent radii, Fanconi's anemia), or a cavernous hemangioma. Examine the placenta to detect a placental chorangioma.

C. Perform a complete blood count, platelet count; review the peripheral blood smear. Anemia (hemolysis, infection, congenital leukemia, or osteopetrosis), polycythemia, extreme leukocytosis (congenital leukemia, Down syndrome), or neutropenia (infection) may all be clues to the etiology of the thrombocytopenia. The peripheral smear may suggest infection or disseminated intravascular coagulation (DIC) (red cell fragmentation), extramedullary hematopoiesis (extreme nucleated erythrocytosis), or Wiskott-Aldrich syndrome (small platelet size in a boy). Any platelet count between 100,000 and 150,000 is worrisome and should be repeated. Any platelet count <100,000 is definitely abnormal, and an explanation should be sought.

D. Any infant with clinical bleeding other than skin petechiae or with other signs of systemic illness (lethargy, irritability, poor feeding, temperature instability) is considered symptomatic.

E. Perform a coagulation screen (PT, PTT, fibrinogen) to determine whether a diffuse coagulopathy is present. Symptomatic infants with thrombocytopenia are frequently septic. Infants with thrombocytopenia and CNS symptoms should be evaluated for intracranial hemorrhage with a CT or ultrasound examination of the head. Bloody stools or abdominal distention suggest necrotizing enterocolitis (NEC).

F. Infants with clinical bleeding secondary to thrombocytopenia should be given 10 cc/kg platelet-rich plasma. This should result in the cessation of bleeding and a marked rise in the platelet count. An inadequate response suggests either rapid platelet consumption (DIC, NEC) or the presence of antiplatelet antibodies (isoimmune, or maternal autoimmune). Bleeding in an infant with isoimmune thrombocytopenia often requires a platelet transfusion from the mother. Bleeding in an infant whose mother has autoimmune thrombocytopenia may require exchange transfusion and/or steroids prior to transfusion with random-donor platelets. Thrombocytopenic infants without clinical bleeding may be observed and not transfused. Systemic heparinization is indicated when thrombocytopenia is secondary to major vessel thrombosis.

G. Perform a platelet count on the mother, and review her history for clues to autoimmune disease. Neonatal thrombocytopenia secondary to maternal autoimmune disease may occur despite a normal platelet count in the mother.

REFERENCES

Gill FM. Thrombocytopenia in the newborn. Sem Perinatol 1983; 7:201.

Naiman JL. Disorders of platelets. In: Oski FA, Naiman JL, eds. Hematologic Problems in the Newborn. 3rd ed. Philadelphia: WB Saunders, 1982; 175.

Newborn THROMBOCYTOPENIA

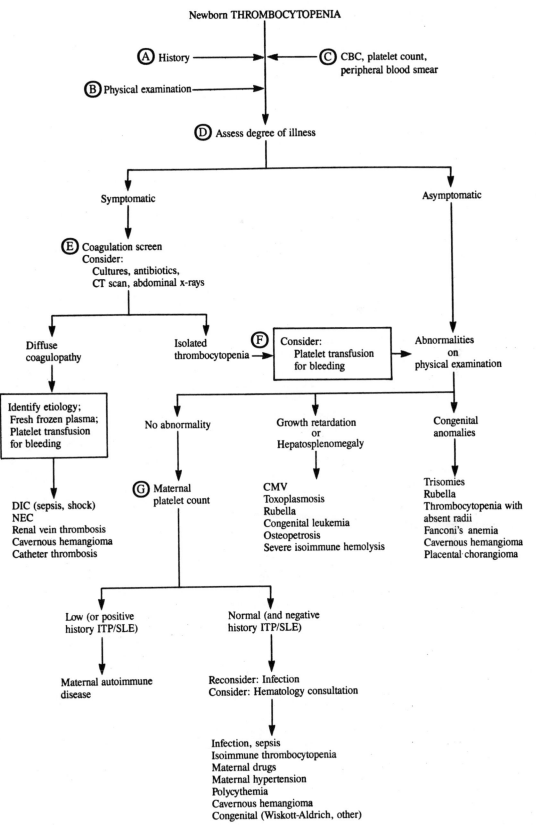

(A) History

(C) CBC, platelet count, peripheral blood smear

(B) Physical examination

(D) Assess degree of illness

Symptomatic

Asymptomatic

(E) Coagulation screen
Consider:
  Cultures, antibiotics,
  CT scan, abdominal x-rays

Diffuse coagulopathy

Isolated thrombocytopenia

(F) Consider:
  Platelet transfusion
  for bleeding

Abnormalities on physical examination

Identify etiology;
Fresh frozen plasma;
Platelet transfusion
for bleeding

No abnormality

Growth retardation or Hepatosplenomegaly

Congenital anomalies

DIC (sepsis, shock)
NEC
Renal vein thrombosis
Cavernous hemangioma
Catheter thrombosis

(G) Maternal platelet count

CMV
Toxoplasmosis
Rubella
Congenital leukemia
Osteopetrosis
Severe isoimmune hemolysis

Trisomies
Rubella
Thrombocytopenia with absent radii
Fanconi's anemia
Cavernous hemangioma
Placental chorangioma

Low (or positive history ITP/SLE)

Normal (and negative history ITP/SLE)

Maternal autoimmune disease

Reconsider: Infection
Consider: Hematology consultation

Infection, sepsis
Isoimmune thrombocytopenia
Maternal drugs
Maternal hypertension
Polycythemia
Cavernous hemangioma
Congenital (Wiskott-Aldrich, other)

213

NEONATAL SEPSIS
Edward R. Berman, M.D.

A. Note the presence of the following high risk factors: prolonged rupture of membranes (>24 hours), maternal fever or infection, amnionitis, septic or traumatic delivery, fetal tachycardia, unexplained preterm labor, or low birth weight (<2500 g).

B. Note nonspecific clinical signs associated with bacterial infection such as temperature instability, lethargy, abdominal distention, poor feeding, respiratory distress (tachynea, apnea), cyanotic spells, jaundice, hepatomegaly, seizures, and shock.

C. Suspect the possibility of sepsis when the initial CBC with differential and platelet count reveals a neutrophil count $<7200/mm^2$ at 12–24 hours or $<3600/mm^2$ at 48 hours and when the ratio of immature to total neutrophils is greater than 1:5 or the platelet count is $<100,000$. Twenty percent of neonates with an immature to total neutrophil ratio greater than 1:5 have sepsis. The value of C–reactive protein, latex haptoglobin, and microsedimentation rate as screens for sepsis in the first 48 to 72 hours of life is unclear.

D. The risk of sepsis in an asymptomatic neonate with an unremarkable CBC with differential and platelet count and one risk factor is minimal ($<1\%$). Patients at low risk have mild, nonspecific signs and symptoms such as poor feeding or mild lethargy with no more than one risk factor. Neonates at moderate risk have multiple risk factors or more than one risk factor associated with nonspecific signs or symptoms. Neonates at high risk for sepsis present with shock, severe respiratory distress, seizures, and marked acidosis without hypoxia.

E. Identify cases of neonatal meningitis. The most frequent bacterial causes are *E. coli* (40%), group *B streptococcus* (30%), followed by *Listeria monocytogenes*, group *A streptococcus*, *S. aureus*, *S. epidermidis*, *Proteus*, *Klebsiella*, *Enterobacter*, and others. Pending culture and sensitivity results, begin ampicillin 200–400 mg/kg/day IV in 3 or 4 divided doses and chloramphenicol 25–50 mg/kg/day *q12 or 24h*. Consider moxolactam 100 mg/kg/day in 2 divided doses as an alternative to chloramphenicol. Treat neonatal meningitis for a minimum f 21 days.

F. Neonatal sepsis is most commonly caused by group *B streptococcus* (30%), *escherichea coli* (30%) followed by *Klebsiella*, *Enterobacter*, *S. aureus*, group *D streptococcus*, *H. influenzae*, *Pseudomonas*, and others. After stabilization to ensure adequate oxygenation (respiratory and circulatory support, correction of acidosis, and maintenance of oxygen-carrying capacity) begin antibiotic therapy with ampicillin 100 to 150 mg/kg/day in 2 to 4 doses IM or IV and gentamicin 2.5 mg/kg/dose every 12 to 24 hours depending on gestational age. In cases of overwhelming sepsis, consider an exchange transfusiion. When sepsis is associated with severe neutropenia, consider a bone marrow aspiration to document depletion of storage pool of neutrophils and granulocyte transfusion. Treat septic infants for 10 to 14 days based upon antibiotic sensitivities of the organisms. If the neonate is unstable, continue the antibiotics for 10 to 14 days despite negative cultures.

REFERENCES

Gnehm H, Klein JO. Management of neonatal sepsis and meningitis. Pediatr Ann 1983; 12:195.

Manroe BL, Weinberg AG, Rosenfeld CR et al. The neonatal blood count in health and disease. Reference values for neutrophilic cells. J Pediatr 1979; 95:89.

Philip AGS. Neonatal sepsis resulting from possible amniotic fluid infection. Clin Pediatr 1982; 21:210.

Squire EN, Reich HM, Merenstein GB, et al. Criteria for the discontinuation of antibiotic therapy during presumptive treatment of suspected neonatal infection. Pediatr Inf Dis 1982; 1:85.

Visser VE, Hall RT. Lumbar puncture in the evaluation of suspected neonatal sepsis. J Pediatr 1980; 96:1063.

Visser VE, Hall RT. Urine culture and the evaluation of suspected neonatal sepsis. J Pediatr 1979; 94:635.

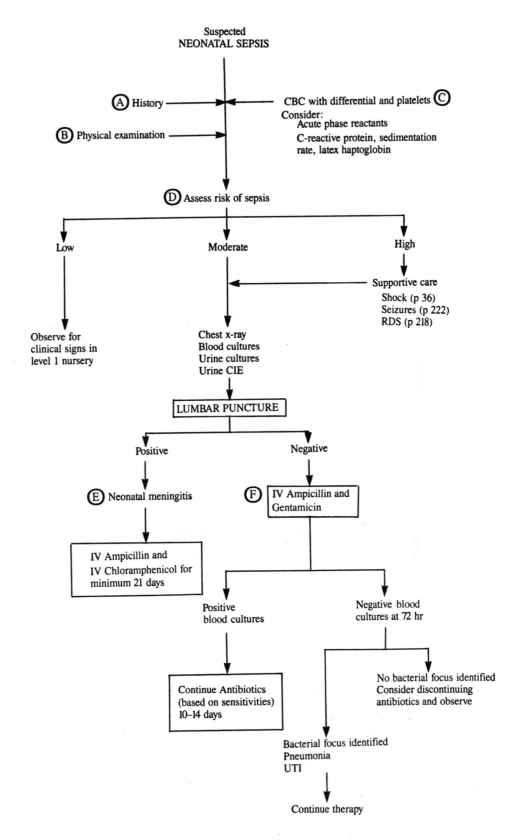

Suspected
NEONATAL SEPSIS

(A) History ——————

(B) Physical examination ——————

CBC with differential and platelets (C)
Consider:
    Acute phase reactants
    C-reactive protein, sedimentation
    rate, latex haptoglobin

(D) Assess risk of sepsis

Low

Moderate

High

Supportive care
  Shock (p 36)
  Seizures (p 222)
  RDS (p 218)

Observe for
clinical signs in
level 1 nursery

Chest x-ray
Blood cultures
Urine cultures
Urine CIE

LUMBAR PUNCTURE

Positive

Negative

(E) Neonatal meningitis

(F) IV Ampicillin and
Gentamicin

IV Ampicillin and
IV Chloramphenicol for
minimum 21 days

Positive
blood cultures

Negative blood
cultures at 72 hr

Continue Antibiotics
(based on sensitivities)
10–14 days

No bacterial focus identified
Consider discontinuing
antibiotics and observe

Bacterial focus identified
Pneumonia
UTI

Continue therapy

CONGENITAL HERPES SIMPLEX INFECTIONS

Edward R. Berman, M.D.

A. Consider the possibility of a congenital herpes infection in infants born to women with genital herpes diagnosed at any time during their pregnancy, women with a prior history of genital herpes, and women who have had sexual contact at any time in the past with a male with genital herpes. Unfortunately 70% of neonates with congenital herpes infection have mothers who have no evidence of maternal herpes infection or exposure to a sexual contact with herpes. Newborns whose mothers have nongenital herpes are not at risk during delivery, and therefore do not require isolation immediately following birth. The mother should cover the nongenital herpes lesions at all times; isolation precautions should be considered after the mother has contact with her infant. The incubation period for neonatal herpes acquired at delivery ranges from 2 to 14 days with most cases becoming apparent within 1 week.

B. Note nonspecific signs of infection such as poor feeding, vomiting, irritability, lethargy, apnea, or respiratory distress. Note the presence of herpetic skin lesions and associated signs of infection including conjunctivitis, altered neurologic status, focal seizures, hepatomegaly and jaundice.

C. Severely ill infants have evidence of localized herpes infection or nonspecific signs and symptoms consistent with disseminated herpes or bacterial sepsis. Infants born vaginally or by cesarean section with membranes ruptured prior to delivery are at moderate risk if their mothers had a positive cervicovaginal culture within 1 week of delivery or a Papanicolaou smear consistent with herpes on the day of delivery. Infants at low risk are those that were delivered by cesarean section with intact membranes to a mother with a positive culture or Pap smear, or babies delivered vaginally by mothers at risk who had a negative Pap smear on the day of delivery and negative cervical vaginal cultures within 1 week prior to delivery.

D. Patients with nonspecific clinical signs and symptoms require a complete septic workup including a lumbar puncture and blood cultures. Begin therapy with ampicillin and an aminoglycoside for presumed sepsis pending culture results after 72 hours.

E. Neonatal herpes simplex infections are classified as localized or disseminated. Infants with localized infection may have involvement of the skin, eyes, oral cavity, or CNS. Initial herpetic skin lesions are likely to progress to involve other sites or proceed to disseminated disease. Disseminated infection presents with nonspecific signs and symptoms, shock, and DIC. Most infants with disseminated herpes do have oral or skin lesions. A lumbar puncture EEG and CT scan identifies CNS involvement (meningoencephalitis) which occurs in half of the cases with localized or disseminated infection. The mortality rate of infants with CNS involvement with local infection is 41%; severe neurologic sequelae and/or ocular sequelae occur in 42% of the survivors. The mortality rate for neonates with disseminated disease is greater than 75%. Obtain an ophthalmology consult to identify eye involvement which produces keratoconjunctivitis and chorioretinitis.

REFERENCES

Kibrick S. Herpes simplex infection at term. JAMA 1980; 243:157.

Overall JC, Whitley RJ, Yeager AS, et al. Prophylactic or anticipatory antiviral therapy for newborns exposed to herpes simplex infection. Pediatr Infect Dis 1984; 3:193.

Whitley RJ, Nahmias AJ, Visintine ASM, et al. The natural history of herpes simplex virus infection of mother and newborn. Pediatr 1980; 66:489.

Whitely RJ, Nahmias AJ, Soong S, et al. Vidarabine therapy of neonatal herpes simplex virus infection. Pediatr 1980; 66:495.

Suspected
CONGENITAL HERPES SIMPLEX INFECTION

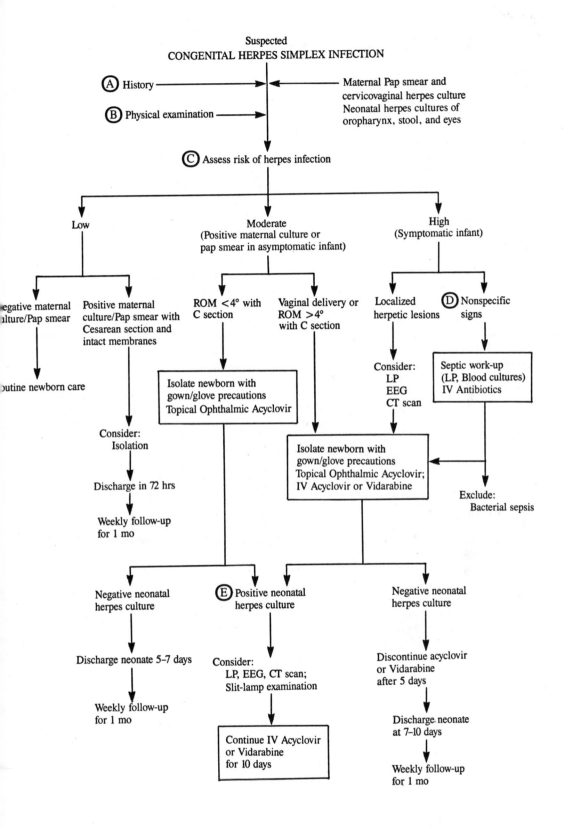

Ⓐ History

Ⓑ Physical examination

Maternal Pap smear and
cervicovaginal herpes culture
Neonatal herpes cultures of
oropharynx, stool, and eyes

Ⓒ Assess risk of herpes infection

Low

Moderate
(Positive maternal culture or
pap smear in asymptomatic infant)

High
(Symptomatic infant)

Negative maternal
culture/Pap smear

Positive maternal
culture/Pap smear with
Cesarean section and
intact membranes

ROM <4° with
C section

Vaginal delivery or
ROM >4°
with C section

Localized
herpetic lesions

Ⓓ Nonspecific
signs

Routine newborn care

Isolate newborn with
gown/glove precautions
Topical Ophthalmic Acyclovir

Consider:
LP
EEG
CT scan

Septic work-up
(LP, Blood cultures)
IV Antibiotics

Consider:
Isolation

Discharge in 72 hrs

Weekly follow-up
for 1 mo

Isolate newborn with
gown/glove precautions
Topical Ophthalmic Acyclovir;
IV Acyclovir or Vidarabine

Exclude:
Bacterial sepsis

Negative neonatal
herpes culture

Ⓔ Positive neonatal
herpes culture

Negative neonatal
herpes culture

Discharge neonate 5–7 days

Consider:
LP, EEG, CT scan;
Slit-lamp examination

Discontinue acyclovir
or Vidarabine
after 5 days

Weekly follow-up
for 1 mo

Continue IV Acyclovir
or Vidarabine
for 10 days

Discharge neonate
at 7–10 days

Weekly follow-up
for 1 mo

217

RESPIRATORY DISTRESS SYNDROME

Edward R. Berman, M.D.

A. Assess the degree of respiratory distress. Severely ill infants are unable to maintain a PaO_2 >50 torr and a $PaCO_2$ <50 torr on 80 to 100% oxygen or have recurrent apnea and shock. Moderately ill infants require an FIO_2 concentration of 60% to 70% to maintain an adequate PaO_2. Mildly ill infants can maintain adequate PaO_2 with less than 60% FIO_2.

B. Continuous positive airway pressure (CPAP) distends alveoli which have collapsed because of deficient surfactant. CPAP can be applied with nasal prongs or an endotracheal tube. A trial CPAP (nasal or tracheal) is worthwhile if the patient is ventilating adequately but oxygenating poorly (FIO_2 >60 to 70%, PaO_2 <60 torr).

C. Consider the possibility of group B streptococcal pneumonia or sepsis associated with other bacterial agents in patients with moderate or severe respiratory distress syndrome. High risk factors for infection include a history of maternal fever, premature rupture of membranes for more than 24 hours, and amnionitis. Laboratory findings which suggest infection include neutropenia, leukocytosis, or a positive C-reactive protein (may not be helpful in first 24–48 hours). Draw blood cultures, consider an LP, perform a urine CIE, and initiate antibiotic therapy with ampicillin and gentamicin.

D. Congestive heart failure secondary to a patent ductus arteriosus (PDA) is common (60%) in premature infants weighing less than 1500 grams. Suspect a PDA when signs of congestive heart failure are associated with a continuous heart murmur, bounding pulses, hepatomegaly, low disastolic blood pressure and a hyperactive precordium. The chest x-ray reveals cardiomegaly with increased pulmonary artery blood flow and/or pulmonary edema. The echocardiogram shows an abnormal ratio of the left atrial size/aortic root size and increased left atrial and left ventricular dimensions. The management of this condition is controversial. Initial management should include fluid restriction and Lasix. Consider recommending the early use of indomethacin. Failure of medical management requires surgical ligation of the PDA.

E. Persistent fetal circulation (PFC) or pulmonary hypertension produces a large right to left shunt through a ductus or patent foramen ovale. Arterial blood gases obtained from a preductal site (right radial artery or temporal artery) have a higher PaO_2 (15–20 torr) than do postductal sites (umbilical artery). Failure to document a difference does not rule out PFC; a closed ductus may exist with a right to left shunt occurring through the foramen ovale. Shunts can be documented by systolic time intervals on echocardiography or by injecting saline in the inferior vena cava with echocardiographic surveillance. Initial management includes correcting metabolic acidosis, hypoxemia and maintaining adequate systemic blood pressure. Consider a trial of tolazoline 1 to 2 mg/kg over 2 to 5 minutes. If this produces a rise in PaO_2 greater than 15 torr, institute a trial of continuous effusion (1 to 2 mg/kg/hr). Continuous tolazoline can cause hypotension, renal insufficiency, GI bleeding, and irritability. Consider the use of dopamine in addition to tolazoline in order to improve cardiac function and maintain blood pressure. Maintaining an adequate circulatory blood volume is essential.

REFERENCES

Bhat R, Fisher E, Raju TN, et al. Patent ductus arteriosus: recent advances in diagnosis and management. Pediatr Clin North Am 1982; 29:1117.

Goetzman BW, Riemenschneider TA. Persistence of the fetal circulation. Pediatr Rev 1980; 2:37.

Hallman M, Gluck L. Respiratory distress syndrome update. Pediatr Clin North Am 1982; 29:1057.

Kitterman JA. Cyanosis in the newborn infant. Pediatr Rev 1982; 4:13.

RESPIRATORY DISTRESS SYNDROME

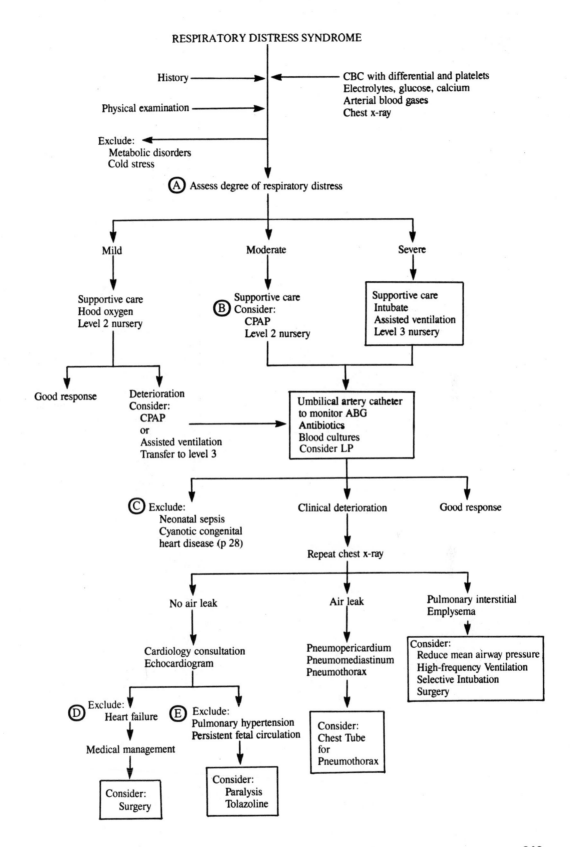

NEONATAL NECROTIZING ENTEROCOLITIS

Edward R. Berman, M.D.

A. Most infants (80%) who develop NEC were born prematurely. Factors related to the development of NEC include intestinal hypoperfusion with ischemia, placement of umbilical artery or umbilical vein catheters, hypertonic feedings, placement of a nasogastric tube, polycythemia, and infection (rotavirus, *E. coli, Klebsiella, Pseudomonas, Salmonella, Clostridium*).

B. Other associated signs include significant residual gastric aspirates or vomiting, hematest/clinitest-positive stools, and nonspecific signs of sepsis such as temperature instability, lethargy, or apnea. Note the presence of abdominal tenderness and erythema; gross gastrointestinal bleeding and shock would suggest acute perforation.

C. The workup for cases of suspected NEC should include a CBC with differential and platelets to look for evidence of sepsis (immature to total neutrophil ratio > 1:5, decreased platelet count, neutropenia), and arterial blood gas for evidence of hypoxia, metabolic acidosis. An abdominal x-ray documents mucosal damage, intramural air (pneumatosis intestinalis) or perforation (free air).

D. Mildly ill patients present with nonspecific signs (mild gastric distention, residual gastric aspirates, hema-positive stools) with an unremarkable initial workup (normal CBC with differential and platelet count, no acidosis on arterial blood gas and normal abdominal films). Moderately ill infants have more specific signs of NEC such as abdominal tenderness or erythema, gross gastrointestinal bleeding, and/or abnormal abdominal x-rays. The severely ill child presents with evidence of acute perforation and peritonitis (shock, unremitting acidosis, DIC, or massive GI hemorrhage).

E. Manage mildly ill patients by discontinuing feedings until the abdominal examination returns to normal. Consider a nasogastric tube for decompression and a glycerine suppository if the infant has not been stooling normally. Failure to respond adequately in 6 to 12 hours is an indication for a repeat abdominal x-ray. Observe closely for ongoing signs and symptoms. Progression is an indication for more aggressive management as described for moderately ill patients.

F. Manage moderately ill patients by discontinuing feeding, placing a nasogastric tube, and initiating antibiotic therapy pending culture results. Infants should be kept NPO a minimum of 7 to 10 days. Intravenous peripheral hyperalimentation should be started as soon as possible. Obtain abdominal x-rays every 6 to 12 hours until films have returned to normal or the abdominal examination has improved. Treat DIC and thrombocytopenia with fresh frozen plasma and platelet transfusions. The neonate may "third space" significant volumes of fluid in the intestinal tract; closely monitor vital signs and urine output, and maintain the circulatory blood volume. Indications for surgical exploration include evidence of intestinal perforation, peritonitis, unremitting acidosis or DIC, and a rapid clinical deterioration.

G. After an episode of NEC, the intestinal mucosa may be damaged and friable. Reintroduce enteric feedings with a dilute elemental formula, and slowly advance the volume and strength. Obtain a barium enema 6 to 8 weeks following the episode in all cases regardless of surgery in order to diagnose any stricture. Consider a barium enema earlier if signs of intestinal obstruction develop.

REFERENCES

Burg FD, Polin MD. A workbook exercise on necrotizing enterocolitis. Pediatr Rev 1981; 3:121.

Thilo EH, Lazarte RA, Hernandez JA. Necrotizing enterocolitis in the first 24 hours of life. Pediatrics 1984; 73:476.

Wilson R, Portillo M, Schmidt E, et al. Risk factors for necrotizing enterocolitis in infants weighing more than 2000 grams at birth: a case-control study. Pediatrics 1983; 71:19.

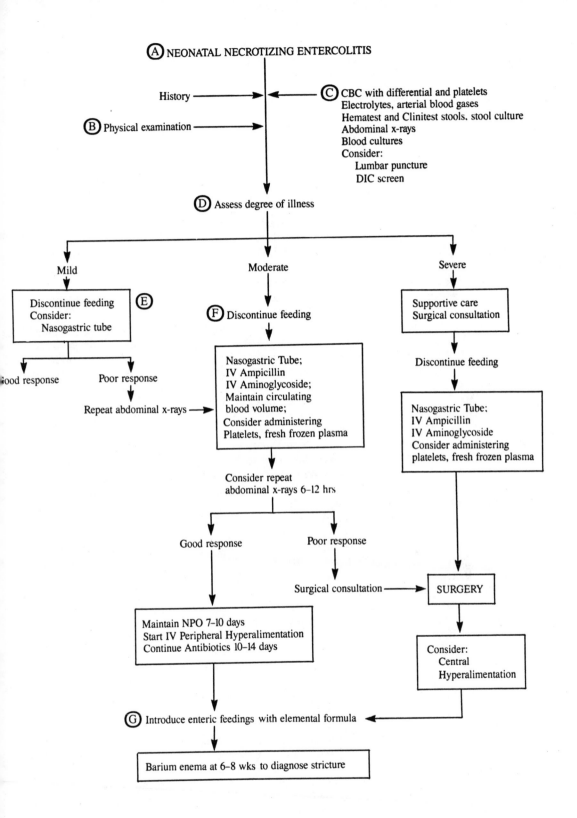

(A) NEONATAL NECROTIZING ENTERCOLITIS

History

(B) Physical examination

(C) CBC with differential and platelets
Electrolytes, arterial blood gases
Hematest and Clinitest stools, stool culture
Abdominal x-rays
Blood cultures
Consider:
    Lumbar puncture
    DIC screen

(D) Assess degree of illness

Mild

Moderate

Severe

Discontinue feeding (E)
Consider:
    Nasogastric tube

(F) Discontinue feeding

Supportive care
Surgical consultation

Good response

Poor response

Repeat abdominal x-rays

Nasogastric Tube;
IV Ampicillin
IV Aminoglycoside;
Maintain circulating
blood volume;
Consider administering
Platelets, fresh frozen plasma

Discontinue feeding

Nasogastric Tube;
IV Ampicillin
IV Aminoglycoside
Consider administering
platelets, fresh frozen plasma

Consider repeat
abdominal x-rays 6–12 hrs

Good response

Poor response

Surgical consultation

SURGERY

Maintain NPO 7–10 days
Start IV Peripheral Hyperalimentation
Continue Antibiotics 10–14 days

Consider:
    Central
    Hyperalimentation

(G) Introduce enteric feedings with elemental formula

Barium enema at 6–8 wks to diagnose stricture

NEONATAL SEIZURES
Edward R. Berman, M.D.

A. Note maternal medication taken during pregnancy, the possibility of use of illicit drugs during pregnancy, type of anesthesia used during delivery, and any history of perinatal asphyxia. Ask about the family history of previously affected newborns.

B. Describe the seizure activity. Signs of "subtle" seizures include horizontal deviation of the eyes, eye blinking or fluttering, abnormal oral-buccal movements, peddling or bicycling movements, and apneic spells. Other types of seizures include tonic seizures, multifocal clonic seizures, focal clonic seizures, and myoclonic seizures. Distinguish jitteriness from seizure activity. Jitteriness involves rhythmic movements of equal rate and amplitude (tremors) that are sensitive to stimuli and cease with passive flexion; no abnormal eye movements are present. Jitteriness is more common than seizures and occurs frequently in infants with hypocalcemia, hypoglycemia, drug withdrawal, and asphyxia.

C. Obtain a Dextrostix test immediately if seizures are suspected. Transient hypoglycemia can be associated with asphyxia, low birth weight, infant of a diabetic mother, a small-for-gestational-age infant, polycythemia, sepsis, cold stress, adrenal hemorrhage, and respiratory distress syndrome. Persistent hypoglycemia is much less common and is caused by defects in carbohydrate metabolism, amino acid/organic acid metabolism, hormonal deficiency, and hyperinsulinism. When the Dextrostix determination is less than 30, obtain a serum glucose and give 2 to 4 cc of D10W as an IV bolus followed by a constant infusion of 6 to 8 mg/kg/min of glucose. If an IV is not present, consider giving glucagon IM.

D. Begin anticonvulsive therapy with phenobarbital; an initial loading dose of 20 mg/kg IV or IM followed by a daily maintenance dose of 4 to 5 mg/kg/day. If the phenobarbital level is therapeutic and seizures continue, administer phenytoin (Dilantin) 15 to 20 mg/kg IV at an IV rate not to exceed 50 mg/min followed by a maintenance dose of 3 to 5 mg/kg/day. Do not give Dilantin IM or PO. If seizures persist, consider giving paraldehyde IV or per rectum. Diazepam (Valium) is not recommended for neonatal seizures; it enhances respiratory depression and hypotension and can displace bilirubin from albumin.

E. Perinatal asphyxia is the most frequent cause of neonatal seizures. From 20 to 60% of asphyxiated infants develop seizures, from as early as 6 to 18 hours of age. Ultrasonography and CT scan will diagnose intracranial hemorrhage, a common cause of seizures, especially in preterm infants of less than 32 weeks gestation. Intracranial hemorrhage may occur in the subarachnoid space, subdural space, or peri-intraventricular area. Bacterial and viral infections are associated with approximately 12% of neonatal seizures. Less common causes include developmental defects, local anesthetic administered by accident into the infant's scalp, and metabolic abnormalities.

F. Persistence of continuous seizures of unknown origin despite therapeutic levels of anticonvulsant medications indicates a trial of pyridoxine. Pyridoxine deficiency is diagnosed when an infant's EEG has profoundly abnormal paroxysmal electrical activity that ceases following the IV injection of pyridoxine.

G. The neurologic outcome of infants with neonatal seizures is related to the etiology of the seizure. Perinatal asphyxia or intraventricular hemorrhage are likely (80–85%) to cause permanent neurologic sequelae. Permanent sequelae also often accompany intracranial infections (30–75%), significant and prolonged hypoglycemia (50%), and early onset hypoglycemia (50%). An EEG done 4 to 7 days after the onset of seizures in term infants may help predict outcome. Infants with a normal EEG and neurologic examination usually have a favorable outcome (85%). An abnormal EEG with an abnormal neurologic examination is a poor prognostic sign; only 10 to 50% of such infants will have subsequent normal development.

NEONATAL SEIZURES

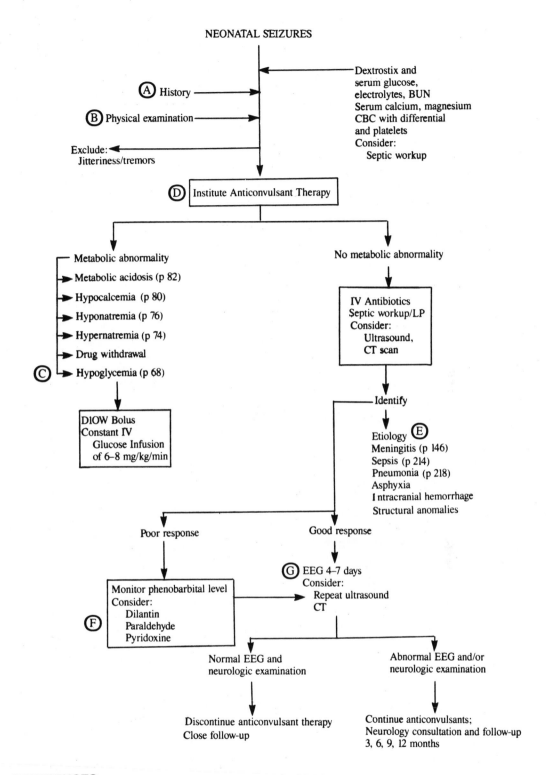

(A) History

(B) Physical examination

Dextrostix and
serum glucose,
electrolytes, BUN
Serum calcium, magnesium
CBC with differential
and platelets
Consider:
   Septic workup

Exclude:
Jitteriness/tremors

(D) Institute Anticonvulsant Therapy

Metabolic abnormality

Metabolic acidosis (p 82)

Hypocalcemia (p 80)

Hyponatremia (p 76)

Hypernatremia (p 74)

Drug withdrawal

(C) Hypoglycemia (p 68)

D10W Bolus
Constant IV
   Glucose Infusion
   of 6–8 mg/kg/min

No metabolic abnormality

IV Antibiotics
Septic workup/LP
Consider:
   Ultrasound,
   CT scan

Identify

Etiology (E)
Meningitis (p 146)
Sepsis (p 214)
Pneumonia (p 218)
Asphyxia
Intracranial hemorrhage
Structural anomalies

Poor response

Good response

(G) EEG 4–7 days
Consider:
   Repeat ultrasound
   CT

Monitor phenobarbital level
Consider:
   Dilantin
(F) Paraldehyde
   Pyridoxine

Normal EEG and
neurologic examination

Abnormal EEG and/or
neurologic examination

Discontinue anticonvulsant therapy
Close follow-up

Continue anticonvulsants;
Neurology consultation and follow-up
3, 6, 9, 12 months

REFERENCES

Bergman I, Pointer MT, Cumrine PK. Neonatal seizures. Sem Perinatol 1982; 6:54.
Lombroso CT, Rose AL. Neonatal seizure states. Pediatrics 1970; 45:404.
Volpe JJ. Neurology of the Newborn. Philadelphia: WB Saunders 1981; 111.

INDEX